Exploring

ELECTRONIC
Health Records

Second Edition

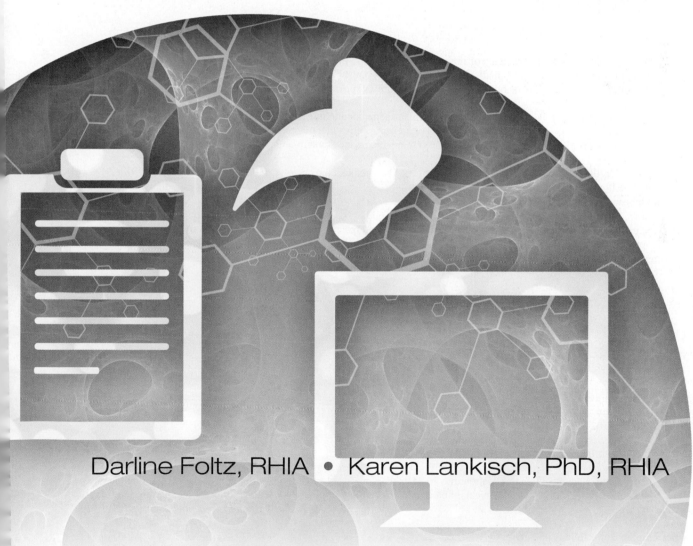

Darline Foltz, RHIA • Karen Lankisch, PhD, RHIA

PARADIGM
EDUCATION SOLUTIONS

St. Paul

Division President: Linda Hein
Vice President, Content Management: Christine Hurney
Managing Editor: Carley Fruzzetti
Developmental Editor: Stephanie Schempp
Director of Production: Timothy W. Larson
Production Editor: Carrie Rogers
Design and Production Specialist: Jaana Bykonich
Copy Editor: Suzanne Clinton
Proofreader: Lori Michelle Ryan
Indexer: Terry Casey
Vice President, Digital Solutions: Chuck Bratton
Digital Projects Manager: Tom Modl
Digital Solutions Manager: Gerry Yumul
Digital Production Manager: Aaron Esnough
Vice President, Sales and Marketing: Scott Burns
Director of Marketing: Lara Weber McLellan
Product Marketing Manager: Selena Hicks

ISBN 978-0-76388-130-6 (print)
ISBN 978-0-76388-129-0 (ebook)

© 2018 by Paradigm Publishing, Inc.
875 Montreal Way
St. Paul, MN 55102
Email: CustomerService@ParadigmEducation.com
Website: ParadigmEducation.com

Printed in the United States of America

26 25 24 23 22 21 20 19 18 17   1 2 3 4 5 6 7 8 9 10

Brief Contents

Contents

Chapter 4 Administrative Management   105

Chapter 5 Scheduling and Patient Management   131

Chapter 6 Privacy, Security, and Legal Aspects of the EHR   153

Chapter 7 Clinical Documentation and Reporting   181

Exploring Electronic Health Records, Second Edition, is an up-to-date, accurate, and approachable courseware that introduces students to the concepts and features of electronic health record systems. This courseware was designed to help students learn about the functionality of the electronic health record (EHR) as it applies to the many careers within the fields of health information management, health information technology, and allied health. Students gain an awareness of how the electronic health record supports efficiencies and accuracy within both inpatient and outpatient facilities, and how EHRs contribute to the goals of increased patient safety and security.

In addition to this book, the courseware also includes tutorials and assessments from Paradigm's EHR Navigator, a live, web-based application. Paradigm designed and developed this system based on the best features of many industry EHR systems. The EHR Navigator provides students with 50 interactive tutorials that teach the principles of EHR software. In addition, each tutorial is supported by corresponding practice assessments. For each tutorial there are several corresponding practice assessments. These tutorials and practice assessments supply a depth of activity practice to ensure that students build skills that are transferable to the variety of EHR systems they will encounter in their careers. Students are then assessed on these important EHR activities within the EHR Navigator.

The EHR Navigator interactive tutorials and assessments can be found on Paradigm's Navigator+. Navigator+ is a learning management system that contains many interactive learning tools, such as case studies, quizzes, critical thinking assignments, exams, and flashcards.

Chapter Features: A Visual Walk-Through

Each chapter contains features that aid student learning. These features, as outlined below, teach students the fundamentals of EHRs, challenge them to think critically, and give them additional online learning opportunities. The features of each chapter are designed to address different learning styles and stress the importance of professionalism and soft skills.

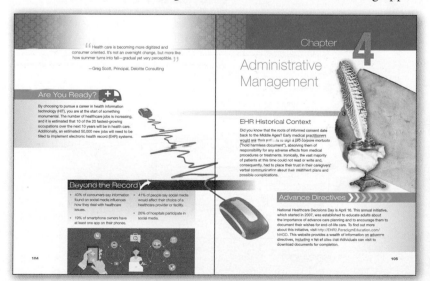

Engaging **two-page openers** provide students with learning opportunities that supplement each chapter's core content. This feature includes fun facts about EHRs, historical background, quotations from government officials, notes from workers in the field, and professionalism tips to prepare students for careers in health information technology or management, and allied health.

1 **Learning Objectives** establish a clear set of goals for each chapter.

2 **Key terms** are set in bold contextually defined, and reinforced with flash cards in the Navigator+ learning management system.

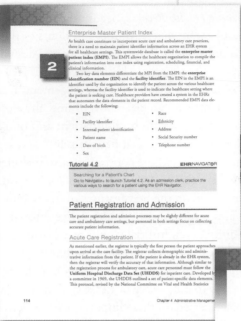

3 **Expand Your Learning** margin features speak to digitally savvy students and integrate Internet resources and online learning opportunities.

What's the Buzz margin features focus on hot topics in HIT and allied health.

Make an Impact margin tips describe how your job in healthcare matters.

Practice Professionalism features advise on soft skills.

4 **Consider This** feature boxes provide real-life scenarios and challenge students to think critically.

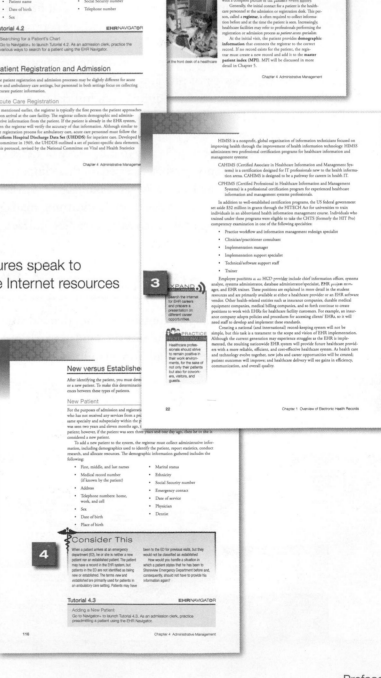

5 **Checkpoint** activities give students periodic stopping points to test their learning within each chapter. To encourage independent study, the answers are provided in Appendix A.

6 **Tutorials** from the EHR Navigator point students to the Navigator+ learning management system to launch interactive tutorials. These tutorials give students hands-on practice in an EHR system.

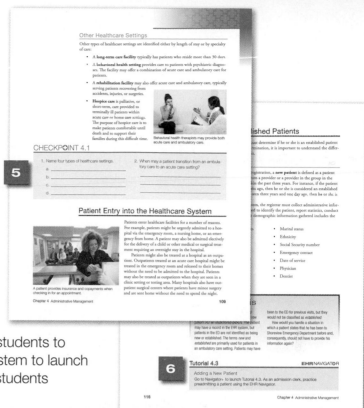

7 **Photographs** reinforce the text and help students to visualize EHR concepts and real-world patient interactions.

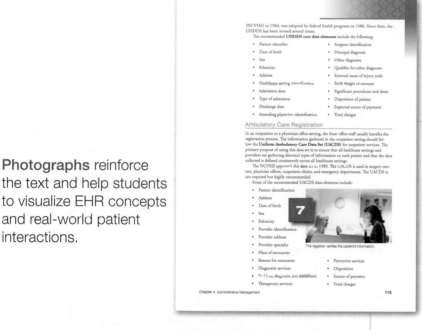

8 **Screenshots** from the EHR Navigator illustrate key components of an EHR system as they relate to chapter content.

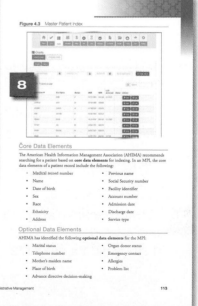

9 **Figures** in the form of flowcharts help students understand crucial workflow concepts.

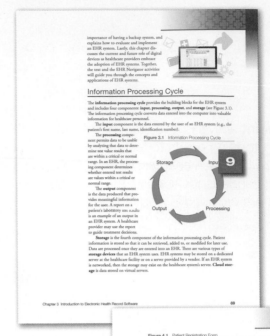

10 **Figures** in the form of healthcare documents and forms provide additional detail and visual reinforcement of chapter topics.

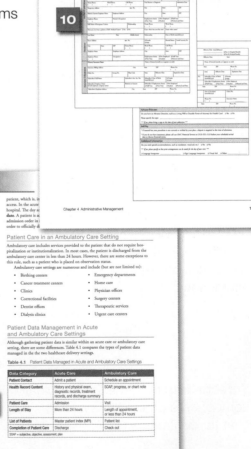

11 **Tables** encapsulate pertinent information related to the chapter and serve as a study aid for students.

12 **Chapter Summary** boxes offer an overview of the key points of each chapter.

13 **EHR Review** sections provide multiple-choice and true/false questions, a list of acronyms from the chapter, and direct students to flash cards available on Navigator+.

14 **EHR Application** sections supply short-answer and critical-thinking activities.

15 **EHR Evaluation** sections provide activities that require students to think critically, demonstrate their understanding of key chapter concepts, and reminds them to complete the practice activities that align to the EHR tutorials from the chapter.

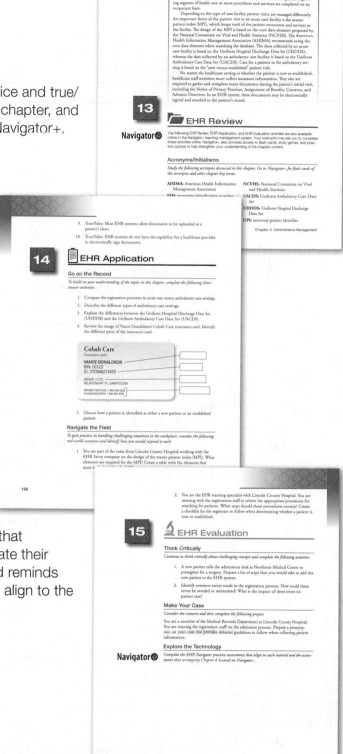

Features and Navigator+

To support their study of the textbook, students have access to additional print and electronic resources. These resources were provided to enhance students' skills and develop their ability to apply these skills within a range of healthcare roles. Paradigm provides all students, regardless of their preferred learning styles, a variety of exercise types.

Appendices

Appendix A contains the answers to chapter Checkpoints. **Appendix B** contains a handwritten medical record that illustrates the components of a typical paper record and is referenced as a learning tool in end-of-chapter and online activities.

Navigator+

Navigator+ is a learning management system that contains the EHR Navigator tutorials, practice assessments, and final assessments, as well as flash cards, quizzes, and other interactive learning materials from the text. Through the Navigator+ site at https://NavPlus.ParadigmEducation.com, instructors can set up an *Exploring Electronic Health Records*, Second Edition, course. The Navigator+ site requires students to log in with an enrollment key, which students will receive from instructors, and a Navigator+ access code, which can be purchased with the textbook or eBook.

For instructors using their own learning management system, Navigator+ allows LTI connectivity, so instructors have the ability to export digital course content into their school's LMS (Blackboard, Canvas, D2L, or Common Cartridge). This means student work is instantly captured and reported, while grades are seamlessly updated into the school's LMS. Instructors can create, delete, modify, and schedule assignments.

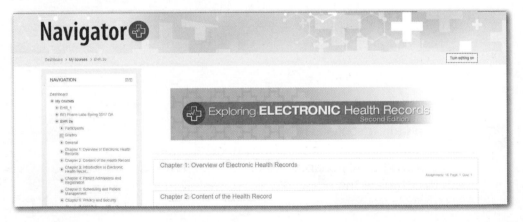

EHR Navigator

Access to the EHR Navigator is included as part of the Navigator+ learning management system. The EHR Navigator is a live program that replicates professional practice and prepares students for today's workplace.

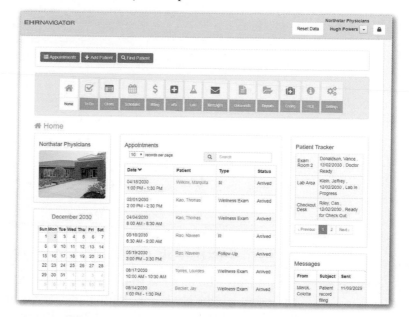

The EHR Navigator provides experience in all areas of EHRs, including adding and scheduling patient appointments, adding clinical data to patient charts, coding, medical billing, managing patient data, and e-prescribing. The EHR Navigator gives students practice in both inpatient and outpatient settings.

The EHR Navigator's interactive tutorials offer students practice in a format that is easy to navigate, colorful, and user friendly. Each chapter contains interactive tutorials based on the core content and EHR system principals. The tutorials train students by stepping them through a variety of inpatient, outpatient, and personal health records activities.

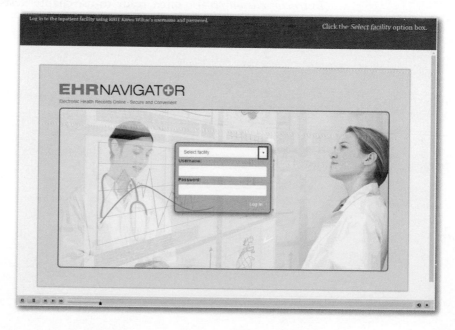

The EHR Navigator also includes assessments that are graded and reported to the instructor. There are multiple practice assessments that correspond to each tutorial, and then a final assessment to test student's understanding of the EHR Navigator.

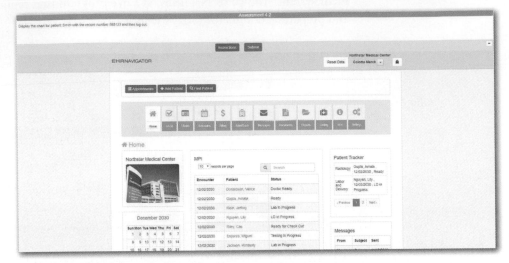

Digital Textbook Content Delivery

For students who prefer to study electronically, the textbook content is delivered seamlessly through the Navigator+ learning management system. Content can be accessed by individual chapter, or at the book level. It is web-based and always available. It can also be accessed for offline use via an iOS app, available for free on iTunes.

Instructor eResources

Exploring Electronic Health Records, Second Edition, provides instructors with helpful tools for planning and delivering their courses and assessing student learning. In addition to course planning tools and syllabus models, the *Instructor eResources* provides chapter-specific teaching hints and answers for all end-of-chapter exercises. The *Instructor eResources* also offers ready-to-use chapter tests and PowerPoint® presentations.

About the Authors

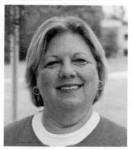 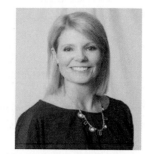

Darline Foltz, RHIA   Karen Lankisch, PhD, RHIA

Darline Foltz is an assistant professor at the University of Cincinnati–Clermont College. She holds bachelor's degrees in both Health Information Management and Information Processing Systems, and is currently working to achieve her master's degree in Educational Studies. Foltz is a Registered Health Information Administrator (RHIA), has more than 30 years of experience in the health information field, and has held multiple hospital management positions. She also holds the CHPS (Certified in Healthcare Privacy and Security) credential. As owner and president of Foltz & Associates, Healthcare Consulting Firm, Foltz has provided health information management and information systems consulting services to many clients, including hospitals, long-term care facilities, dialysis clinics, and mental health agencies. Active in professional and community service, she is a past-president of the Ohio Health Information Management Association and former chairperson of the long-term care section of the American Health Information Management Association (AHIMA).

Dr. Karen Lankisch is a professor and program director of Health Information Systems Technology at the University of Cincinnati–Clermont College. She is certified through the American Health Information Management Association (AHIMA) as a Registered Health Information Administrator and has more than ten years of experience in the field of health information. In addition, she serves as a support faculty member for the Instructional Design Technology Graduate Program, as well as an external mentor in the University of Cincinnati's New Faculty Institute Initiative. Dr. Lankisch is a Quality Matters Master Peer Reviewer and has completed reviews both nationally and internationally. In addition to being an author, she has served as a national consultant for Paradigm Education Solutions, giving workshops and presentations to instructors on Paradigm's technology learning solutions. Her research interests are emerging technology, online course design, and constructivist approaches to adult education. In 2013, she received the University of Cincinnati Faculty Award for Innovative Use of Technology in the Classroom. In 2016, she was selected for membership to the University of Cincinnati Academy of Fellows for Teaching and Learning.

Acknowledgments

The quality of this body of work is a testament to the feedback we have received from the many contributors and reviewers who participated in the development of *Exploring Electronic Health Records*, Second Edition.

We would like to thank the following reviewers who have offered valuable comments and suggestions on the content of this textbook.

Desantila Sherifi, MBA, RHIA
Devry University
Ambler, PA

Debra Slusarczyk
Camden County College
Woodbury, NJ

Special thanks to the members of Paradigm's Health Information Technology Advisory Board for providing valuable and thoughtful advice throughout the development of this text.

Additional thanks go to the exam and PowerPoint writers and testers, as well as to the programmers, writers, and testers of the EHR Navigator software. In particular, we thank Jessica Lindfors, Jeri Novalany, Meaghan Raleigh, Timothy Niccum, and Dayne Smith.

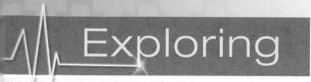

Exploring

ELECTRONIC
Health Records

Second Edition

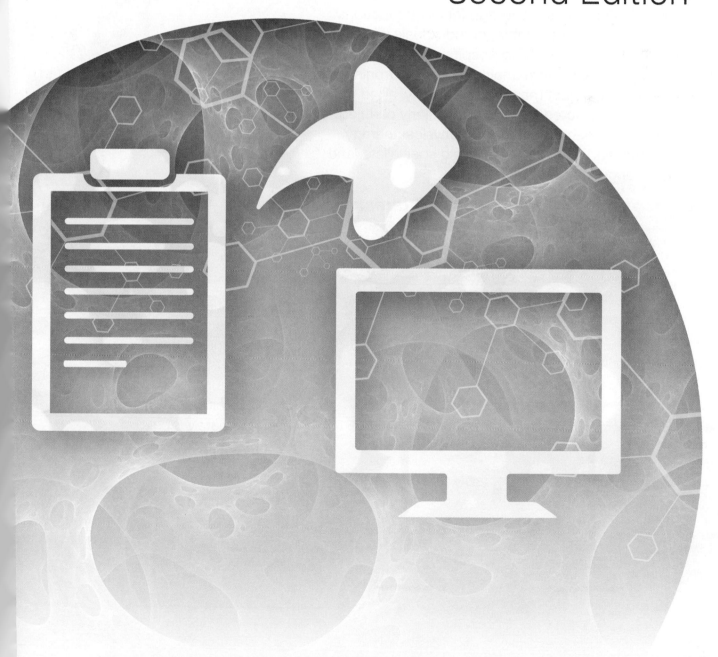

> " Today three-fourths of doctors are using EHRs. There is now a digital care footprint for almost everyone in the country. "

— US Department of Health and Human Services (HHS) Secretary Sylvia Burwell at the Health Information Management Systems Society conference in 2016

Are You Ready?

Employment of health information technicians is projected to grow 15% from 2014 to 2024, which is much faster than the average for all occupations. Myriad careers are available for individuals with an HIM background, including hospital chief executive officers, coders, system analysts, and electronic health record project managers. Similarly, allied health careers are predicted to grow, particularly certified occupational therapy assistants, physical therapy assistants, audiologists, hearing aid specialists, and speech language pathologists.

What aspect of the field most interests you?

Beyond the Record

- Outpatient facilities that adopt and use electronic health records (EHRs) for 15 years could save as much as $42 billion each year.

- Inpatient facilities that adopt and use EHRs for 15 years could experience a net savings of $371 billion.
- As of September 2016, nearly all hospitals (96%) and approximately 8 in 10 physicians used certified EHRs.

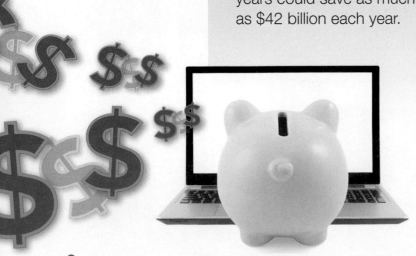

Overview of Electronic Health Records

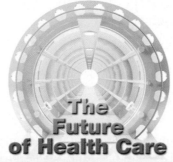

The Future of Health Care

How will implementing electronic health records (EHRs) change the healthcare field? Patient safety is likely to improve because EHRs eliminate one of the most common causes of medical errors: illegible handwriting. EHRs will also improve communication between patients and the healthcare team once healthcare providers are able to more easily access their patients' complete medical histories.

1.1 Define the terms *electronic medical record (EMR)* and *electronic health record (EHR)* and understand their distinctions.

1.2 Explain the concept of interoperability and its importance in the EHR environment.

1.3 Understand the difference between *syntactic interoperability level* and *semantic interoperability level*.

1.4 Define computer protocol and discuss the most common communication protocol, Health Level 7 International (HL7).

1.5 Understand the health IT ecosystem.

1.6 Describe a learning healthcare system (LHS).

1.7 Describe the Health Information Technology for Economic and Clinical Health Act and the federal incentive program for implementing EHRs.

1.8 Understand the concept of meaningful use and identify the main components of each stage.

1.9 List and discuss the benefits and barriers to implementing EHRs.

1.10 List and discuss the evolving potential roles in the EHR environment.

EXPAND
YOUR LEARNING

To hear how access to your medical records improves the quality of care you receive, view this video:

http://EHR2.Paradigm Education.com/ ITVideos.

Most providers of health care in the United States are required to use **electronic health records (EHRs)**. EHRs replace traditional paper medical records that have been used for centuries, making health information accessible to healthcare providers across the world with only a few keystrokes. This nearly instantaneous access to health information increases facility efficiency, improves patient outcomes, and results in a healthier population.

Never before have healthcare delivery and technology met at such a pivotal point. US federal regulations and incentives have motivated many hospitals, physicians, dentists, nursing homes, outpatient clinics, and other providers to implement EHRs.

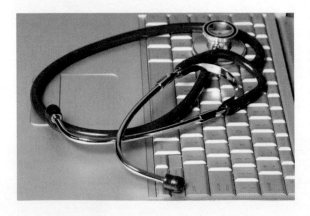

The **American Recovery and Reinvestment Act of 2009 (ARRA)** authorized the **Centers for Medicare & Medicaid Services (CMS)** to award incentive payments to eligible professionals who demonstrated meaningful use of a certified EHR. The healthcare providers that participated in EHR implementation in 2011 were eligible for the maximum financial incentives. Financial incentives for healthcare providers continued through 2014. On January 1, 2015, the US government began reducing Medicare payments to healthcare providers without EHR systems that complied with federal standards. (The specifics of these regulations and the healthcare providers affected will be discussed later in this chapter.)

EMR versus EHR

The terms *electronic medical record (EMR)* and *electronic health record (EHR)* are often confused with one another. EMRs and EHRs are similar concepts but different in both scope and relationship. The EMR belongs to a single healthcare provider or organization, whereas the EHR integrates EMRs from multiple providers. In other words, EMRs are individual data sources that inform and populate collected patient information to form the global EHR system.

Electronic Medical Record

An **electronic medical record (EMR)** is an electronic version of patient files within a single organization, and it allows healthcare providers to place orders, document results, and store patient information for one facility, commonly called the **healthcare delivery (HCD) system**. For example, Hope Hospital in Cincinnati, Ohio, might implement an EMR to replace its separate order entry, results reporting, and documentation computer systems. Implementing a complete EMR will replace the paper medical record and can be used by physicians, nurses, other clinicians, and clerical staff. The EMR becomes the facility's legal record of the treatment course provided to patients while they are in the care of the facility. The EMR is owned by the HCD system, a concept that is discussed further in Chapter 2. Figure 1.1 represents an EMR and illustrates how each facility's EHR is a separate, stand-alone record.

Figure 1.1 Electronic Medical Records from Different Healthcare Facilities

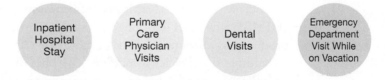

These scenarios indicate possible EMR usage:

- Dr. Schwartz enters an order at the bedside terminal of patient Ellie Smith for a complete blood count laboratory test to rule out anemia.

- Nurse Holloway scans the barcode on patient Susan Miller's identification band followed by the barcode on the medication prior to administering the drug. This procedure helps to guarantee the accuracy of the medication's type, dose, and route of administration and helps verify that the patient is not allergic to this medication.

- Admission Clerk Shika Nadal registers a patient for admission, creating a new account number that links to the patient's EMR.

- Dental Hygienist Sarah Alvaro obtains dental X-rays of patient Lashonda Johnson with a camera that interfaces with the dental office's EMR.

- Dr. Blatt enters his hospital patient visits into his mobile device as he performs patient rounds and then syncs the device with his practice's EMR.

- Linda Agee, practice manager for Cardiology Associates, ensures that all physicians and staff members document services provided and copays collected so that the practice's billing staff can automatically generate accurate bills as a by-product of the data.

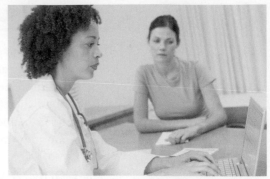

A patient and her doctor review information in the patient's EMR during an office visit.

- Carol Matta, psychologist for Family Mental Health Associates Inc., electronically documents her clients' visits after the end of each therapy session so that the records will be available to the on-call psychologists in the event of an emergency.

Although the EMR helps these healthcare providers electronically document their patient encounters, it generally does not allow them access to patient files from another healthcare facility.

Electronic Health Record

The EHR contains patient health information gathered from the EMRs of multiple HCD organizations and is electronically stored and accessed. EHRs differ from EMRs because they contain subsets of patient information from each visit that a patient has experienced, possibly at many different HCD systems (see Figure 1.2). EHRs are interactive and can share information among multiple healthcare providers.

According to the **Healthcare Information and Management Systems Society (HIMSS)**, the EHR is a "longitudinal electronic record of patient health information produced by encounters in one or more care settings. The EHR system automates and streamlines the clinician's workflow….[It] has the ability to independently generate a complete record of a clinical patient encounter and possesses sufficient data granularity to support clinical decision support systems (CDSSs), quality management, clinical reporting, and interoperability."

Figure 1.2 Electronic Health Record

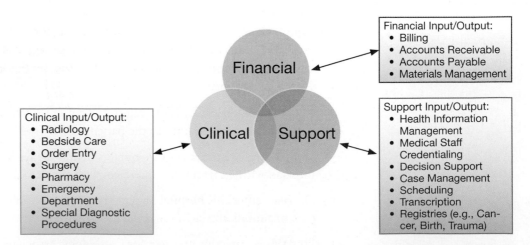

CHECKPOINT 1.1

1. What is the definition of an electronic medical record (EMR)? _____

   _____

   _____

2. What is the definition of an electronic health record (EHR)? _____

   _____

   _____

   _____

3. List three major differences between an EMR and an EHR.

   a. _____

   b. _____

   c. _____

Consider This

Kim Singh visits the emergency department of Hope Hospital complaining of chest pain. Kim mentions that she had an echocardiogram and an electrocardiogram (ECG) performed at the office of cardiologist Dr. Carruthers approximately one month ago. The emergency department physician is able to immediately view Kim's echocardiographic and ECG results.

Kim's health record is located in a central repository of health information in which Hope Hospital, Cincinnati Dental Care, Dr. Carruthers's office, and Happy Knoll Nursing Home all participate. How might Kim's care have differed if the emergency department and the cardiologist did not have electronic health records that communicate with one another? How might her care have differed in a paper health record environment?

The term **longitudinal** indicates that a patient's EHR will continue to develop over the course of care. Every medical event and document can be accessed within the EHR, regardless of facility, country, or time period.

Kim Singh's longitudinal EHR is represented in Figure 1.3 and now contains both her visit to Dr. Carruthers's office and her emergency department visit to Hope Hospital. Notice that patient information can be freely shared among different HCD settings. This patient's longitudinal EHR will continue to grow as she has additional encounters with providers such as an optometrist, surgeon, outpatient surgery center, nursing home, dentist office, or mental health professional.

In the preceding example, the EHR central data repository stores all patient data for the participating healthcare facilities on a privately owned server, which is one method of storing EHRs.

Figure 1.3 Longitudinal Electronic Health Record

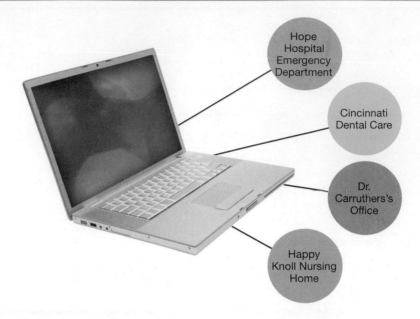

Hope Hospital Emergency Department

Cincinnati Dental Care

Dr. Carruthers's Office

Happy Knoll Nursing Home

Interoperability

The success of the EHR primarily rests on **interoperability**, which is the ability of one computer system to communicate with another computer system. Similar to how individuals must speak the same language to share information and understand what is being communicated, computers must also speak the same language to communicate. Additionally, the systems must be able to operate at a high enough level of interoperability to share and process data.

Levels of Interoperability

With healthcare computer systems, there are three different levels of interoperability that demonstrate a range of communication ability. Computer systems unable to exchange information are considered Level 0, whereas computer systems with Level 3 interoperability can share and manipulate data to the degree needed to support EHR systems. See Figure 1.4 for an illustration of the levels of interoperability. Each level is defined as follows:

- **Level 0:** Stand-alone systems have **no interoperability**.

- **Level 1:** This level (also known as **technical interoperability**) is considered a basic or foundational level of communication. This level of communication infrastructure allows systems to exchange bits and bytes of data without any ability to interpret the shared data.

- **Level 2:** This level is called the **syntactic interoperability level**. This level provides a common data format for data exchange; the data can be interpreted, but the meaning of the data may not be understood.

- **Level 3:** The **semantic interoperability level** is a high level of interoperability that allows the meaning of the data to be shared. The data and information may also be interpreted, allowing EHR systems to function.

Figure 1.4 Levels of Conceptual Interoperability Model

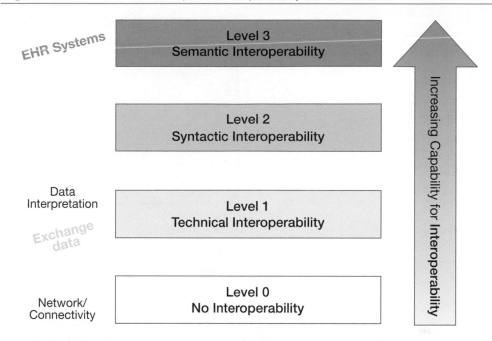

The focus when referring to interoperability in relation to the EHR is on syntactic and semantic interoperability (Levels 2 and 3). A minimally successful EHR system must at least use a common data format that can exchange information, and that format must meet the definition of syntactic interoperability (Level 2). However, ideally an EHR system will meet the definition of semantic interoperability (Level 3) so that health information can be understood and interpreted, not merely shared.

For example, if the EHR of Children's Hospital wants to share data with the EHR of Dr. Allen, a primary care physician, then both EHR systems must have a common technical foundation and, at the very least, syntactic interoperability. Syntactic interoperability facilitates the basic communication and exchange of information between EHRs, enabling the EHR system at Children's Hospital to send the laboratory reports of a patient to Dr. Allen's EHR system. The semantic interoperability of both EHRs allows Dr. Allen to understand the meaning of the laboratory results.

The concept of interoperability is not unique to EHRs. For example, fire and police communication systems must have interoperability to effectively communicate with each other and to respond to emergencies in a fast, organized fashion.

Computer Protocols

For EHRs to be useful and beneficial, *all* participating EMRs need one standard set of interoperability computer protocols. A **computer protocol** is a standardized method of communicating or transmitting data between two computer systems. The most common healthcare communication protocol in use today is **Health Level Seven International (HL7)**, which focuses on the exchange of clinical and administrative data. HL7 is also the name of an international group of collaborating healthcare subject-matter experts and information scientists. Figure 1.5 provides an example of an immunization record written using HL7 protocol.

Figure 1.5 Health Level Seven International Protocol

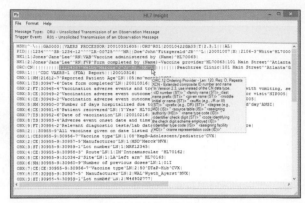

Courtesy of Steve Hart, Senior IT Consultant, HL7 2.X Certified, http://www.hartsteve.com/creations/hl7insight

This is the challenge facing the health information technology (IT) stakeholders today—choosing one language or set of protocols that all EHRs will use, thus enabling access for proper use of health information within the health IT ecosystem.

A **health IT ecosystem** (illustrated in Figure 1.6) is a collection of individuals and groups that are interested in health information technology. Included in a health IT ecosystem are clinicians, hospitals, various healthcare providers, public health workers, technology developers, payers, researchers, policy makers, individual patients, and many others. All of these stakeholders in the health IT ecosystem are interested in interoperability. As you can see in Figure 1.6, the patient is the starting point of the ecosystem. Health information is accessed and shared for quality and safety in care delivery, population health management, regional information exchange, and analytics for research. Data can then be used to establish or update clinical guidelines to support public health policy and to update CDS systems.

Figure 1.6 Health IT Ecosystem

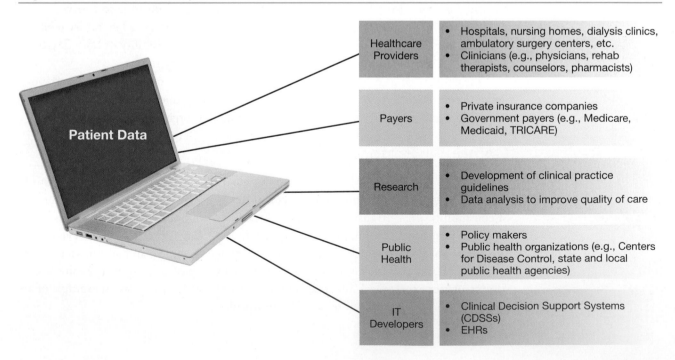

The **Office of the National Coordinator for Health Information Technology (ONC)** is the US federal body that recommends policies, procedures, protocols, and standards for interoperability. The ONC is part of the US Department of Health and Human Services (HHS) and was created by the ARRA. The mission of the ONC is "to improve health and health care for all Americans through use of information and technology." In its work to improve health and health care through the use of information and technology, the ONC has been working on interoperability with interested stakeholders of health IT. The ONC published "A 10-Year Vision to Achieve an Interoperable Health IT Infrastructure" that is to be accomplished by achieving the following three goals:

- **2015–2017:** Send, receive, find, and use priority data domains to improve health quality and outcomes.

- **2018–2020:** Expand data sources and users in the interoperable health IT ecosystem to improve health and lower costs.

- **2021–2024:** Achieve nationwide interoperability to enable a learning health system in which the patient is at the center of a system that can continuously improve care, public health, and science through real-time data access.

A **learning healthcare system (LHS)** is an approach to improving the quality of health care by using patient clinical data from EHRs to drive medical research and by using medical research to influence clinical practices. An LHS has patients at the center of a system that continually collects and processes data, working toward goals of improved quality of care.

The ONC has funded a number of health IT programs, including the development of the **Nationwide Health Information Network (NwHIN)**. The NwHIN is a set of standards, services, and policies that enables health information to be securely exchanged over the Internet and that will help create an environment in which healthcare information is stored and shared securely and electronically. To help facilitate the move from paper medical records to an EHR, the ONC created a forum, the Standards and Interoperability Framework (S&I Framework), in which healthcare providers and stakeholders can focus on solving real-world interoperability challenges.

CHECKPOINT 1.2

1. What is the definition of interoperability?

_____

_____

_____

2. What level of interoperability is needed for electronic health records to interpret data?

_____

_____

3. What is the most common type of healthcare communication protocol in use today?

_____

_____

Federal Regulations

Members of the US Congress demonstrated their commitment to nationwide implementation of EHR technology by enacting the **Health Information Technology for Economic and Clinical Health (HITECH) Act** in February 2009, which was part of the ARRA. This legislation set aside $19.2 billion to achieve the following goals:

- To encourage physicians, hospitals, and other providers to implement the EHR by offering financial incentives. The HITECH Act defined different stages of EHR implementation and funding to healthcare providers. For example, physicians could receive up to $44,000 in incentive payments under Medicare and even more if they treated Medicaid patients. A hospital could receive up to $2 million as a base payment.

- To create the Health Information Technology Extension Program, which was designed to help small- and medium-sized physician practices implement an EHR system

- To establish a national Health Information Technology Research Center (HITRC) and Regional Extension Centers (RECs) to work with each other to share best practices for implementing EHRs and act as resources for physicians and other healthcare providers

Incentive Programs

After a provider implemented an EHR system that met the established government requirements, that provider upon submission of an application would receive incentive funds under the Medicare and/or Medicaid programs. Eligible healthcare providers that implemented "meaningful use" (described further in the next section) of a certified EHR received up to $44,000 over five years under the Medicare EHR Incentive Program and up to $63,750 over six years under the Medicaid EHR Incentive Program. Figure 1.7 illustrates the professionals who were eligible for the Medicare EHR Incentive Program and the Medicaid EHR Incentive Program.

Providers who did not implement an EHR system by January 1, 2015, have been receiving reduced reimbursement from Medicare. For example, physicians who had not adopted certified EHR systems or could not demonstrate meaningful use by the beginning of 2015 saw their Medicare reimbursements reduced by 1%, a rate that was increased to 2% in 2016 and 3% in 2017. If less than 75% of eligible providers (EPs) have become meaningful users of EHRs by 2018, the adjustment will change by one percentage point each year to a maximum of 5%. Obviously, most healthcare facilities desire full reimbursement and cannot afford to not implement an EMR/EHR system.

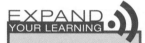

EXPAND YOUR LEARNING

You can find more information regarding meaningful use and incentive programs on the Centers for Medicare & Medicaid Services website:

http://EHR2.Paradigm Education.com/ CMSprograms.

Figure 1.7 Eligible Providers (EPs) under Medicare and Medicaid EHR Incentive Programs

---

EPs under the Medicare EHR Incentive Program include:

- Doctors of medicine or osteopathy
- Doctors of dental surgery or dental medicine
- Doctors of podiatry
- Doctors of optometry
- Chiropractors

EPs under the Medicaid EHR Incentive Program include:

- Physicians (primarily doctors of medicine and doctors of osteopathy)
- Nurse practitioners
- Certified nurse-midwives
- Dentists
- Physician assistants who furnish services in a federally qualified health center or rural health clinic led by a physician assistant

Meaningful Use

Meaningful use (see Figure 1.8) is the set of standards defined by the **Centers for Medicare & Medicaid Services (CMS)** Incentive Programs that govern the use of EHRs. Meaningful use is defined as using certified EHR technology to:

- Improve quality, safety, and efficiency and reduce health disparities
- Engage patients and family
- Improve care coordination and population and public health
- Maintain privacy and security of patient health information

Ultimately, it is hoped that the meaningful use compliance will result in:

- Better clinical outcomes
- Improved population health outcomes
- Increased transparency and efficiency
- Empowered individuals
- More robust research data on health systems

Healthcare providers must prove that they have implemented EHR technology and are thus eligible for incentive funds by meeting the requirements of meaningful use. Meaningful use is included in the HITECH Act and defines the accepted levels of EHR implementation and qualifications to receive federal incentives. These definitions can be measured in quality and quantity.

Figure 1.8 Stages of Meaningful Use

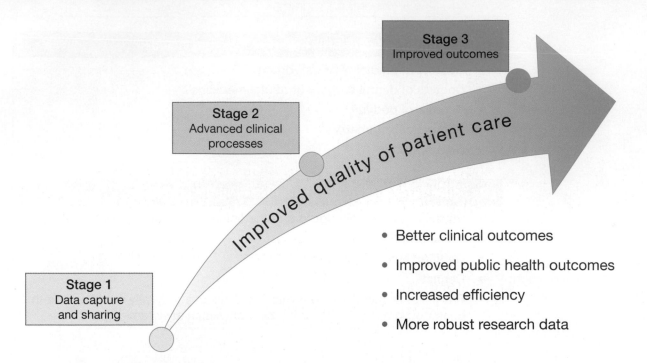

Meaningful use requirements evolved in three stages. Stage 1 requirements focused on data capture and sharing and were implemented during 2011–2012. Stage 2 requirements focused on advancing clinical processes and were implemented in 2014. Stage 3 requirements focused on improved outcomes and were implemented in 2016.

Stage 1

Stage 1 set the foundation for the EHR incentive programs by establishing requirements for the electronic capture of clinical data, including providing patients with electronic copies of health information. There are three main components of Stage 1 meaningful use:

- Use of certified EHR technology in a meaningful manner, such as electronic prescribing (eRx)

- Use of certified EHR technology for the electronic exchange of health information to improve the quality of health care

- Use of certified EHR technology to submit clinical quality measures (CQM) and other measures

Stage 2

Stage 2 expanded upon the Stage 1 criteria and encouraged the use of health IT for continuous quality improvement at the point of care and the exchange of information. There are seven topic areas of objectives and measures included in Stage 2. These include the following:

- Protect electronic protected health information (ePHI)

- eRx

- Health information exchange

- Patient-specific education (e.g., diabetes education, diet and exercise education)

- Medication reconciliation (comparing a patient's medications taken at home with hospital medications)

- Patient electronic access

- Public health reporting

A few examples of meeting the criteria included in Stage 2 include generating and transmitting electronic prescriptions upon the discharge of a patient; providing patients the ability to view online, download, and transmit their health information within 36 hours of discharge; and having the hospital send a summary care record for each patient who transitions to another institution or provider for care.

Stage 3

Stage 3 continued to expand on Stages 1 and 2 by requiring providers to meet criteria that demonstrate coordination of care through patient engagement and participation in a health information exchange and public health reporting. There are eight topic areas of objectives and measures included in Stage 3. These objectives and measures include the following:

- Protect ePHI

- eRx

- CDSSs (provide information regarding a particular diagnosis or treatment to clinicians to enhance decision-making in the clinical workflow of the patient)

- Computerized provider order entry (CPOE) (orders for medications and treatment are entered directly into the EHR)

- Patient electronic access

- Coordination of care (the organization of a patient's healthcare treatment to improve the quality of care and eliminate duplication of tests and procedures)

- Health information exchange

- Public health reporting

Examples of meeting the criteria included in Stage 3 include implementing CDSSs interventions focused on improving performance on high-priority health conditions and using CPOE for medication, laboratory, and diagnostic imaging orders directly entered by the ordering provider.

An important change to meaningful use in 2018 is that all providers will be required to participate in Stage 3 regardless of their prior participation in the meaningful use program. The government is moving all providers to the same stage of meaningful use to simplify reporting requirements and to have everyone focused on the same objectives and criteria.

Benefits of EHRs

The transition to EHRs requires monumental effort on the part of doctors, healthcare staff, regulators, government officials, and everyone working in the healthcare industry. The final goals of the transition are higher-quality healthcare services, more effective and efficient communication, and healthier patients. Advocates of the transition cite many potential and already realized benefits as reasons to approach this work with excitement and a sense of opportunity. The most obvious benefits (all leading to improved patient care and safety) include:

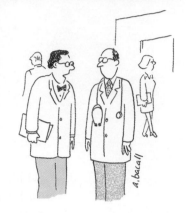

"Another advantage of switching to electronic health records is that it will make your indecipherable handwriting obsolete."

- Improved documentation

- Streamlined and rapid communication

- Immediate and improved access to patient information

Improved Documentation

A classic complaint about doctors is their terrible handwriting. Many medication errors are the result of illegible and misinterpreted physician notes. Staff members waste time and become frustrated trying to read and interpret clinician notes, and the clinician often needs to be contacted to clarify meaning. Figures 1.9 and 1.10 illustrate the difference between handwritten and electronic progress notes, respectively.

EHRs use standardized templates that capture data by typing, scanning, and using drop-down menus, among other features. Physicians can enter complex prescriptions, and typically, patients can electronically fill out forms and questionnaires without incident. A doctor can record patient visit notes directly into the EHR without transcribing tape-recorded or handwritten notes. Not only will daily documentation be more accurate, but medical studies may also be more effectively conducted. For example, a

Figure 1.9 Handwritten Progress Note

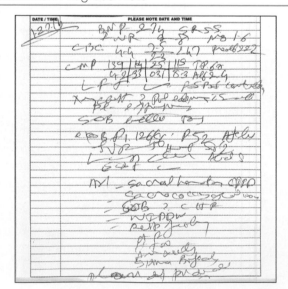

Figure 1.10 Electronic Progress Notes

Progress Note

Patient name:	McDowell, Terrence	**Medical Record Number:**	585067
Date of Birth:	07/19/58	**Patient Number:**	1772518
Location:	Northstar Medical Center	**Admission Date:**	02/18/30
Provider:	Gertz, Lester MD	**Room/Bed:**	567-1
Date/Time:	02/19/30 14:00		

SUBJECTIVE: Yesterday, this patient was worked up on the ER and subsequently admitted to 567-1 when he was diagnosed with community-acquired pneumonia along with COPD exacerbation. Review of the ER and admission documentation reveals that the patient is a 72-year-old male Caucasian patient with a long-standing history of COPD.

OBJECTIVE:

VITAL SIGNS: The patient's max temperature over the past 24 hours has been 101.3F; his blood pressure at present is 148/90, his pulse is 93. His O2 sats are 95% on 2L via nasal cannula.

HEART: Regular rate and rhythm without murmur, gallop, or rub.

LUNGS: Lungs are very tight. Wheezes bilaterally and rhonchi on the right mid base. Nurses report that he has a productive cough of green purulent sputum.

ABDOMEN: Soft and nontender. Bowel sounds x4 are normoactive.

NEUROLOGIC: Patient is alert and oriented x3. His pupils are equal and reactive.

ASSESSMENT:

1. Chronic COPD with acute exacerbation.

2. Community-acquired pneumonia, awaiting sputum culture report.

3. Generalized weakness and deconditioning secondary to the above.

---

new drug can be closely monitored, and a hospital's effort to track patterns like smoking cessation or overall diet improvement may be much easier. Data can be collected, identified, and sorted within a single database, leading to more accurate and innovative research.

Streamlined and Rapid Communication

The implementation of an EHR system streamlines the patient documentation process. The provision of patient care in any HCD system is complex because of the coordination of staff members and workflow processes in such areas as medications, procedures, testing, decision-making, and communication. When documenting patient care using a paper record, healthcare personnel must enter patient information multiple times on multiple forms. However, when documenting patient information electronically, personnel enter the information once, which saves time, allows an easy database search, and helps maintain the consistency and integrity of the patient record.

EHR technology also allows for streamlined and rapid communication of information. For example, instead of waiting for a patient's test results to pass among several staff members, healthcare providers using an EHR system can be automatically alerted when the laboratory technicians file the reports.

EHR technology also streamlines the medication-dispensing process and improves medication safety. For example, a patient's paper prescription typically travels from the doctor to the nurse, from the nurse to the clerk, and then from the clerk to the pharmacist. An EHR system allows a physician to use e-prescribing, a process that transmits the prescription directly to the pharmacist. This transmittal process eliminates the need for a nurse or other staff member to enter the medication order into the computer, a clerical step that impedes patient care. E-prescribing also allows direct communication between the pharmacist and the prescriber to resolve any prescription errors. An EHR system has an automatic feature that alerts prescribers to drug incompatibilities, a step that may take several hours to determine when filling a paper prescription.

Immediate and Improved Access to Patient Information

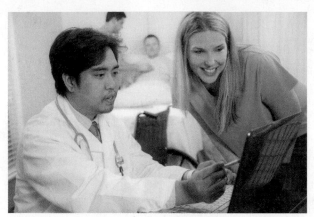

Staff members access a patient's information quickly and efficiently when using an EHR system.

With a robust, interoperable EHR system, healthcare organizations can nearly instantaneously access a patient's entire health history by viewing a patient's dental records, home healthcare visits, psychiatry records, and any other necessary history. The significance of this ability cannot be overstated. Healthcare staff can spot medical errors and inconsistencies more quickly and can instantly view the results of medical procedures performed across the globe. They can easily track and measure years of patient outcomes without having to search for misplaced records.

Healthcare facilities are not the only ones benefiting from this access. Patients who cannot remember past procedures, diagnoses, or allergies can be protected from hasty and underinformed medical decisions. Patients can monitor personal health goals and even report glucose readings or progress during their exercise routines from home, and patients with an allergic reaction or injury presenting to a different hospital while on vacation will not have to worry. All of their health records will be accessible, thus allowing any healthcare provider the ability to make informed and safe choices.

Barriers to EHR Implementation

To best assist with the transition to EHRs and to ensure an efficient, successful program, it is important to understand the reservations held by some patients, physicians, staff, and agencies. Many of these barriers are valid concerns in the emerging EHR field. Overcoming such barriers will be critical for developing effective policies and technologies and for educating everyone within the healthcare industry. Some common criticisms of the EHR system include the following:

- High cost

- Insufficient privacy and security

- Inexperience in implementation and training

- Significant daily process changes

High Cost

High cost is the most common barrier described by healthcare leadership. Whether the cost is $15,000 to implement an EHR system for a small physician or dental practice or several million dollars for a large hospital, the costs can be a relative burden for most healthcare providers. Although federal financial incentives have helped offset the costs of implementing EHR systems, healthcare providers did not receive the incentive funds until *after* the systems were implemented and proven to meet US federal standards. For a small nursing home, mental health center, or even a small hospital, the required large investment in adopting and implementing EHR technology can be a significant deterrent.

Insufficient Privacy and Security

One of the biggest benefits to an EHR system—easy access to patients' medical records—is also one of the public's biggest concerns. Unlimited access requires facilities and providers to install secure firewalls (specialized computer programs that prevent unauthorized access) and to implement privacy policies and procedures, access monitoring, and privacy breach enforcement. Violations of online security involving credit card companies, banks, and gaming systems have alerted the public to the risk of storing and distributing personal information online, so the thought of such personal information being only a few clicks away can be troubling, possibly discouraging patients from being honest about their medical histories.

Inexperience in Implementation and Training

US federal regulations requiring HCD systems to implement EHRs have spawned the growth of many EHR systems and vendors. Faced with a great variability of the products and service levels in the EHR market, physicians, dentists, hospital chief executive officers (CEOs), and others are justifiably reluctant to select an EHR company that may leave its clients with little to no support. Such lack of software support could mean that the healthcare provider would have to implement an entirely new EHR system, resulting in increased costs and disruption of services.

CEOs and office managers are also concerned about hiring the right staff to implement and maintain the EHR. Employers must ensure that new staff members will be qualified to handle the move away from paper records. The US federal government recognized this issue and passed legislation to create certification programs for health information technology (HIT) careers. (This subject is discussed in greater detail later in this chapter.)

EXPAND
YOUR LEARNING

To learn more about topics such as consumer engagement, EHR adoption, health information exchange, health IT workforce, and more, go to http://EHR2.Paradigm Education.com/Buzz-Blog, click the Tag you are interested in reading more about, and you will be directed to a government-sponsored site.

Significant Daily Process Changes

Doctors and staff may also be reluctant to embrace a system that requires an overhaul of their daily duties and tasks. A physician might argue that using EHRs will take *longer* to process patients and their information. For example, after a patient checkup, the physician might typically jot down notes or dictate into a tape recorder, then pass that information along to a staff member for transcription. With the EHR, the doctor must log on to the system, locate the patient's chart, enter the information, and then save it to the patient's files. All employees of a healthcare facility will experience similar changes to a system they might have been using for several years or decades. This change in routine could easily feel frustrating and unnecessary, thus creating barriers to change and difficulties in the successful implementation of an EHR system. It may take years for staff members to buy into the new technology. Offices might also see staff turnover as a result of duty and task changes.

CHECKPOINT 1.3

1. List three benefits of implementing an electronic health record (EHR) system.

   a. _____

   b. _____

   c. _____

2. List four barriers to successfully implementing an EHR system.

   a. _____

   b. _____

   c. _____

   d. _____

Moving Forward

In the same way that building a new subway system or highway is expensive to implement and may cause traffic delays while being built, investment in the EHR is a temporary burden. The savings from replacing inefficient paper medical records will inevitably pay off the initial investment, and healthcare providers can switch to a more efficient system.

Future Challenges to EHR Implementation

Privacy and security problems are not specific to EHRs; rather, these problems are similar to those of any company or industry that maintains an online presence. Although efforts must—and will—be made to protect personal health records, the world is just beginning to understand the true risks of managing personal information online. Because of increasing awareness of identity theft, many people have learned not to post the names and birth dates of their children on personal websites, and others have learned not to email credit card and Social Security numbers based on unsolicited requests. In the same way, industries are using significant resources to create security programs and procedures to address past breaches and anticipate future issues. Chapter 6 will discuss privacy and security issues in greater detail.

Interoperability will continue to be a challenge for many years while IT vendors work toward achieving a standard computer protocol and Level 3, semantic interoperability.

Having adequate support for the EHR system, both from the EHR vendor and from qualified staff, will be an important piece of the puzzle for healthcare facilities. Given time, quality EHR vendors are likely to rise to the top, giving healthcare providers confidence in their chosen EHR companies. As the field of HIT grows, more students will graduate with the appropriate knowledge and experience to implement, use, and maintain an EHR system. The inconveniences experienced by doctors and other clinical staff early on in the process are essential steps toward the dramatic improvement to the US healthcare system.

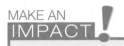

MAKE AN IMPACT

Professionals with proper education and credentials assist healthcare providers with proper implementation of EHR systems.

Evolving Roles in the EHR Environment

Managing the transition from paper to electronic records requires individuals with special skills and education. The US Department of Labor, Bureau of Labor Statistics reports that the demand for **health information management (HIM)** professionals will increase 15% from 2014 to 2024, much faster than the average for all occupations, and it acknowledges that the "increasing use of electronic health records will continue to broaden and alter the job responsibilities of health information technicians. For example, with the use of EHRs, technicians must be familiar with EHR computer software, maintaining EHR security, and analyzing electronic data to improve healthcare information."

The **American Health Information Management Association (AHIMA)** provides many opportunities for credentialing health information professionals interested in implementing and managing EHRs, such as the following:

RHIT: registered health information technician (associate's degree) RHITs perform the technical procedures related to the management of health information, frequently working in positions of medical coding, billing, and data management.

RHIA: registered health information administrator (bachelor's degree) The RHIA works as a liaison between healthcare providers, organization staff, payers, and patients. The RHIA is an expert in managing health information and the professionals responsible for managing health information.

CHTS: certified healthcare technology specialist This certification denotes proficiency in certain health IT roles and is intended for professionals with various education backgrounds who are interested in working with EHRs.

Certified in Healthcare Privacy and Security (CHPS) is a certification that identifies an individual's competence in privacy and security protection programs in all types of healthcare organizations.

Having this certification denotes competence in designing, implementing, and administering comprehensive privacy and security protection programs in all types of healthcare organizations.

HIMSS is a nonprofit, global organization of information technicians focused on improving health through the improvement of health information technology. HIMSS administers two professional certification programs for healthcare information and management systems:

CAHIMS (Certified Associate in Healthcare Information and Management Systems) is a certification designed for IT professionals new to the health information arena. CAHIMS is designed to be a pathway for careers in health IT.

CPHIMS (Certified Professional in Healthcare Information and Management Systems) is a professional certification program for experienced healthcare information and management systems professionals.

In addition to well-established certification programs, the US federal government set aside $32 million in grants through the HITECH Act for universities to train individuals in an abbreviated health information management course. Individuals who trained under these programs were eligible to take the CHTS (formerly the HIT Pro) competency examination in one of the following specialties:

- Practice workflow and information management redesign specialist
- Clinician/practitioner consultant
- Implementation manager
- Implementation support specialist
- Technical/software support staff
- Trainer

Employee positions at an HCD provider include chief information officer, systems analyst, systems administrator, database administrator/specialist, EHR project manager, and EHR trainer. These positions are explained in more detail in the student resources and are primarily available at either a healthcare provider or an EHR software vendor. Other health-related entities such as insurance companies, durable medical equipment companies, medical billing companies, and so forth continue to create positions to work with EHRs for healthcare facility customers. For example, an insurance company adopts policies and procedures for accessing clients' EHRs, so it will need staff to develop and implement these standards.

Creating a national (and international) record-keeping system will not be simple, but this task is a testament to the scope and vision of EHR implementation. Although the current generation may experience struggles as the EHR is implemented, the resulting nationwide EHR system will provide future healthcare providers with a more reliable, efficient, and cost-effective healthcare system. As health care and technology evolve together, new jobs and career opportunities will be created; patient outcomes will improve; and healthcare delivery will see gains in efficiency, communication, and overall quality.

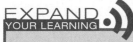

EXPAND YOUR LEARNING

Search the Internet for EHR careers and prepare a presentation on different career opportunities.

PRACTICE PROFESSIONALISM

Healthcare professionals should strive to remain positive in their work environments, for the sake of not only their patients but also for coworkers, visitors, and guests.

Chapter Summary

With 75% of physicians using EHRs today, almost everyone in the United States has a digital healthcare footprint. This digital footprint is in the form of an EMR.

EMRs are individual data sources that belong to a single healthcare provider or organization. EMRs inform and populate EHRs.

The EHR is a longitudinal electronic record of patient health information produced by encounters in one or more care settings. The EHR system automates and streamlines the clinician's workflow. The EHR can independently generate a complete record of a clinical patient encounter, and it possesses sufficient detail of the data to provide clinical decision support, quality management, clinical reporting, and interoperability.

Interoperability is the ability of one computer system to communicate with another computer system and is one of the overarching challenges facing successful EHR implementation. The syntactic interoperability level provides a common data format for the exchange of data, but the meaning of the data cannot be understood. The semantic level of interoperability is a high level of interoperability that allows the meaning of the data to be shared and interpreted, allowing EHR systems to function. For EHRs to be useful and beneficial, all participating EMRs need one standard set of interoperability computer protocols. A computer protocol is a standardized method of communicating or transmitting data between two computer systems. The most common communication protocol in use today is called Health Level Seven International (HL7), which focuses on the exchange of clinical and administrative data. HL7 is also the name of an international group of collaborating healthcare subject-matter experts and information scientists.

A health IT ecosystem is a collection of individuals and groups that are interested in health information technology. Included in a health IT ecosystem are clinicians, hospitals, various healthcare providers, public health workers, technology developers, payers, researchers, policymakers, individual patients, and many others. A learning healthcare system (LHS) is an approach to improving the quality of health care by using patient clinical data from EHRs to drive medical research and by using medical research to influence clinical practices.

In February 2009, the US Congress demonstrated its commitment to a nationwide implementation of EHR technology by enacting the Health Information Technology for Economic and Clinical Health (HITECH) Act. The HITECH Act defined different stages of EHR implementation and incentive funding to encourage providers to begin using EHRs. Meaningful use is defined as using a certified EHR System to improve healthcare quality, safety, efficiency, care coordination, and health outcomes; to improve the access to health care across all racial, ethnic, and socioeconomic groups; to engage patients and families in the provision and coordination of their health care; and to increase the transparency and efficiency of the provision of health care while maintaining the privacy and security of patient health information.

The benefits of implementing an EHR system include improved documentation, streamlined and rapid communication, and immediate and improved access to patient information. The barriers to implementing an EHR system include the high cost of implementation, concerns regarding privacy and security, inexperience in implementation and training, and significant daily process changes for healthcare providers.

There are many professional roles in the EHR environment. The US Department of Labor, Bureau of Labor Statistics reports that the demand for health information management professionals will increase 15% from 2014 to 2024. There are also many other emerging roles, such as a practice workflow and information management redesign specialist, clinician/practitioner consultant, implementation manager, implementation support specialist, technical/software support staff, and trainer.

Navigator ✚

The following EHR Review, EHR Application, and EHR Evaluation activities are also available online in the Navigator+ learning management system. Your instructor may ask you to complete these activities online. Navigator+ also provides access to flash cards, study games, and practice quizzes to help strengthen your understanding of the chapter content.

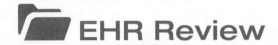

EHR Review

Acronyms/Initialisms

Study the following acronyms discussed in this chapter. Go to Navigator+ for flash cards of the acronyms and other chapter key terms.

AHIMA: American Health Information Management Association

ARRA: American Recovery and Reinvestment Act of 2009

CMS: Centers for Medicare and Medicaid Services

CPHIMS: Certified Professional in Healthcare Information and Management Systems

EHR: electronic health record

EMR: electronic medical record

HCD: healthcare delivery system

HHS: US Department of Health and Human Services

HIM: health information management

HIMSS: Healthcare Information and Management Systems Society

HIT: health information technology

HITECH: Health Information Technology for Economic and Clinical Health

HITRC: Health Information Technology Research Center

HL7: Health Level Seven International

LCIM: Levels of Conceptual Interoperability Model

LHS: Learning Healthcare System

NwHIN: Nationwide Health Information Network

ONC: Office of the National Coordinator for Health Information Technology

REC: Regional Extension Center

RHIA: registered health information administrator

RHIT: registered health information technician

Check Your Understanding

To check your understanding of this chapter's key concepts, answer the following questions.

1. What is the most common communication protocol?

   a. Syntactic

   b. Semantic

   c. Health Level Seven International

   d. NwHIN

2. What is the US federal body that recommends policies, procedures, protocols, and standards for interoperability?

   a. Office of the National Coordinator for Health Information Technology

   b. Centers for Medicare & Medicaid Services

   c. Health Information Technology for Economic and Clinical Health

   d. US Department of Health and Human Services

3. What is an EHR that continues to develop over the lifelong course of care?

   a. Vertical EMR

   b. Longitudinal EHR

   c. Personal health record

   d. Interoperable health record

4. Interoperability is

   a. a communication protocol.

   b. the ability of one computer system to communicate with another system.

   c. a longitudinal protocol.

   d. another name for an EMR.

5. The individual data sources that inform and populate the collected patient information of the global EHR are

   a. personal health records.

   b. physician office billing records.

   c. hospital records.

   d. EMRs.

6. True/False: The abbreviations EHR and EMR can be interchangeably used because they represent the same type of electronic record.

7. True/False: Electronic health records (EHRs) are interactive and can share information among multiple healthcare providers.

8. True/False: The ONC has funded the Nationwide Health Information Network (NwHIN) for the secure exchange of health information over the Internet.

9. True/False: The S&I Framework is a forum of healthcare providers and stakeholders.

10. True/False: Healthcare providers that did not implement an EHR system by 2014 were assessed fines by the US federal government.

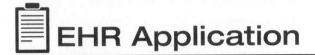 EHR Application

Go on the Record

To build on your understanding of the topics in this chapter, complete the following short-answer activities.

1. When members of the US Congress enacted the HITECH Act, they set specific goals the act would accomplish. List and briefly explain these goals.

2. List the three main components of Stage 1 meaningful use.

3. List the six levels of interoperability.

4. Briefly discuss the demand for health information management professionals that will be created by the increased use of EHRs.

5. Name two credentials offered by AHIMA for health information professionals.

Navigate the Field

To gain practice in handling challenging situations in the workplace, consider the following real-world scenarios and identify how you would respond to each.

1. North City Medical Associates is a physician practice that has struggled over the past 10 years with a tremendous growth in new patients and a lack of technology to keep up with the additional record keeping, billing, and scheduling. Jackie Lee, office manager at North City Medical Associates, decided to take advantage of incentive funds offered by the US federal government and implemented an EHR system 18 months ago. Jackie now reports that the EHR system has paid for itself several times over through practice efficiency and cost savings. Describe some specific ways in which you believe North City Medical Associates made its practice more efficient and may have experienced cost savings following its implementation of the EHR system.

2. As the health information manager at Wellness Hospital, you have been asked to research what the hospital must prove to meet meaningful use guidelines. Describe what the hospital can do to meet these guidelines.

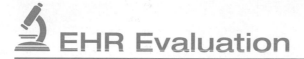

EHR Evaluation

Think Critically

Continue to think critically about challenging concepts and complete the following activities.

1. Interview a health information manager at a hospital regarding the challenges of managing a health information department in a hospital that uses an EHR system.

2. Investigate an entry-level position at http://EHR2.ParadigmEducation.com/EHRCareerAppx.

   a. Select an entry-level position that you might be interested in pursuing.

   b. Describe the position along with the promotional and transitional career pathways.

Make Your Case

Consider the scenario and then complete the following project.

You work at a medium-sized hospital with an attached physicians clinic. Your boss is considering implementing an EHR system. Create a presentation describing the benefits of and barriers to EHR implementation.

Explore the Technology

To expand your mastery of EHRs, explore the technology by completing the following online activities.

1. Perform an Internet search and name three EHR software systems commonly used by physician offices.

2. Conduct an Internet job search to identify five different types of EHR positions located in your area.

3. Locate a website sponsored by the US federal government that provides information and resources regarding EHRs.

4. Locate two certifications other than RHIT and RHIA that can be awarded to individuals in the EHR field.

Are You Ready?

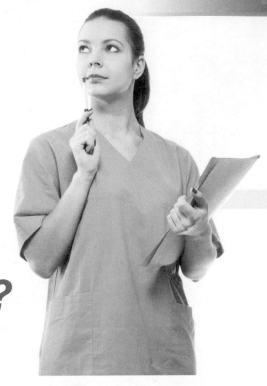

The workflow of a paper-based medical office is more employee intensive than an office that uses an electronic health record (EHR) system.

How do EHRs change the day-to-day responsibilities if you are part of the health administrative staff?

How might your role evolve as more of your duties are electronically performed?

Beyond the Record

- Each patient visit requires approximately 10–13 pieces of paper.

- The healthcare industry uses thousands of tons of paper every year.

- A physician accumulates approximately 975 new pages of paperwork each week and spends about eight hours per week processing it.

EHR Time Line

- **Between 206 BCE and 8 ADE**—Chunyu Yi keeps the first known medical record.

- **Between 1790 and 1821**—Some of America's earliest hospitals begin keeping patient records, including New York Hospital, Pennsylvania Hospital, and Massachusetts General Hospital.

- **1860s**—Physicians treating Civil War soldiers keep standardized records.

- **1917**—The American College of Surgeons (ACS) develops a hospital standardization program.

2

Content of
the Health Record

Maintaining a Legal Health Record

The health record, whether paper or electronic, is the legal record for a healthcare organization. Thus, there are many standards a health record should follow to protect the healthcare organization.

For a health record to be used as evidence in a court case, it needs to follow four basic principles. The record must be:

- documented following normal routines;
- kept in the regular course of healthcare business;
- recorded during or close to the time the event happened;
- recorded by a person with knowledge of the events.

Healthcare facilities must routinely assess policies and procedures regarding record keeping to ensure their records are legally sound.

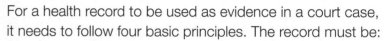

- **1970s**—Dr. Lawrence L. Weed and Jan Schultz develop a medical record software program called PROMIS (Problem-Oriented Medical Information System).

- **1990s**—The US Department of Veterans Affairs' Computerized Patient Record System (CPRS) is the first large-scale deployment of electronic health records (EHRs).

- **2009**—The American Recovery and Reinvestment Act of 2009 (ARRA) outlines federal incentives for adopting EHRs.

- **2016**—Patient medical records are comprehensive, portable, and accessible.

2.1 Examine the history of the health record.

2.2 Define the term *health record* and examine its multiple purposes.

2.3 Describe the primary and secondary uses of an EHR system.

2.4 Differentiate the types of data in the health record.

2.5 Describe the purpose, format, and features of both the paper and electronic health record (EHR).

2.6 Explain the importance of proper documentation in the health record.

2.7 Describe the requirements and standards for the health record.

2.8 Explain ownership and stewardship of the heath record.

2.9 Describe the transition from the paper health record to the electronic health record.

2.10 Compare and contrast the workflow of the paper health record versus the EHR.

The concept of electronic health records (EHRs) has emerged from the growing partnership between health care and technology. The integration of EHRs in the healthcare practice is built on the foundation of health record content. Health records contain essential elements of clinical, administrative, financial, and legal information that play key roles in a patient's current and future health care. The healthcare field uses health records to manage and research improvements and innovations. Healthcare settings are required to maintain health records for every patient, and they must all follow the licensing, accrediting, and other regulatory body requirements.

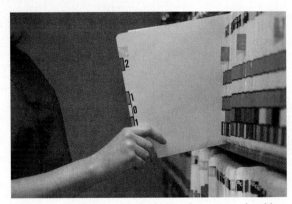

Whether on paper or in an electronic system, health records play key roles in a patient's current and future health care.

History of the Health Record

According to the US National Library of Medicine, a **healthcare facility** "includes hospitals, clinics, dental offices, outpatient surgery centers, birthing centers, and nursing homes." Each facility creates individual health records for its patients. These records reflect all episodes of care that patients receive. Throughout history, providers have kept health records for their patients. Although the methods of documentation have changed, the importance of keeping and recording patient information has not.

Early Health Records

Hippocrates, considered one of the most important figures in medical history, and his followers were among the first to describe and document many diseases and medical conditions. However, Chunyu Yi, a famous Chinese physician of the Han dynasty who died around 8 CE, kept the first known health record. He tracked his patients' names, residences, occupations, disease information, diagnoses, and prognoses. This record provides valuable historic data.

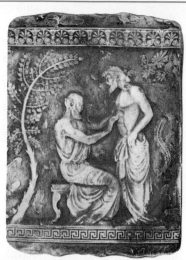

Hippocrates was one of the first healthcare practitioners to document diseases.

Between 1790 and 1821, some of America's earliest hospitals began keeping patient records, including New York Hospital, Pennsylvania Hospital, and Massachusetts General Hospital. Health records, historically restricted by the documentation habits of each individual healthcare provider, began to evolve in the United States during the Civil War. During this time, doctors began to record medical information in an increasingly standardized form, as social and physical mobility meant that they might treat patients they had never seen before. This trend continued as health records were established for immigrants to America at the advent of the 20th century.

In 1917, the **American College of Surgeons (ACS)** developed a hospital standardization program that established the **minimum standards**, which identified the elements required for reporting care and treatment. Minimum standards ensured that the health record communicated an accurate account of the healthcare information as well as the status of the patient. Some of the suggested standards for maintaining the patient record included patient identification, personal and family history, reason for encounter, history of current illness, physical examination, diagnosis, treatment, progress notes, and discharge. These standards are still being used almost a century later.

Evolution of Electronic Health Records

Beyond traditional shelf filing of handwritten paper records, few advances in medical records storage have been noted. Microfilm was used in the 1950s and optical scanning in the 1980s, but no real advancements in actual record keeping were made until the birth of the EHR.

Dr. Lawrence L. Weed is considered to be one of the pioneers in the EHR movement. Dr. Weed, a medical doctor specializing in internal medicine, along with his colleague Jan Schultz,

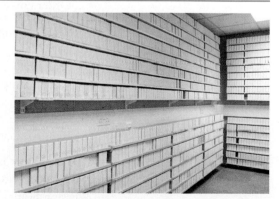

Medical records were often stored on microfilm starting in the 1950s.

developed the **problem-oriented medical record (POMR)**, a systematic approach to the documentation of medical records. In the 1970s, they also developed a software program called **Problem-Oriented Medical Information System (PROMIS)** at the University of Vermont under a federal grant. Healthcare providers did not embrace PROMIS, primarily because too much information was needed to complete the required fields, so physicians felt that they spent too much time focusing on documentation rather than patient care.

In the 1990s, the US Department of Veterans Affairs (VA) developed the first EHR that was used on a large scale, called VistA. VistA is still in use today at hundreds of VA medical centers and outpatient clinics across the United States. VistA software is available to any healthcare provider, individual, or organization at no cost through the public domain.

In 1991, the Health and Medicine Division (HMD) of the National Academics of Sciences, Engineering, and Medicine, formerly the Institute of Medicine (IOM), issued a report calling for the elimination of paper-based patient records within 10 years. In the report, it noted that implementing an EHR infrastructure for health care was imperative to improving the quality of care in the United States by making patient health information readily available to healthcare providers.

Then, in May 2003, HMD provided guidance to the US Department of Health and Human Services (HHS) on the key capabilities of an EHR System. HMD stated that an EHR System should include the following:

- A longitudinal record (discussed in Chapter 1)

- Immediate electronic access to patient data, accessible by only authorized users

- A clinical decision support component to enhance the quality, safety, and efficiency of patient care

- Support for efficient processes in the delivery of health care

To achieve these four key capabilities of an EHR system, the HMD further recommended that all EHR systems should have the following eight core functionalities:

- Health information and data

- Clinical results management

- Order entry and management

- Decision support

- Electronic communication and connectivity

- Patient support

- Administrative processes

- Reporting and population health management

HMD's report provided further detail and specifications of these eight core functionalities by location of the delivery of health care, including hospitals, ambulatory care, nursing homes, and care in the community. HMD also outlined the time period under which these core functionalities should be implemented. The time frames were 2004–2005, 2006–2007, and 2008–2010, therefore fully functional EHR systems by 2010. As we learned in Chapter 1, this time frame was adjusted by the federal government so that EHRs would be implemented by 2015.

Refer to Figure 2.1 for an example of the detailed specifications for the fourth core component, Decision Support.

The American Recovery and Reinvestment Act of 2009 (ARRA) outlines federal incentives for adopting EHRs. Included in the ARRA was the Health Information Technology for Economic and Clinical Health (HITECH) Act, which required the timely implementation of EHRs. Without the requirements and incentives of ARRA and the HITECH Act, providers may not have implemented EHRs.

Today, healthcare providers focus on documenting both the patient's past and present care. The health record is an essential part of a patient's health care because it helps providers make informed and accurate diagnostic and treatment decisions and is a tool for communication among caregivers.

Figure 2.1 Decision Support

Core Functionality	Hospitals			Ambulatory Care			Nursing Homes			Care in the Community (Personal Health Record)		
	2004-5	2006-7	2008-10	2004-5	2006-7	2008-10	2004-5	2006-7	2008-10	2004-5	2006-7	2008-10
4. Decision Support												
Access to knowledge sources												
-Domain knowledge	X			X				X		X		
-Patient education	X			X					X	X		
Drug alerts												
-Drug dose defaults	X			X			X			NA		
-Drug dose checking		X			X			X		NA		
-Allergy checking	X			X			X			NA		
-Drug interaction checking												
-Drug-lab checking	X	X		X	X		X		X	NA		
-Drug -condition checking		X			X				X	NA		
-Drug-diet checking		X			X				X	NA		
Other rule-based alerts (e.g., significant lab trends, lab test because of drug)		X			X			X		NA		
Reminders												
-Preventive services	X			X				X		X		
Clinical guidelines and pathways												
-Passive	X			X				X		X		
-Context-sensitive passive		X			X				X		X	
-Integrated		X			X				X	NA		
Chronic disease management	NA					X			X		X	

Purposes of the Health Record

The **health record** is an accumulation of information about a patient's past and present health. The primary purpose of the health record, whether recorded electronically or on paper, is to document the health history of the patient. The health record is composed of **data**, which includes the descriptive or numeric attributes of one or more variables. Data collected and analyzed becomes **information**. A **record** is a collection, usually in writing, of an account or an occurrence.

Documenting in the Health Record

Typically, the health record begins at the first visit or admission. A patient may have different records with each healthcare provider, such as a primary care physician, cardiologist, dermatologist, or dentist. Each provider must accurately enter the information in the record, such as who provided the health services; what, when, and why the services were provided; and the outcome. The information in the health record is essential when tracking the patient's illnesses along with the treatments, communication, and continuity of care among healthcare providers.

Primary and Secondary Uses of an EHR System

There are five primary uses of an EHR system. As discussed previously, the delivery and the management of patient care are arguably the most important primary uses of the EHR. Other primary uses include financial processes such as billing and reimbursement, administrative processes such as quality improvement and legal documentation, and patient self-management such as the personal health record and the patient portal.

There are four secondary uses of an EHR system, including education, regulation, research, and public health.

Health Record Data

There are four major categories of data in the health record: administrative, clinical, legal, and financial. **Administrative data** includes demographic information about the patient, such as the patient's name, address, date of birth, race, primary language, religion, and marital status. **Clinical data** is information such as admission dates, office visits, laboratory test results, evaluations, and emergency visits. **Legal data** is composed of consents for treatment and authorizations for the release of information. The last category, **financial data**, includes the patient's insurance and payment information for healthcare services (see Figure 2.2).

Administrative Data

Administrative data is information that the patient provides or populates in the health record. The administrative information typically found in the health record includes the following:

- Patient's name
- Address
- Telephone number
- Place of birth
- Date of birth

- Age
- Sex
- Marital status
- Ethnic origin
- Emergency contact information

The healthcare staff collects administrative information to verify the patient's identity and to help create a patient's demographic profile. See Figure 2.3 for an example of a form used to collect administrative information.

Figure 2.2 Types of Health Record Data

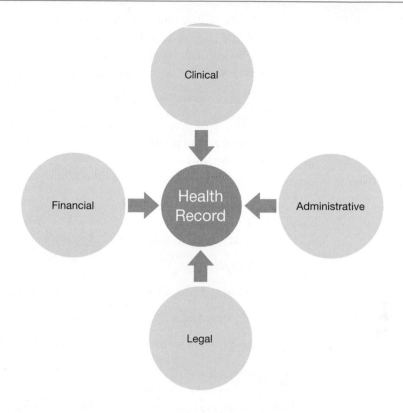

Figure 2.3 Admission Face Sheet

**Center City Outpatient Program
ADMISSION FACE SHEET**

Patient Name: Last _____ First _____ Middle _____

Are you known by a previous name? ❏ No   ❏ Yes: _____

Patient Address: _____

Home Phone:_____ Work Phone:_____ Cell Phone:_____

Date of Birth: _____

Sex: ❏ M   ❏ F

Occupation: _____

Marital Status: ❏ Single   ❏ Married   ❏ Separated   ❏ Divorced   ❏ Widowed   ❏ Partner

Clinical Data

Clinical data includes the medical information taken and recorded by the healthcare provider. The clinical data should be detailed, complete, precise, timely, and accurate, because the information plays a large role in the overall health plan of the patient. The clinical data includes documentation such as the following:

- Pathology and laboratory reports
- History and physical assessments
- Allergies
- X-rays
- List of medications
- Surgeries
- Hospital admissions
- Progress notes

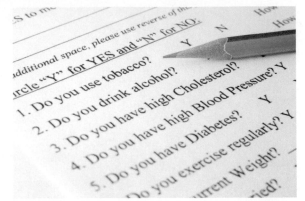

A questionnaire taken by the patient can provide clinical data.

Figure 2.4 provides an example of clinical data.

Legal Data

Legal data in the health record may be found on a variety of forms that are also considered legal documents. These documents include the following:

- Release of records: written request to release patient's health information to another healthcare provider or other entity in need of the patient's information
- Health Insurance Portability and Accountability Act (HIPAA) forms: HIPAA notice of privacy authorization
- General consent for care: agreement to general treatment and care
- Informed consent: agreement to a procedure
- Advance directives: written statement describing a patient's wishes regarding medical treatment in the event that the individual is no longer able to make such decisions because of illness or incapacity

Figure 2.5 illustrates an example of a form considered to be a legal document. Chapter 6 further explores legal documents in more detail, describing how they are added to and released from the EHR.

Health records are considered legal documents. A court of law may use the health record in many different types of legal proceedings. The healthcare facility protects itself by requiring proper documentation and ensuring accurate information where and whenever it is required.

Figure 2.4 Clinical Data Form

PATIENT NAME: Mulligan, Tyler
MR #: 785093
ROOM: Exam Room 1
DATE: February 15, 2030

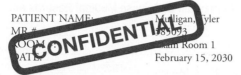

TREADMILL STRESS TEST

INDICATION
The patient was admitted to Northstar Medical Center complaining of mild chest pains. He is a 26-year-old white male who is actually quite athletic but has been noted on several occasions to have borderline hypertension. He has a family history of coronary artery disease in the father (who, incidentally, was a smoker), who died at the age of 54 secondary to coronary artery disease.

TECHNIQUE
The patient was exercised according to standard Bruce protocol for a total of 9 minutes and 30 seconds, at which time the test was stopped because he had obtained the target heart rate.

FINDINGS
He has a maximal heart rate of 181, which was approximately 93% of the predicted maximum of 195. He developed some clear up-sloping ST- and T-wave segment changes of 1–2 mm, specifically in leads V3, aVF, and anterior leads V3 through V6, but this resolved in the rest period. He developed only a mild blood pressure rise to a maximum of 146/90 at maximal exercise. Blood pressure returned to his resting normal quickly in recovery.

IMPRESSION
Negative treadmill stress test, with negative hypertensive response.

PLAN
Patient was given signs and symptoms of cardiac chest pain, including pressing substernal chest pain, shortness of breath, sweating, nausea or vomiting, or increase of pain with activity.

ADDENDUM
Patient was given extensive cardiovascular precautions, including the possibility of significant cardiac disease despite a seemingly negative treadmill stress test. The patient voiced understanding of this fact and also the need to seek immediate clinical attention should chest pain or other cardiovascular symptoms appear.

_____
Patrick Chaplin, MD

DF/DL
D:
T:

Financial Data

Financial data consists of insurance and employer information. A copy of the patient's insurance coverage, when available, may also be included. There may be times when a patient pays for healthcare services with a payment plan or another type of financial arrangement. The financial data section of the health record would note this agreement. Figure 2.6 shows a financial data form that a patient may be asked to complete at the time of the visit. Financial data is often combined with administrative data, meaning that both types of data are collected on the same form.

Figure 2.5 Legal Data Form

Authorization to Release Medical Records and Billing Information

Name: _____

Address: _____

City: _____ State: _____ ZIP: _____

Date: _____ (MM/DD/YYYY)

Name of Hospital or Physician: _____

Address: _____

City: _____ State: _____ ZIP: _____

I, _____, hereby authorize _____ (hospital or physican name) to release to _____ (name of person to receive records), any information in my personal medical records, including all X-rays, computed tomography scans, and any other information pertinent to my treatment, along with all billing information while under the care of _____ during the time period from _____. I give my permission for this medical information to be used for insurance claim purposes. I do not, however, give permission for any other use or for any redisclosure of this information.

Signature: _____

Patient Name (Printed): _____

Date: _____

This authorization will expire one year from the date of the signature above. I understand that I can revoke this authorization at any time by writing to the healthcare provider, but that revoking this authorization will not affect disclosures made or actions taken before the revocation is received.

I also understand that:

–I am not required to sign this authorization, and my health care or payment for care will not be affected by my refusal.

–Federal privacy regulations will no longer apply to the information disclosed, and the entity receiving the records may not be subject to patient privacy laws and may redisclose the records.

–I am entitled to receive a copy of this authorization.

–A copy of this authorization may be utilized with the same effectiveness as an original.

Figure 2.6 Financial Data Form

Patient Insurance Information

Primary Policyholder Information

Insurance Plan: _____

Policyholder's Name: _____

Address: _____

_____

Home Phone: _____ Work Phone: _____ Cell Phone: _____

Birth Date: _____

Relationship to Patient: _____

Employer Name: _____

Employer Address: _____

Consider This

The electronic health record (EHR) must meet the same requirements of a paper health record to be considered a legal document. Healthcare providers must accurately document vital signs, chief complaints, history, orders, plans, and prescriptions. The procedures and tools must also comply with the state's and organization's requirements. Documentation must be original, corrected, clarified, and amended. The EHR must maintain clinical messages, reports, and auditing tools. In addition, healthcare organizations must implement policies to include how unique health records are created and maintained; how content is chosen to be required; how they are authenticated and accessed; how privacy, confidentiality, and security are maintained; and how amendments and corrections are made. Healthcare organizations must create policies for record retention, archiving, destruction, abstracting, and reporting. Healthcare organizations should work with vendors to ensure that their EHR software adheres to the regulations to maintain a legal health record. What else can healthcare organizations do to maintain the legal health record in an EHR system? What might EHR vendors do to help healthcare organizations maintain a legal health record?

National Committee on Vital and Health Statistics Core Data Elements

In 1996, the **National Committee on Vital and Health Statistics (NCVHS)** completed a review of core health data elements and developed a list and definitions of the 42 core elements that can be used in a variety of healthcare settings. The patient provides the patient/enrollment data at the initial visit with the healthcare provider or facility, not at subsequent visits. Table 2.1 lists these core data elements and their definitions.

In addition to the core data elements proposed by NCVHS, other data sets have been proposed as national guidelines to encourage the exchange of information across healthcare providers and settings. The American Health Information Management Association (AHIMA) developed a core data set for the physician practice EHR, with its core elements divided into demographic and administrative information, vital signs, reason for visit, present illness, medical history, physical examination, problem and medication list, screenings, immunization, summary, referrals, and authentication.

Table 2.1 National Committee on Vital and Health Statistics Core Data Elements

Core Data Element	Definition
Patient/Enrollment Data	
Personal/Unique Identifier	Two options: A. Name—Last, first, middle, suffix B. Numeric identifier Without a universal unique identifier or a set of data items to form a unique identifier, it is challenging to link data across healthcare facilities and providers.
Date of Birth	MM/DD/YYYY
Sex	M/F

Race and Ethnicity	Recommendation to be self-reported
	Race
	  1. American Indian/Eskimo/Aleut
	  2. Asian or Pacific Islander
	  3. Black
	  4. White
	  5. Other
	Ethnicity
	  1. Hispanic origin
	  2. Not of Hispanic origin

Residence	Full address and ZIP code

Marital Status	1. Married—married (currently married; classify common-law marriage as married)
	   a. Living together
	   b. Not living together
	2. Never married—never married or annulled
	3. Widowed—person widowed and not remarried
	4. Divorced—person divorced and not remarried
	5. Separated—person legally separated
	6. Partner—civil unions (some forms now include this option)

Living/Residential Arrangement	Living Arrangement
	  1. Alone
	  2. With spouse (alternate: with spouse or unrelated partner)
	  3. With children
	  4. With parent or guardian
	  5. With relatives other than spouse, children, or parents
	  6. With nonrelatives
	Residential Arrangement
	  1. Private residence/household
	  2. Homeless shelter
	  3. Housing with services or supervision
	  4. Jail/correctional facility
	  5. Healthcare institutional setting
	  6. Homeless
	  7. Other residential setting

Core Data Element	Definition
Self-Reported Health Status	There is no consensus on how to define health status, but a common measure is the following: Excellent Very good Good Fair Poor
Functional Status	The functional status of a person is an increasingly important health measure shown to be strongly related to medical care utilization rates. Many scales have been developed that include both (a) self-report measures such as limitations of activities of daily living and instrumental activities of daily living, and National Health Interview Survey age-specific summary, and (b) clinical assessments such as the International Classification of Impairments, Disabilities, and Handicaps, and the Resident Assessment Instrument. Self-report measures and clinical assessments are both valuable and informative.
Years of Schooling	Years of schooling completed by the enrollee/patient as a proxy for socioeconomic status. This core data element is highly predictive of health status and healthcare use.
Patient's Relationship to Subscriber/Person Eligible for Entitlement	1. Self 2. Spouse 3. Child 4. Other
Current or Most Recent Occupation/Industry	Used to track occupational diseases
Encounter Data	
Type of Encounter	1. Inpatient 2. Outpatient 3. Emergency department 4. Observation 5. Ambulatory 6. Other
Admission Date (inpatient)	Format MM/DD/YYYY
Discharge Date (inpatient)	Format MM/DD/YYYY
Date of Encounter (ambulatory and physician services)	Format MM/DD/YYYY
Facility Identification	Identifier for hospitals, ambulatory surgery centers, nursing homes, and hospices, among others
Type of Facility/Place of Encounter	Identifier for type or place of encounter; part of the National Provider Identifier (NPI)
Healthcare Provider Identification (outpatient)	The NPI enables each provider to have a universal unique number across the system
Provider Location or Address of Encounter (outpatient)	Full address and ZIP code for the location of the provider
Attending Physician Identification (inpatient)	The unique national identification assigned to the clinician of record at discharge
Operating Physician Identification (inpatient)	The unique national identification assigned to the clinician who performed the principal procedure
Provider Specialty	Part of the NPI system that identifies the provider's specialty
Principal Diagnosis (inpatient)	The condition determined to be chiefly responsible for patient admission

Core Data Element	Definition
Primary Diagnosis (inpatient)	The diagnosis responsible for the majority of the care given to the patient
Other Diagnoses (inpatient)	Conditions should be coded that affect patient care in terms of requiring the following: 1. Clinical evaluation 2. Therapeutic treatment 3. Diagnostic procedures 4. Extended length of hospital stay 5. Increased nursing care/monitoring
Qualifier for Other Diagnoses (inpatient)	The following should be applied to each diagnosis coded under *other diagnoses* 1. Onset prior to admission 2. Onset not prior to admission 3. Onset uncertain
Patient's Stated Reason for Visit or Chief Complaint (ambulatory)	Reason at the time of the encounter for seeking attention or care
Diagnosis Chiefly Responsible for Services Provided (ambulatory)	Contains the code(s) for the diagnosis, condition, problem, or the reason for encounter/visit chiefly responsible for the services provided
Other Diagnoses (ambulatory)	Additional code(s) that describe any conditions coexisting at the time of the encounter/visit that require management
External Cause of Injury	Code for the external cause of an injury, poisoning, or adverse event; completed whenever there is a diagnosis of an injury, poisoning, or adverse event
Birth Weight of Newborn (inpatient)	Specific birth weight of the newborn recorded in grams or in pounds and ounces
Principal Procedure (inpatient)	The principal procedure is one that was performed for definitive treatment, rather than one performed for diagnostic or exploratory purposes, or necessary to take care of a complication. If there appear to be two procedures that are principal, then the one most related to the principal diagnosis should be selected as the principal procedure. 1. Is surgical in nature 2. Carries a procedural risk 3. Carries an anesthetic risk 4. Requires specialized training
Other Procedures (inpatient)	All other procedures that are considered significant. A significant procedure is one of the following: 1. Is surgical in nature 2. Carries a procedural risk 3. Carries an anesthetic risk 4. Requires specialized training
Dates of Procedures (inpatient)	MM/DD/YYYY
Services (ambulatory)	Describe all diagnostic services of any type, including history and physical examinations, laboratory studies, X-rays, and others performed and pertinent to the patient's reasons for the encounter; all therapeutic series; all preventive services and procedures at time of encounter
Medications Prescribed	All medications prescribed by the healthcare provider at the time of the encounter. Include dosage, strength, and amount prescribed.

Core Data Element	Definition

Disposition of Patient (inpatient)	1. Discharge status
	  a. Discharged alive
	  b. Discharged dead
	  c. Status not stated
	2. Discharge setting
	  a. Discharged to home or self-care
	  b. Discharged to acute care hospital
	  c. Discharged to a nursing facility
	  d. Discharged to other healthcare facility
	  e. Discharged home to be under care of a home health services agency
	  f. Left against medical advice

Disposition (ambulatory)	Provider's statement of the next steps in care of patient. The following are the suggested classifications: 1. No follow-up planned 2. Follow-up planned or scheduled 3. Referred elsewhere
Patient's Expected Sources of Payment	Name of each source of payment including primary and secondary sources
Injury Related to Employment	Yes or No
Total Billed Charges	Copayment or update payment data when available

CHECKP⊕INT 2.1

1. Define *data*, *information* and *record*.

_____

_____

_____

2. Describe several types of information that may be found within a health record.

_____

_____

_____

Health Record Format

Format is related to the arrangement of a paper health record. There are no specific requirements on how paper health records are formatted, as long as an organization uses the same format throughout its facility. There are three organizational formats used in paper health records: source-oriented record, integrated health record, and problem-oriented record.

Source-Oriented Record

The **source-oriented record (SOR)** is the most common format used by healthcare facilities. This format organizes the health documents into sections that contain information collected from a specific department or type of service; for example, all progress notes, laboratory reports, and radiology reports are assembled together in their respective sections. Within each section, the health record content is organized in chronologic order. (Most healthcare facilities using the source-oriented format keep the health content in chronologic rather than reverse chronologic order.) SORs permit rapid retrieval of health content, although the format can make it challenging to view the complete health status of the patient.

Integrated Health Record

The second format type is the **integrated health record**, which is organized either in chronologic or reverse chronologic order. The health content is not separated by department or type of service; therefore, health documentation is viewed by date. Healthcare facilities may use the integrated health record format in several ways. The medical chart may place all forms together or be organized by healthcare setting (e.g., all dental forms in one section, all primary care documents in another). The integrated health record provides a complete view of the health status of the patient, although this format makes it difficult to compare findings from the same type of service, such as comparing two radiology reports completed at the beginning and at the end of a patient's stay.

Problem-Oriented Record

The third format type is the **problem-oriented record (POR)**. As discussed previously, Dr. Lawrence L. Weed developed this type of record because the SOR did not provide a complete view of the patient's health status. The POR focuses on assessment of the clinical documentation by healthcare providers and the creation of a plan that addresses the patient's health concerns. This type of format promotes a team approach to documentation through the use of the SOAP format progress notes.

- S (Subjective): the reason the patient is at the healthcare facility for care, as well as comments from the patient or patient's family about the existing condition

- O (Objective): specific notes such as results from a laboratory test completed during the patient's visit

- A (Assessment): the healthcare provider's opinion on the condition or diagnosis

- P (Plan): the healthcare provider's plan to diagnose or treat the patient

The SOAP format is used in both paper and electronic records.

CHECKPOINT 2.2

1. Describe the source-oriented health record format.

   _____

   _____

   _____

   _____

2. What are the four components of the SOAP progress note format?

   a. _____

   b. _____

   c. _____

   d. _____

Health Record Content

The content of a health record will vary depending on the type of healthcare facility. Chapter 4 will go into greater detail on the different types of healthcare facilities. In this chapter, the health record content of patients in acute and ambulatory settings will be discussed. Note the variances in the patient records of these two types of facilities.

Acute Care Setting

Facilities that provide acute care include acute care hospitals and long-term care hospitals (LTCH). Patients who are admitted to these facilities are called inpatients. **Inpatients** occupy a hospital bed for at least one night in the course of treatment, examination, or observation.

Record Content

For an inpatient admitted to an acute care setting, a health record usually contains the following content:

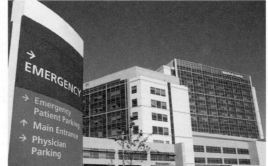

A hospital is an acute care facility.

- Admission record: state of the patient when he or she is admitted to an acute care facility

- History and physical: information regarding the patient's past and current health condition, assessment, and treatment or diagnostic work-up plan

- Progress notes: entries of the patient's care and progress reported by the healthcare providers

- Laboratory tests: test and laboratory results ordered by healthcare providers

- Diagnostic tests: medical tests that assist in the diagnosis of the patient's health issue

- Operative notes: notes immediately written after surgery that document the procedure and results

- Pathology reports: detailed information on the review of specimens from tissue or cell biopsy

- Physician orders: orders given by the physician for medications, fluids, patient testing, etc.

- Consents: authorizations for treatment

- Consultations: reports provided by other healthcare providers that review the patient's health issues

- Emergency department encounters: documentation of visits or encounters in the emergency department

- Discharge summary: summary of the patient's course of care signed by the attending physician

The content in each record may be supplied in different formats but typically contains similar data.

Ambulatory Care Setting

Ambulatory care is an increasingly popular mode of healthcare delivery. Some ambulatory care settings include:

- Physician offices

- Clinics

- Surgery centers

- Dental offices

- Imaging centers

- Occupational health centers

- Oral and maxillofacial offices

- Podiatrist offices

- Pain management

- Community or college health centers

- Urgent care centers

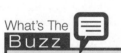

A dental office is an example of an ambulatory care facility.

The term *ambulatory* is used for medical care, including diagnosis, observation, treatment, and rehabilitation services. Patients receiving treatment in an ambulatory setting are called outpatients. **Outpatients** are patients who do not spend more than 24 hours in a healthcare facility and/or are not admitted to the hospital.

Record Content

What's The Buzz

Digital signatures have made many other industries more efficient. But they can be more controversial in the healthcare industry. Although e-signatures can be used under HIPAA, some legal and security mechanisms must be put in place.

Each facility, unless part of an organization, creates and maintains its own health record for a patient. The ambulatory care record typically contains the following content:

- Demographic information: patient's name, address, date of birth, and other patient information not medical in nature

- Contact information: various telephone numbers and email addresses, as well as emergency contacts

- History and physical: health history, a review of vital signs, and a complete organ-specific physical examination

- Immunization records: comprehensive list of dates and types of vaccines received as a child, as well as additional vaccines such as flu, tetanus, and hepatitis

- Problem lists: list of patient's current health issues

- Allergy lists: list of medications, food, and other items to which a patient is allergic

- Prescription lists: list of current medications, including dosages

- Progress notes: updates to the patient's healthcare issues; may be in a SOAP format

- Assessment: summary of the likely causes of the patient's current health issues; provides course of action to address health issues

- Consultations: documentation of a patient's visit to another healthcare provider and what that healthcare provider recommends or concludes

- Referrals: permission or suggestions for the patient to be seen by another healthcare provider

- Treatment plans: plan for treatment of the patient's health issues

- Patient instructions: directions and orders to be followed by the patient to help with his or her health issues

- Laboratory tests and results: test and laboratory results ordered by the healthcare provider

- Consents: authorizations for treatment

- Communication: letters, emails, telephone messages, or any other documented communication

- External correspondence: communication between the healthcare provider and any other provider or carrier that provides information about the patient

- Financial information: payment arrangements and insurance information

Each specialty practice may provide the health information in a slightly different way, but the concept and purpose of each category is the same.

CHECKP⊕INT 2.3

1. Name five content areas found in an acute care health record.

   a. _____

   b. _____

   c. _____

   d. _____

   e. _____

2. Name five content areas found in an ambulatory care health record.

   a. _____

   b. _____

   c. _____

   d. _____

   e. _____

Documentation in the Health Record

The healthcare facility is responsible for the quality of care provided to its patients. Direct documentation of this care must be provided in a paper record or EHR system and is the responsibility of the healthcare provider. This documentation must be accurate, timely, and complete, reflecting all procedures, treatments, medications, tests, assessments, observations, and communications involved with patient care. Remember the saying, "If it's not documented, it didn't happen."

The maintenance and accuracy of the health record are important responsibilities of health information staff, whose duty is to ensure that healthcare records are readily available when patients arrive for care. The staff must also ensure that all forms are in each patient's record, verify that the healthcare provider has documented care, validate the accuracy of the coding of service, and adhere to established healthcare data standards.

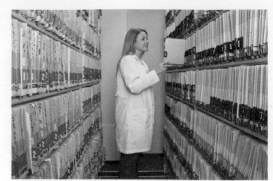

Paper medical records must be pulled from shelves and be readily available when patients arrive at a healthcare facility.

Practice Professionalism

A medical scribe is a profession that has come about because of EHRs. A medical scribe performs documentation in the EHR, gathers information for the patient's visit, and assists physicians.

Documentation Guidelines

Every healthcare organization should establish policies and procedures specifying health record documentation guidelines, for both paper and electronic health records, to ensure that health record documentation is accurate, timely, and supportive of assessment, diagnoses, and treatment. These documentation guidelines are established based on the laws, rules, and standards of licensing agencies, accrediting bodies, and payers of healthcare treatment and services. Some of the typical documentation guidelines for paper and electronic records are compared and listed in Table 2.2.

Table 2.2 Documentation Guidelines for Paper and Electronic Health Records

Paper Health Records	Electronic Health Records
A separate, physical paper record is established for each patient	A separate, electronic record is established for each patient
Paper documents are assembled in an established chart order, including chronological or reverse chronological order	Electronic documents are organized in an organized fashion that promotes fast, easy retrieval of information
Proper authentication (all documents signed/initialed with pen)	Proper authentication (electronic signatures on all documents)
All documentation dated and timed, including signatures authenticating verbal and telephone orders	All documentation dated and timed, including signatures authenticating verbal and telephone orders
Timely documentation handwritten or dictated/transcribed (i.e., history and physical documented within 24 hours of admission, progress notes documented at the time of the visit/treatment, etc.)	Timely documentation typed or dictated/transcribed (i.e., history and physical documented within 24 hours of admission, progress notes documented at the time of the visit/treatment, etc.)
Legible handwriting	N/A
Complete documentation to support diagnoses and procedures	Complete documentation to support diagnoses and procedures
Patient identifiers on each piece of paper (i.e., patient name, medical record number, patient account number, date of birth, etc.)	Patient identifiers on each electronic document (i.e., patient name, medical record number, patient account number, date of birth, etc.)
Results of all tests and procedures are filed in the paper medical record in a timely fashion	Results of all tests and procedures are electronically filed in the EHR in a timely fashion
Correction of errors: single ink line through the documentation with date and initials of author. Documentation is NEVER obliterated or destroyed from a paper record.	Correction of errors: strike through documentation in error and include the date and author initials or documentation moved to a separate, retrievable electronic file. Information/documentation is NEVER completely deleted from the EHR.

When working with health records, healthcare personnel need to be aware of three areas of concern that affect patient safety: the legibility of the entries, the use of only approved abbreviations and acronyms in the documentation, and the protocol for changing or correcting documented entries. Specifics of these safety concerns are outlined next.

Legibility of Entries

When working with paper record entries, interpreting the handwriting of healthcare providers may be difficult (see Figure 2.7). Consequently, healthcare personnel must query the appropriate staff members about any unclear entries. This verification protects both the safety of the patient and the liability of the healthcare worker and the facility.

Figure 2.7   Handwritten Physician Order

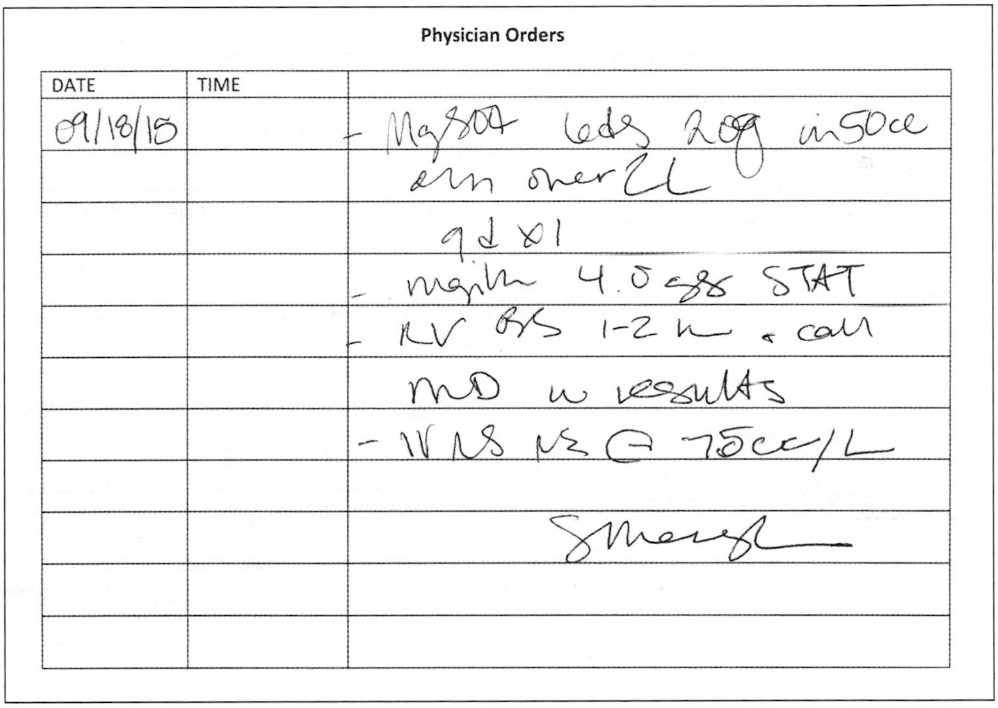

The Use of Abbreviations and Acronyms

Abbreviations and acronyms are often used in the health record. Therefore, to ensure clear communication, there are standards for abbreviations and symbols that should be followed when documenting information. Some examples of approved abbreviations are provided in Table 2.3. Healthcare facilities can place additional rules in their bylaws that indicate other acceptable abbreviations per facility preference.

The Joint Commission developed an official "Do Not Use" List of abbreviations as part of its information management standards that healthcare organizations must follow. In addition, the commission has proposed a list for possible future inclusion in the official "Do Not Use" List. The "Do Not Use" List is found in Figure 2.8.

Table 2.3 Health Record Abbreviations and Acronyms

Abbreviation	Meaning	Abbreviation	Meaning
ABN	Advanced beneficiary notice	MD	Medical doctor
BMI	Body mass index	MMR	Measles, mumps, and rubella
BP	Blood pressure	MS	Musculoskeletal
CV	Cardiovascular	Neuro	Neurologic
DOB	Date of birth	NPP	Notice of privacy practices
DPT	Diphtheria, pertussis, and tetanus	O2	Oxygen
ENMT	Ears, nose, mouth, and throat	OR	Operating room
ETOH	Alcohol	p.o.	By mouth
GI	Gastrointestinal	PCP	Primary care provider
GYN	Gynecologic	PRN	As needed
HPI	History of present illness	ROS	Review of systems
IM	Intramuscularly	Temp	Temperature
LMP	Last menstrual period	VIS	Vaccine information sheet

Figure 2.8 The Joint Commission's Official "Do Not Use" List of Abbreviations

Facts about the Official "Do Not Use" List of Abbreviations

June 9, 2017

The Joint Commission's "Do Not Use" List is part of the Information Management standards. This requirement does not apply to preprogrammed health information technology systems (for example, electronic medical records or CPOE systems), but this application remains under consideration for the future. Organizations contemplating introduction or upgrade of such systems should strive to eliminate the use of dangerous abbreviations, acronyms, symbols, and dose designations from the software.

Official "Do Not Use" List[1]

Do Not Use	Potential Problem	Use Instead
U, u (unit)	Mistaken for "0" (zero), the number "4" (four), or "cc"	Write "unit"
IU (International Unit)	Mistaken for IV (intravenous) or the number 10 (ten)	Write "International Unit"
Q.D., QD, q.d., qd (daily) Q.O.D., QOD, q.o.d, qod (every other day)	Mistaken for each other Period after the Q mistaken for "I" and the "O" mistaken for "I"	Write "daily" Write "every other day"
Trailing zero (X.0 mg)* Lack of leading zero (.X mg)	Decimal point is missed	Write X mg Write 0.X mg
MS MSO_4 and $MgSO_4$	Can mean morphine sulfate or magnesium sulfate Confused for one another	Write "morphine sulfate" Write "magnesium sulfate"

[1] Applies to all orders and all medication-related documentation that is handwritten (including free-text computer entry) or on preprinted forms.

*Exception: A "trailing zero" may be used only where required to demonstrate the level of precision of the value being reported, such as for laboratory results, imaging studies that report size of lesions, or catheter/tube sizes. It may not be used in medication orders or other medication-related documentation.

Development of the "Do Not Use" List

In 2001, The Joint Commission issued a *Sentinel Event Alert* on the subject of medical abbreviations. A year later, its Board of Commissioners approved a National Patient Safety Goal requiring accredited organizations to develop and implement a list of abbreviations not to use. In 2004, The Joint Commission created its "Do Not Use" List to meet that goal. In 2010, NPSG.02.02.01 was integrated into the Information Management standards as elements of performance 2 and 3 under IM.02.02.01.

For more information, contact the Standards Interpretation Group at 630-792-5900, or complete the Standards Online Question Submission Form.

© The Joint Commission, 2017. Reprinted with permission.

Changing or Correcting Documented Entries

Healthcare personnel need to follow established procedures when changing or correcting documented entries in a paper health record. Information must not be erased.

When correcting information in an EHR, authors strike through documentation in error and include the date and author initials or they move the documentation to a separate, retrievable electronic file. Information/documentation is never completely deleted from the EHR. Healthcare personnel may also document an addendum to clarify documentation. Information may not be deleted from an entry.

Health Record Standards

Several accreditation, professional, and federal organizations provide guidelines and support on maintaining the integrity of patient health records. By affiliation with these organizations and meeting their professional standards and goals, healthcare facilities can distinguish their services from others as well as reduce the number of state and federal reviews. A focus of all of these organizations is to improve the quality of patient care and health record documentation.

Accreditation Organizations

Accreditation organizations affiliated with healthcare quality include the Commission for Accreditation of Rehabilitation Facilities (CARF), The Joint Commission, the National Committee for Quality Assurance (NCQA), the Community Health Accreditation Program (CHAP), and the Accreditation Association for Ambulatory Health Care (AAAHC).

The **Commission for Accreditation of Rehabilitation Facilities (CARF)** is an independent, nonprofit organization that focuses on aging services, behavioral health, child and youth services, employment and community services, medical rehabilitation, and opioid treatment programs. **The Joint Commission**, formerly known as the Joint Commission on Accreditation of Healthcare Organizations (JCAHO), is an independent, not-for-profit organization that accredits and certifies a variety of healthcare organizations, ranging from dental to behavioral health to acute care facilities. Health record content standards are addressed in each field of health care.

The **National Committee for Quality Assurance (NCQA)** is an independent, nonprofit organization that focuses on healthcare quality. Healthcare organizations such as individual or group healthcare providers and health plans that seek NCQA accreditation do so voluntarily.

The **Community Health Accreditation Program (CHAP)** and the **Accreditation Association for Ambulatory Health Care (AAAHC)** are two examples of specialty accrediting organizations.

Professional Organizations

The Association for Healthcare Documentation Integrity (ADHI), the American Health Information Management Association (AHIMA), and the Healthcare Information and Management Systems Society (HIMSS) are three professional organizations that support healthcare information personnel in maintaining quality assurance of health records.

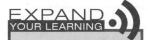

EXPAND YOUR LEARNING

Search for these organizations on the Internet to learn more about how they promote high standards in documenting health information.

The **Association for Healthcare Documentation Integrity (AHDI)** has vowed "to set and uphold standards for education and practice in the field of clinical documentation that ensure the highest level of accuracy, privacy, and security for the US healthcare systems in order to protect public health, increase patient safety, and improve quality of care for healthcare consumers." The **American Health Information Management Association (AHIMA)** is a professional organization that provides resources, education, and networking with other professionals. AHIMA focuses on the quality of health information used in the delivery of health care. Initially, the organization focused on hospital records, but it now supports ambulatory, community health, and many other health care delivery (HCD) organizations.

The **Healthcare Information and Management Systems Society (HIMSS)** focuses on using information technology and management systems to improve the quality and delivery of health care.

Federal Organizations

Lastly, the federal organizations actively involved in setting standards for health records are the Agency for Healthcare Research and Quality (AHRQ), the Centers for Medicare & Medicaid Services (CMS), the Health Resources and Services Administration (HRSA), and the Quality Improvement Organizations (QIO).

The AHRQ agency focuses on improving the safety and quality of health care.

Centers for Medicare & Medicaid Services (CMS) is a federal government agency that oversees federal healthcare programs, including Medicare Conditions of Participation (CoPs). In 2009, CMS expanded its role to include the implementation of EHR incentive programs, meaningful use of certified EHR systems, drafting standards for certified EHR technology, and updating privacy and security regulations under HIPAA. The **Health Resources and Services Administration (HRSA)** is an agency of the US Department of Health and Human Services. This agency focuses on improving health and health equity through innovative programs and a skilled health workforce and providing access to services to those who are economically or medically vulnerable.

A **Quality Improvement Organization (QIO)** is a group of health experts, providers, and consumers who are dedicated to improving the quality of care for people with Medicare.

Ownership and Stewardship of Health Records and Health Information

Health record and health information ownership and stewardship are controversial topics that have grown increasingly complex as healthcare facilities transitioned from paper health records to EHRs.

Ownership of Health Records

Historically, state laws and healthcare professional associations have accepted that the healthcare facility that created the health record owns the physical health record. For example, a sole practitioner (a single, independent healthcare practice) owns the record created in his or her practice just as a hospital or other inpatient facility owns records for all patients admitted or treated at the facility.

Ownership of Health Information

Historically, there have also been discussions and attempts to separate the ownership of the physical health record from the ownership of the health data contained in the record. Is the patient the owner because he or she is the subject of the record? Or, is the healthcare facility the owner because it generated the information and physically has possession of the record? Many leaders in health information management anticipate that future legislation will address the subject of the ownership of health information, ultimately creating a uniform definition of ownership.

Ownership versus Stewardship

While clarification of the ownership of health records and health information is needed, the concept of stewardship is a way to address the responsibilities of retention, privacy, and maintenance of health records and health data without having to solve the issue of ownership. Since stewardship implies careful and responsible management, as stewards, all healthcare providers and staff involved in the creation, use, maintenance, and retention of health records and data are responsible for ensuring that health data is generated, used, and stored in a manner that complies with all required laws, rules, standards, and guidelines.

Obtaining a Health Record

EXPAND YOUR LEARNING

To see how your state handles the ownership of health information, visit http://EHR2 .ParadigmEducation .com/ MedRecordOwner.

Patients have the right to access and/or obtain a copy of their health records, whether paper or electronic, depending on federal and/or state laws. To request a copy of the health record from the healthcare provider, typically a patient provides a written request, signs a HIPAA-compliant release of records form, and then pays the necessary fees. The cost of a copy, paper or electronic, of the health record varies depending on the provider and facility. See Figure 2.9 for an example of a release of information authorization form for a patient's health record. As EHRs have developed, new ways to authorize the release of medical records have evolved, including digital download and electronic sharing and access.

Now that more health records are housed in an EHR system, an increasing number of patients request an electronic copy of their records. The ability to receive electronic records is discussed in more detail in Chapter 6.

Figure 2.9 Release of Information

EMC Medical Center MRN/Chart #________________

PATIENT INFORMATION

Name ________ Address ________ City ________ State ________ ZIP ________

Date of Birth ________ Daytime Phone ________ Previous Name (if applicable) ________

AUTHORIZES

Name of Healthcare Provider/Plan ________________

Address ________________

TO DISCLOSE TO

❑ Self

Delivery Options: ❑ Pick Up ❑ View on Site ❑ Mail to Address Above

❑ To Be Picked Up By Another Person

I hereby authorize ________________ to pick up my records.

Send to: ❑ ________________
Name of Healthcare Provider/Plan

Address ________________ Fax Number ________________

DATE(S) OF INFORMATION TO BE DISCLOSED: From ________ to ________. If left blank, only information from the past two (2) years will be disclosed.

INFORMATION TO BE DISCLOSED:
❑ All medical records related to (specify condition, treatment, etc.): ________________
❑ All billing records related to (specify condition, treatment, etc.): ________________
❑ Radiology films/images (specify test): ________________
❑ Other records: ________________

DO NOT DISCLOSE THE FOLLOWING INFORMATION:
❑ Alcohol/drug use ❑ HIV test results ❑ Mental health status ❑ Developmental disabilities

PURPOSE (check all that apply):
❑ Further Medical Care ❑ Legal ❑ Insurance ❑ Personal ❑ Other:________

YOUR RIGHTS WITH RESPECT TO THIS AUTHORIZATION
I am aware that I have the right to inspect and receive a copy of the health information I have authorized to be used and/or disclosed by this authorization. I understand that I may be charged a fee for record copies. In addition, I understand that I do not need to sign this authorization in order to receive treatment. I understand that I may revoke this authorization by notifying the disclosing medical records/health information department in writing. However, I understand that my revocation will not be effective as to uses and/or disclosures: (1) already made in reliance upon this Authorization; or (2) needed for an insurer to contest a claim/policy as authorized by law if signing the Authorization was a condition to obtaining insurance coverage. I realize that the information used and/or disclosed pursuant to this Authorization may be subject to redisclosure and no longer protected by federal privacy law.

SIGNATURE OF PATIENT/LEGAL REPRESENTATION
________________________________ DATE: ________________

Importance of EHR Transition

Unfortunately, it took a natural disaster to underscore the importance of transitioning from paper health records to EHRs.

On Monday, August 29, 2005, Hurricane Katrina made landfall in southeastern Louisiana. The impact of the hurricane caused the levee system in New Orleans to fail, and many parts of the city flooded significantly as a consequence. This disaster washed away thousands of paper records, and many residents of the greater New Orleans area lost all of their medical information. In addition, many healthcare providers fled New Orleans, which left many patients adrift in their healthcare needs. These patients had no record of their health histories, current health status, or information regarding their

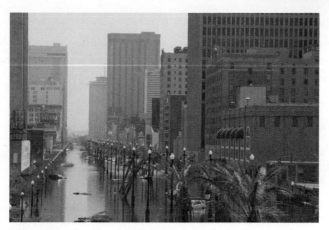

Many paper health records were destroyed in Hurricane Katrina.

medications and had no way to contact their healthcare providers. In response, the federal government, along with public and private organizations, created the KatrinaHealth.org website to help healthcare providers and pharmacies obtain access to patients' prescription information. Although this service helped many New Orleans residents, one segment of the city's population still had access to their medical records: veterans. The Veterans Health Administration uses VistA, which is an EHR system that was created in the 1970s to assist with HCD for veterans and their families. Because this information was electronic, displaced veterans were able to access their records no matter where they chose to relocate.

Hurricane Katrina highlighted the necessity for health information to withstand natural disasters, an important lesson that supports the initiative for the development of EHRs.

Conversion from Paper Health Records to EHRs

The transition from paper health records to EHRs is slowly building momentum as healthcare providers are experiencing the challenges of working with a records management system that cannot keep pace with changing technology.

Consider This

St. John's Hospital in Joplin, Missouri, converted its medical records from paper to electronic data on May 1, 2011, three weeks before

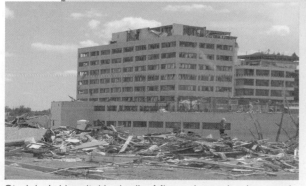

St. John's Hospital in Joplin, Missouri, was back up and running quickly after a 2011 tornado because the facility had recently implemented an EHR system.

a devastating tornado hit the area. Because the hospital had an electronic health record (EHR) system, it was able to recover patient information and send it to other healthcare facilities. In addition, St. John's set up mobile surgical and scanning equipment in its parking lot to provide further patient services. The only glitch in accessing the EHR system was a temporary loss of electrical power. However, once power was restored, healthcare providers could continue to care for their patients because the data had not been lost.

Since then, many healthcare facilities using EHRs have addressed the loss of electrical power. What measures could circumvent this issue?

Limitations of Paper Records

Paper health records have served an important role in patient health care for many decades. However, they also present many challenges to healthcare providers, including the following:

- Increasing complexity of healthcare delivery
- Single location of records
- Restricted access, allowing only one user to view records at a time
- Inconsistent documentation
- Unsecured storage in the event of a natural disaster or human error

In addition, the paper health record is time-consuming and labor-intensive. Figure 2.10 shows a typical workflow for a paper health record in an ambulatory care setting.

Due to the challenges presented by this time-consuming workflow, and the increasing amount of patient and provider information required to be documented, the concept of using an EHR system became increasingly embraced by healthcare practitioners.

Figure 2.10 Paper Health Record Workflow

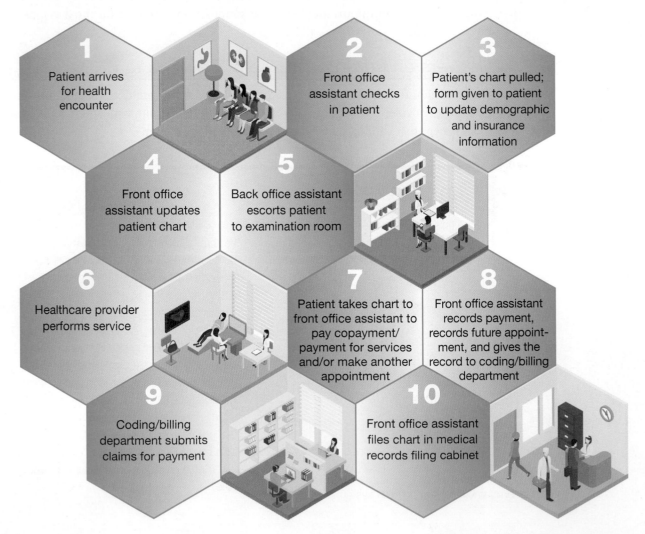

1 Patient arrives for health encounter

2 Front office assistant checks in patient

3 Patient's chart pulled; form given to patient to update demographic and insurance information

4 Front office assistant updates patient chart

5 Back office assistant escorts patient to examination room

6 Healthcare provider performs service

7 Patient takes chart to front office assistant to pay copayment/payment for services and/or make another appointment

8 Front office assistant records payment, records future appointment, and gives the record to coding/billing department

9 Coding/billing department submits claims for payment

10 Front office assistant files chart in medical records filing cabinet

Advantages of EHRs

As discussed in Chapter 1, an EHR is not just an electronic version of a paper record, although the two have common data elements. Rather, an EHR begins with a database populated with health content from the patient's healthcare encounters. It includes demographic information, progress notes, assessments, results, consultations, and many of the other documents found in a paper health record. The database of the patient's healthcare encounters is updated each time the patient seeks medical care. Figure 2.11 demonstrates how data flows and is accessed in an EHR.

Healthcare providers can enter information in an EHR using laptops, desktop computers located in patient examination rooms, or wireless devices used during patient encounters. This easy accessibility to a patient's health record is certainly a key advantage over a paper record that must be accessed from one location. The provider can log in to the EHR using a unique username and a secure password. Once the record is accessed by the provider, his or her activities within the record are tracked by the system.

The record itself offers a standardized format containing drop-down menus, lists, icons, and free-text areas for practitioners to enter health information into the database. Because of this standardization, EHRs can be easily searched for specific patient information as well as automatically prompt clinicians to send reminders and follow up with patients. Lastly, the electronic data format provides users with a complete picture of a patient's overall health status.

The workflow of an EHR differs from the pathway of a paper health record. As shown in Figure 2.12, the process is more streamlined for healthcare personnel.

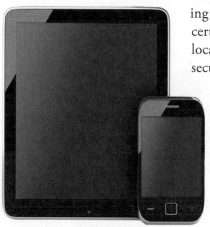

Health information can be entered on laptops, desktop computers, or wireless devices such as tablets or mobile phones.

Figure 2.11 EHR Data Flowchart

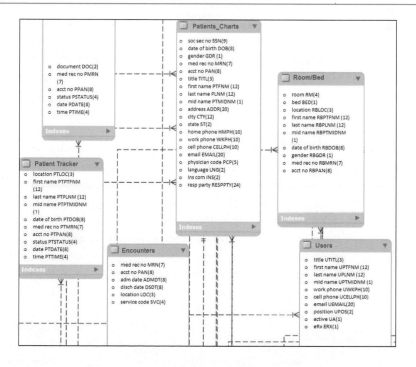

Figure 2.12 EHR Patient Encounter

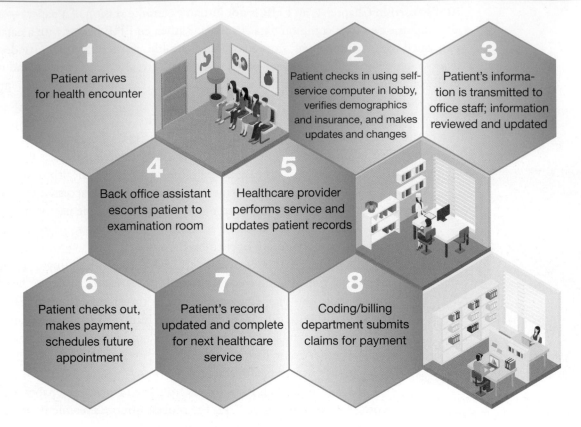

1
Patient arrives
for health encounter

2
Patient checks in using self-service computer in lobby, verifies demographics and insurance, and makes updates and changes

3
Patient's information is transmitted to office staff; information reviewed and updated

4
Back office assistant escorts patient to examination room

5
Healthcare provider performs service and updates patient records

6
Patient checks out, makes payment, schedules future appointment

7
Patient's record updated and complete for next healthcare service

8
Coding/billing department submits claims for payment

Challenges of EHR Transition

Implementing an EHR system also presents some challenges. Converting the paper records into an electronic format is both time-consuming and costly. As HCD systems convert from paper to an electronic format, portions of patient records will be stored electronically and on paper, resulting in a **hybrid health record**. Healthcare providers with small patient populations are likely to be able to convert to EHRs in a shorter time frame than healthcare providers with large patient populations, such as major hospitals. For these larger facilities, the conversion may take several years and, consequently, hybrid health records will need to be implemented.

There may be additional challenges in converting from paper health records to EHRs, such as dealing with duplicate records, establishing the identities of patients/unique patient identifiers, detecting insurance fraud, and identifying questionable identities of patients in various components in the EHR system.

Once all the records have been converted, healthcare workers must review records to ensure accuracy. Even with EHRs, there is room for error during the data entry or data conversion process. Removing erroneous information from an EHR is not allowed, and doing so may be seen as fraud if it is attempted.

Training all users of the EHR system to use EHR content can be difficult. Employees may lack the necessary technologic skills, and some users may be reluctant to learn a new system.

The goal of an EHR system is to improve patient health care by allowing access to multiple providers across all aspects of health care and involving the patient more directly, so that all players have current information of the patient's past and present health status. Having accurate and accessible EHRs will result in improved patient care and outcomes.

Chapter Summary

Some of America's earliest hospitals began keeping patient records in the early 1800s, although the first known health record was kept by Chunyu Yi, a famous Chinese physician, around 8 CE. In 1917, the American College of surgeons developed a hospital standardization program that established the minimum standards for elements that should be included in health records to report care and treatment. These standards are still being used today. Paper health records continued to be used for many years with the first EHR implementation occurring in the 1990s by the US Department of Veterans Affairs. EHR implementations have occurred and continue to occur in most healthcare facilities nationwide.

A health record is an accumulation of information about a patient's past and present health. The primary purpose of the health record, whether recorded electronically or on paper, is to document the health history of the patient. The health record is composed of data that includes the descriptive or numeric attributes of one or more variables. Data collected and analyzed becomes information. A record is a collection, usually in writing, of an account or an occurrence.

There are five primary uses of an EHR system, including the delivery of patient care, the management of patient care, financial processes, administrative processes, and patient self-management.

There are four secondary uses of an EHR system, including education, regulation, research, and public health.

There are four major categories of data in the health record, including administrative, clinical, legal, and financial data. The data in the health record is based on elements developed by the National Committee on Vital and Health Statistics. The information in the paper health record follows one of three formats: the source-oriented record, the integrated health record, or the problem-oriented record. Different formats of the health record are used depending on the healthcare setting.

Every healthcare organization should establish policies and procedures specifying health record documentation guidelines, for both paper and electronic health records, to ensure that health record documentation is accurate, timely, and supportive of assessment, diagnoses, and treatment. Documentation guidelines for data entries must be followed by healthcare personnel.

There are several organizations that provide standards for health records, including The Joint Commission, National Committee for Quality Assurance, Community Health Accreditation Program, Accreditation Association for Ambulatory Health Care, American Health Information Management Association, and the Association for Healthcare Documentation Integrity.

Health record and health information ownership is a controversial topic that has grown increasingly complex as healthcare facilities transitioned from paper health records to EHRs. Historically, state laws and healthcare professional associations have accepted that the healthcare facility that created the health record owns the physical health record. The concept of stewardship is a way to address the responsibilities of retention, privacy, and maintenance of health records and health data without having to solve the issue of ownership. As stewards, all healthcare providers and staff involved in the creation, use, maintenance, and retention of health records and data are responsible for ensuring that health data is generated, used, and stored in a manner that complies with all required laws, rules, standards, and guidelines.

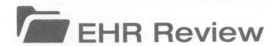

EHR Review

Navigator✚

The following EHR Review, EHR Application, and EHR Evaluation activities are also available online in the Navigator+ learning management system. Your instructor may ask you to complete these activities online. Navigator+ also provides access to flash cards, study games, and practice quizzes to help strengthen your understanding of the chapter content.

Acronyms/Initialisms

Study the following acronyms discussed in this chapter. Go to Navigator+ for flash cards of the acronyms and other chapter key terms.

AAAHC: Accreditation Association for Ambulatory Health Care

ACS: American College of Surgeons

AHDI: Association for Healthcare Documentation Integrity

AHIMA: American Health Information Management Association

ARRA: American Recovery and Reinvestment Act of 2009

CHAP: Community Health Accreditation Program

CMS: Centers for Medicare & Medicaid Services

CoPs: Medicare Conditions of Participation

CPRS: Veterans Health Administration's Computerized Patient Record System

HCD: healthcare delivery

HIMSS: Healthcare Information and Management Systems Society

HIPAA: Health Insurance Portability and Accountability Act of 1996

HMD: Health and Medicine Division

NCQA: National Committee for Quality Assurance

NCVHS: National Committee on Vital and Health Statistics

NPI: National Provider Identifier

POMR: problem-oriented medical record

POR: problem-oriented record

PROMIS: Problem-Oriented Medical Information System

SOAP format: subjective, objective, assessment, plan

SOR: source-oriented record

Check Your Understanding

To check your understanding of this chapter's key concepts, answer the following questions.

1. An ambulatory healthcare facility may be all of the following except

    a. a surgery center.

    b. an intensive care unit.

    c. a dental office.

    d. a psychologist office.

2. The four major categories of information in the health record include administrative, clinical, financial, and

    a. demographic.

    b. diagnostic.

    c. procedural.

    d. legal.

3. The acronym POMR means

    a. problem-oriented medical record.

    b. progress-oriented medical record.

    c. patient-oriented medical record.

    d. patient-oriented medication record.

4. The treatment plan is

    a. an itemized list of the patient's health problem(s).

    b. an organized collection of the patient's health problem(s).

    c. a list of reasons why the patient is at the healthcare facility.

    d. a plan for treatment of the patient's health problem(s).

5. Information standards include an official "Do Not Use" List of abbreviations. Which organization developed this list?

    a. American College of Surgeons

    b. The Joint Commission

    c. National Committee for Quality Assurance

    d. Association for Healthcare Documentation Integrity

6. True/False: The health record is limited to a patient's acute care health information.

7. True/False: An advantage of an electronic health record (EHR) is accessibility by multiple healthcare providers.

8. True/False: The second step in the workflow of an EHR is that the patient checks in using a self-service computer, verifies demographics and insurance information, and makes updates and changes to his or her record.

9. True/False: Abbreviations and acronyms are often used in the medical record. The abbreviation for "by mouth" is p.o.

10. True/False: An ambulatory care setting is where the patient stays longer than 24 hours.

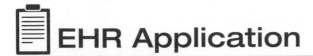 # EHR Application

Go on the Record

To build on your understanding of the topics in this chapter, complete the following short-answer activities.

1. Discuss the importance of the workflow of paper health records and EHRs. Include in your discussion what would happen if a paper or electronic record missed a step in the workflow process.

2. Explain the purpose of the health record.

3. Compare and contrast the various accreditation, professional, and regulatory organizations involved in paper health records and EHRs.

4. Identify the four types of data found in the health record. Provide an example of each type of data.

5. Explain the concept of the health record ownership.

Navigate the Field

To gain practice in handling challenging situations in the workplace, consider the following real-world scenarios and identify how you would respond to each.

1. You are in charge of the medical records department. Your healthcare facility is preparing for a state department of health review, and you want to ensure that your facility's health records follow the suggested standards. There are several organizations that provide accreditation standards as well as guidance on the content and format of the health record. Select two of the following organizations and prepare a report on the importance of the organization: The Joint Commission, National Committee for Quality Assurance, Community Health Accreditation Program, Accreditation Association for Ambulatory Health Care, American Health Information Management Association, and Association for Healthcare Documentation Integrity. After researching the two organizations, develop a checklist for reviewing your department's medical records based on the guidelines suggested by the two organizations.

2. As director of Health Information, you are in charge of training the new physicians and nurses on the official "Do Not Use" List of Abbreviations developed by The Joint Commission. Prepare a summary document that the providers can use after the training session.

 EHR Evaluation

Think Critically

Continue to think critically about challenging concepts and complete the following activities.

1. Match the following description of the problem-oriented medical record with the SOAP format.

    a. Subjective

    b. Objective

    c Assessment

    d. Plan

    _____ A. X-rays of the right hand will be ordered. If a fracture is seen, the patient will be referred to the orthopedic surgeon. The patient will be given a tetanus booster because he has not had one in the past 10 years. His wounds will be cleaned today, and antibiotic ointment and light bandages will be applied. He will be restricted from using his right hand at work for the next three days with no gripping. He will keep his wounds clean and watch for infection. He will follow up in the clinic in four days to reassess his injury and hopefully return back to full duty.

    _____ B. Mr. Smith is a 35-year-old man who was operating a cherry picker forklift today at work when he backed up and smashed his right hand in between the handle of his lift and a wooden pallet. He complains of pain in his second, third, and fourth fingers. He notes that his fingers are swollen and that they hurt when he tries to bend them. He has not noted any numbness in the fingers but says they are throbbing in pain. He also states that there are several cuts on his hand. He was seen by the company nurse who cleaned his wounds and put bandages on them. He was sent here by his company for evaluation.

    _____ C. VS BP 120/72 P74 Temp 98.7° F

    Right hand: The second, third, and fourth fingers are swollen from the PIP joints to the MCP joints. Bruising is present. ROM of the PIP joints is limited. There is normal ROM of the DIP and MCP joints. Extensor and flexor tendon strength is intact. Distal sensation is intact. Capillary refill is brisk. There are several abrasions noted on each finger. The remainder of the hand and wrist is free of injury.

    _____ D. 1. Right hand contusion

    2. Abrasions right hand

2. A 56-year-old woman with sudden onset upper back pain presents to the emergency department. This is the patient's first visit to Northstar Medical Center. Use the sample medical record located in Appendix B to identify the components of the medical record.

   A. Demographic information—include the patient name, address, and date of birth

   B. Contact information—home, work, and cell phone numbers and email address

   C. History and physical—health history, review of vital signs, and complete organ-specific physical examination

   D. Problem list—list of current health issues

   E. Allergy list—list of medications, food, and other items, if any, to which a patient is allergic

   F. Prescription list—list of current medications, including dosages

Make Your Case

Consider the scenario and then complete the following project.

This chapter illustrated how Hurricane Katrina affected medical records. Dig deeper into this topic by locating five reputable websites that discuss the impact of the hurricane on the medical records of local citizens. Read and consider the information carefully. Then create a preparedness plan that would prevent a loss of medical information in a future catastrophe.

Explore the Technology

To expand your mastery of EHRs, explore the technology by completing the following online activities.

1. Conduct an Internet search for patient registration/admission forms at two acute and two ambulatory care facilities. Identify and explain the registration/admission process at each type of facility. Is the patient required to complete the forms before admission/visit? If so, are there forms the patient downloads and completes? Does the patient register online? If so, how does the patient do that? Is there a patient portal that requires the patient to create an account? If so, are the instructions clear? What are the advantages and disadvantages of the system the care facility is using?

2. Research the three different formats of the health record. Explain the advantages and disadvantages of each type of format.

3. Locate three websites that provide information and resources on proper health record documentation. Do the three sources provide different guidelines for proper health record documentation? How are they similar and different?

4. Research why the NCVHS list of 42 core elements is important. How will the core elements affect the EHR?

Are You Ready?

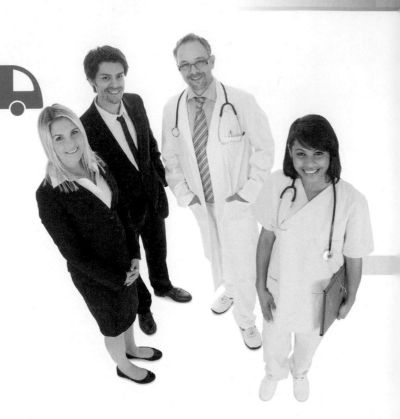

As you begin your studies in health information technology, you probably do not know where your career will take you. One thing is for certain, though: no matter what aspect of health care you plan to pursue, you will come into contact with an electronic health record (EHR). With that in mind, the simulated EHR software accompanying this textbook will teach you the basic skills necessary to master the real-world EHR system that is a future certainty for all healthcare facilities.

Beyond the Record

- In 2015, there were more than 1,100 different EHR software vendors. This number doubled in four years.

- Today more than 80% of healthcare providers use smartphones or tablets to help aid medical decisions.

- A six-character password takes a hacker about 10 minutes to crack, and the most common password is 123456. To ensure security, passwords in an EHR system need to be strong.

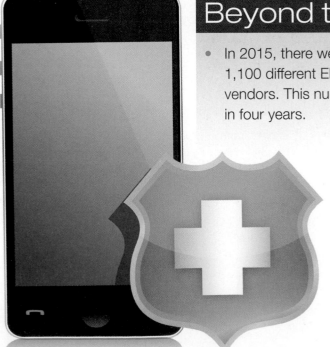

Password ● ● ● ● ● ● ● ● ● ● ● ● ● ●

Chapter 3

Introduction to Electronic Health Record Software

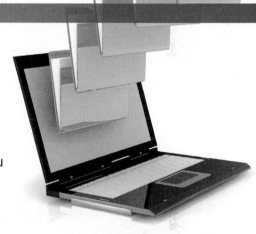

This textbook uses a comprehensive, realistic electronic health records (EHR) system called EHR Navigator. EHR Navigator is designed to introduce and practice the key functions found in EHR systems (e.g., patient admission, registration, scheduling, communication, privacy, security, coding, billing, reimbursement, clinical decision support, and patient portals). Using the EHR Navigator throughout this textbook will help you experience how an EHR system works in the field.

Field Notes

Electronic health records (EHRs) have improved quality of care with regard to documentation, helping to standardize processes throughout our hospitals at a regional level. We can now quickly and effectively analyze patient information to prevent any issues that may arise. Physicians complete charts timely and accurately with fewer medical errors (e.g., poor legibility, unapproved abbreviations). Maintaining an EHR saves money and time by eliminating the cost of storing, retrieving, transporting, and printing records. An EHR also allows practitioners to quickly view records from other hospitals and hospital affiliates, thus improving patient care.

– Misty A. Glasgow, MBA
HIM/Privacy Officer

Learning Objectives

3.1 Understand the terms *input*, *output*, *processing*, *storage*, and *local area network*.

3.2 Demonstrate how to navigate an EHR system.

3.3 Describe the password and security measures of an EHR system.

3.4 Identify menu options in EHR Navigator.

3.5 Examine charting features in EHR Navigator.

3.6 Review the various scheduling features of EHR Navigator.

3.7 Examine secure messaging, document management, laboratory integration, and e-prescribing features of EHR Navigator.

3.8 Explain the importance of backing up the EHR system.

3.9 Examine mobile features in an EHR system.

An electronic health record (EHR) system manages all aspects of a patient visit, from the time a patient contacts the healthcare facility to the time the insurance and billing are both processed. This system can be accessed by healthcare personnel who work in an acute care setting as well as those individuals who work in an ambulatory care facility. As defined in Chapter 2, an acute care facility treats patients who have acute health issues that require inpatient care. An ambulatory care setting services outpatients or patients who do not require admission to acute care facilities. There are many types of ambulatory care facilities such as a physician's office, a hospital emergency department, a dental office, a surgery center, or a health clinic. An EHR system provides interoperability among various healthcare facilities, which allows the facilities to communicate with each other and view the patient's health record. To help you understand how an EHR system operates, you must become familiar with the system's features and have plenty of opportunities for practice. The EHR Navigator will help you do just that.

The EHR Navigator is a comprehensive EHR and practice management system that provides you with hands-on experience within a realistic EHR system. This practice software, accessed through the Navigator+ learning management system, provides you with the necessary skills to work in any EHR system you might encounter in either an acute care or ambulatory care setting. You will become familiar with patient management, scheduling, medical charting, laboratory integrations, medical documents, e-prescribing, clinical collaboration, reporting, coding, and billing. You will also practice patient portal activities.

In addition to the explanation of the features of an EHR system, the text examines the security settings and requirements of a typical EHR system, discusses the importance of having a backup system, and explains how to evaluate and implement an EHR system. Lastly, this chapter discusses the current and future role of digital devices as healthcare providers embrace the adoption of EHR systems. Together, the text and the EHR Navigator activities will guide you through the concepts and applications of EHR systems.

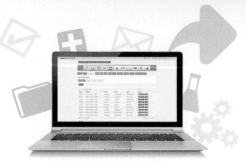

Information Processing Cycle

The **information processing cycle** provides the building blocks for the EHR system and includes four components: **input**, **processing**, **output**, and **storage** (see Figure 3.1). The information processing cycle converts data entered into the computer into valuable information for healthcare personnel.

The **input** component is the data entered by the user of an EHR system (e.g., the patient's first name, last name, identification number).

The **processing** component permits data to be usable by analyzing that data to determine test value results that are within a critical or normal range. In an EHR, the processing component determines whether entered test results are values within a critical or normal range.

The **output** component is the data produced that provides meaningful information for the user. A report on a patient's laboratory test results is an example of an output in an EHR system. A healthcare provider may use the report to guide treatment decisions.

Figure 3.1 Information Processing Cycle

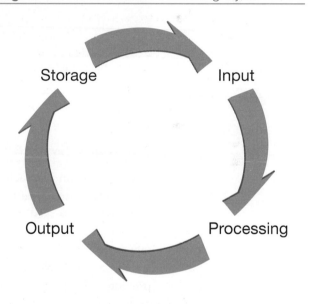

Storage is the fourth component of the information processing cycle. Patient information is stored so that it can be retrieved, added to, or modified for later use. Data are processed once they are entered into an EHR. There are various types of **storage devices** that an EHR system uses. EHR systems may be stored on a dedicated server at the healthcare facility or on a server provided by a vendor. If an EHR system is networked, then the storage may exist on the healthcare system's server. **Cloud storage** is data stored on virtual servers.

As technology continues to develop, EHR systems become easier to use. Internet and intranet technologies will allow you to access and share an EHR system in one building as well as in remote locations. This accessibility can be a liability, which is why an EHR system must be secure and accessed based on necessary functions to perform a specific job. As an additional security measure, the data entered and extracted from the EHR system is encrypted to maintain security and protect patient privacy.

Hardware Support

An EHR system is most commonly accessed through a computer workstation. A typical **workstation** includes a computer and input and output devices. Healthcare providers may also be supplied with digital mobile devices not wired to a workstation. Both computer workstations and digital devices can be found in healthcare facilities

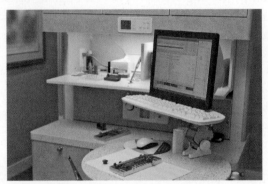

today. An **input device**—such as a keyboard, mouse, scanner, microphone, camera, stylus, or touch screen—is used to enter data into an EHR system. An **output device**—such as a computer monitor, digital device screen, or printer—displays the results from EHRs. Because the printing functionality of an EHR is a security issue, healthcare staff members must adhere to their facilities' policy and procedure manuals for the permissible circumstances for printing a patient's health record.

EHR systems are commonly accessed through a computer workstation.

Network Systems

The workstation also includes access to the Internet and intranet system. Computer workstations are networked through a **local area network (LAN)**. A LAN is a group of computers connected through a network confined to a single area or small geographic area such as a building or hospital campus. The network is secure and reliable, enabling safe transfer of the data among the workstations. The networked computer system allows computer workstations to work and communicate together. The network should provide a great deal of flexibility and should be adaptable to new technologies, such as fiber-optic cables, new software, and wireless communication. The LAN utilizes a dedicated server for the workstations. The network is connected through either wired or wireless connections. The advantage of a wireless connection is that the healthcare provider may be anywhere and have access to an EHR system. Figure 3.2 shows a visual representation of a network system.

A **wide area network (WAN)** is a network that covers a broader area than a LAN. It is a computer network that spans regions, countries, or the world. As health care becomes more global and interoperable, more WANs will be used to connect the LANs of separate healthcare facilities.

Figure 3.2   Network System

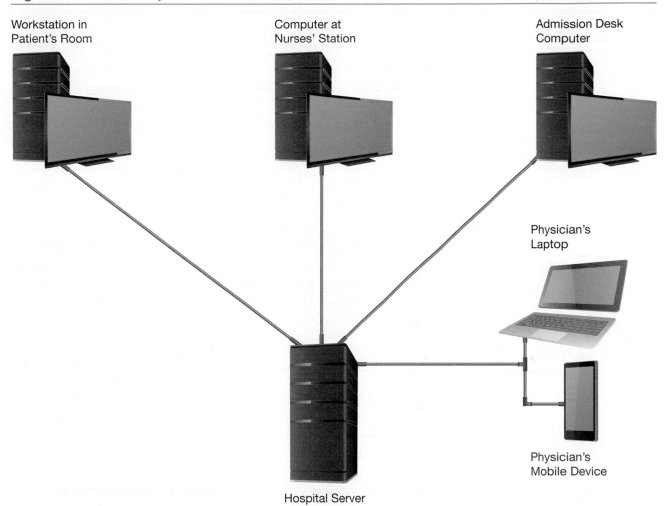

Workstation in Patient's Room

Computer at Nurses' Station

Admission Desk Computer

Physician's Laptop

Hospital Server

Physician's Mobile Device

EHR Accessibility

The expense of having a computer workstation in every service room may prevent providers from expanding an EHR system as widely as necessary for maximum efficiency. However, not having access to a workstation may cause a delay in updating and adding information to an EHR for other healthcare providers to view. One solution for this accessibility issue is the use of mobile and digital devices, which some healthcare providers are beginning to utilize. Mobile and digital devices will be explored later in this chapter.

Data may be entered into EHRs via a keyboard. Some EHR systems have voice recognition software that will adapt to your voice and speech patterns and input data into the system. Electronic handwriting or touch screen input may also be available, depending on the EHR system design. Some EHR systems have templates that allow you to select text options from a drop-down menu, allowing standard data to be quickly added to the patient's record.

1. Name the four components of the information processing cycle.

   a. _____

   b. _____

   c. _____

   d. _____

2. Explain how a LAN affects the use of an EHR system.

   _____

   _____

   _____

   _____

Privacy and Security in the EHR System

The privacy and security settings of an EHR system must conform to Health Insurance Portability and Accountability Act of 1996 (HIPAA) regulations. (For more information on HIPAA regulations, refer to Chapter 6.) These settings include the use of passwords and user permissions.

Password Protection

An EHR system must allow acute and ambulatory care facilities to create, change, and safeguard passwords. Facilities must have policies and procedures in place for managing passwords. Typically, passwords are six to eight characters long, with a combination of alphanumeric characters, and typically contain at least one uppercase letter. When you enter your password, characters appear as dots, asterisks, or other symbols, thus preventing other users from seeing the password. Generally, you must change your password every 90 to 120 days. In addition to using a password to enter the system, specific areas of an EHR system may also be password protected to maintain the privacy and security of patient health records. The password is encrypted in the transmittal process between your workstation and an EHR system. An audit manager or administrator records the user log-ins and log-outs to monitor use of the EHR system. EHR systems allow for backend auditing so there is an objective record available that indicates all users who have accessed a patient's chart. Audit records can be reproduced to address access issues or HIPAA noncompliance.

When you first log in to an EHR system, you key in a default password, then follow the prompts to change your password. Typically, you can attempt to log in three times before being locked out and requiring the password to be reset by the administrator or information technology (IT) manager at the facility.

User Permissions

An EHR contains a patient's **protected health information (PHI)**. If you are an employee of an acute care or ambulatory care facility, you must have a unique user name that registers your identity and tracks your activity in an EHR system. Each user's access to information is based on the type of information he or she will need to view or modify. Therefore, users are assigned access according to their job functions (e.g., healthcare provider, nurse, health information professional, registrar). For example, a registration or admission clerk may not have access to a patient's X-rays but would have access to the patient's insurance information. This assigned access ensures the security and confidentiality of patient records. Figure 3.3 illustrates how an administrator can assign you permission to access various areas of an EHR system based on your job position. These permissions define the areas of the software in which a user may view, add, edit, or delete information. For example, a front desk clerk at an outpatient facility may see a screen similar to the one shown in Figure 3.4 when accessing the EHR Navigator. When admitting a patient, an admission clerk would view a screen similar to the one shown in Figure 3.5.

Figure 3.3 Assign User Permissions

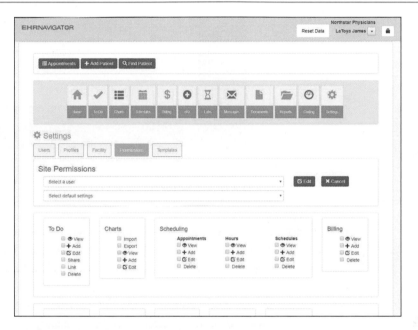

Figure 3.4 Home Screen—Outpatient

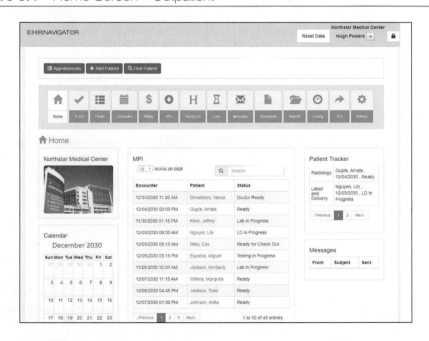

Figure 3.5 Patient Admission—Inpatient

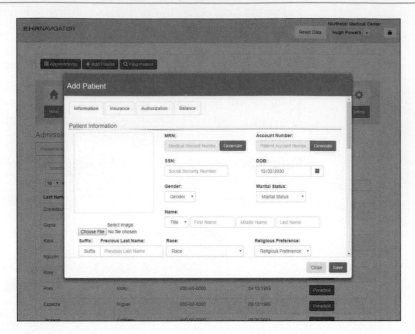

Hibernation Mode

When you must step away from your workstation, an EHR system should be set to **hibernation mode**, a privacy feature that prevents disclosure of PHI. Patients and healthcare providers alike may be able to see a workstation as they pass by, so the information on the screen must be protected. When you are not actively using the EHR system, or if you must step away for a few minutes, it must be in the hibernation mode. If you do not set the hibernation mode manually, it will automatically go into hibernation mode after a period of inactivity. To escape the hibernation mode and reaccess a patient's health record, you must reenter your username and password. Figure 3.6 shows these precautions.

Figure 3.6 Log-in Due to Hibernation

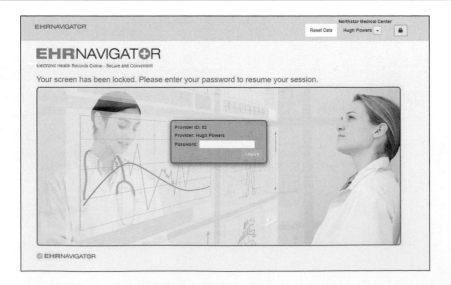

Accessing the EHR Navigator

In this chapter as well as throughout *Exploring Electronic Health Records*, Second Edition, hands-on tutorials, practice assessments, and assessments using the web-based EHR Navigator will provide you with practical experience. Each interactive tutorial is designed to demonstrate an EHR concept. After completing the interactive tutorial, you have the opportunity to practice the skills you just learned by taking a variety of practice assessments. Once you feel you have mastered the skill, you can take the automatically graded assessment that corresponds to each of the tutorials offered throughout the chapters. These tutorials, practice assessments, and assessments are based on a review of many inpatient and outpatient EHR systems and therefore are transferable to a variety of healthcare settings. When you log in to the Navigator+ learning management system to launch the tutorials, you will be guided by an audio recording through each step of the tutorial. The tutorials will begin by reviewing various features and capabilities of the software. Once you have mastered the software, you will begin to apply the EHR concepts presented in the text via the practice assessments. As a final check, there are assessments at the end of each chapter that test your understanding of the chapter concepts and their applications.

Capabilities of EHR Systems

The Office of the National Coordinator for Health Information Technology (ONC) has defined the capabilities that are necessary for the meaningful use of EHR technology. These capabilities were originally defined by the Certification Commission for Health Information Technology (CCHIT), the organization that was previously responsible for certifying EHR systems. These capabilities include functionality, interoperability, and security. **Functionality** is the ability to create and manage EHRs for all patients in a healthcare facility. In addition, functionality includes the ability to automate workflow in a healthcare facility. **Interoperability** is the ability of an EHR system to exchange data with other sources of health information, including pharmacies, laboratories, and other healthcare providers. Interoperability is achieved through standards such as Health Level Seven International (HL7), which aims to facilitate sharing and transferring clinical information from one system to another. **Security** is the standard that prevents data loss and ensures that patient health information is private.

EHR Software Features

This section addresses the software features that improve efficiency in the administrative and clinical components of a healthcare facility. Some of the administrative features examined include messaging, to-do list, scheduling, patient management, billing, and coding. Several features that are used in a clinical setting are also discussed, including medical charting, clinical collaboration, results reporting, clinical decision support, and patient portals.

Using the EHR Navigator

The EHR Navigator encompasses inpatient and outpatient EHR systems. Within each menu are submenu options. Figure 3.7 illustrates the inpatient system, Northstar Medical Center. The outpatient system, Northstar Physicians, is shown in Figure 3.8.

Figure 3.7   EHR Overview—Inpatient

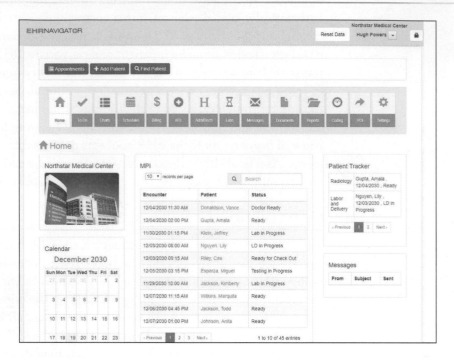

Figure 3.8   EHR Overview—Outpatient

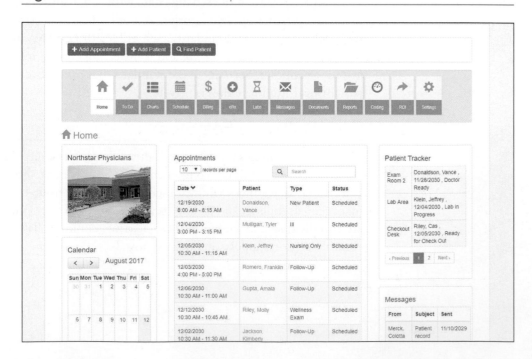

Menus

The menu bar is at the top of the screen. The options on the Northstar Medical Center menu bar are *Home*, *To Do*, *Charts*, *Schedule*, *Billing*, *eRx*, *Admission/Discharge*, *Labs*, *Messages*, *Documents*, *Reports*, *Coding*, *ROI* (release of information), and *Settings* (see Figure 3.9).

Figure 3.9 Menus—Inpatient

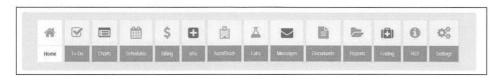

The options on the Northstar Physicians menu bar are *Home*, *To Do*, *Charts*, *Schedule*, *Billing*, *eRx*, *Admission/Discharge*, *Labs*, *Messages*, *Documents*, *Reports*, *Coding*, *ROI*, and *Settings* (see Figure 3.10).

Figure 3.10 Menus—Outpatient

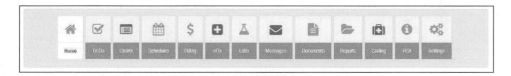

When you click each of the menu options, a list of functions appears below the menu option.

Settings

The EHR Navigator has a *Settings* feature that allows the healthcare facility to add users, edit facility information, grant user permissions, and customize features to meet the needs of the healthcare facility. Figure 3.11 illustrates the *Settings* feature for both inpatient and outpatient facilities.

Figure 3.11 Settings

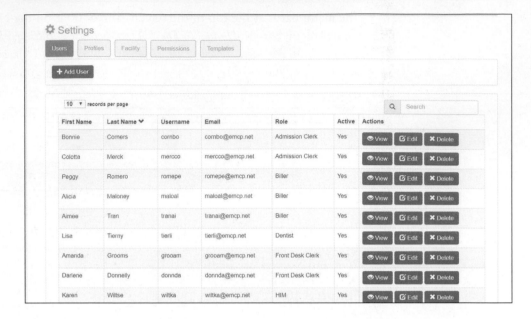

Users

In the *Users* submenu option, all users are listed along with their respective roles (e.g., physician, HIM professional, unit clerk, pharmacist). This site is also where the EHR administrator or office manager can add or edit users (see Figure 3.12).

Figure 3.12 Users Submenu

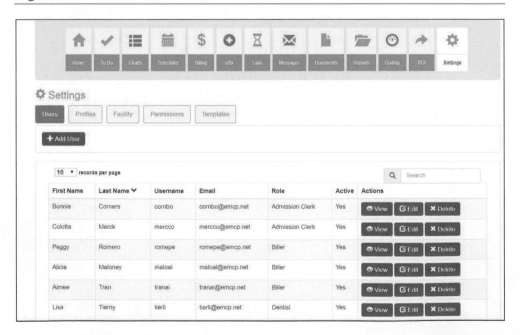

Profiles

By selecting *Profiles*, you may update your basic information (see Figure 3.13).

Figure 3.13   Profiles Submenu

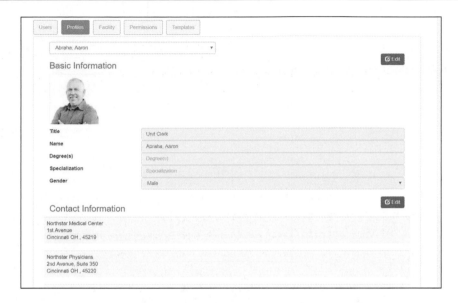

Facility

The *Facility* submenu of the EHR Navigator (see Figures 3.14 and 3.15) allows you to view basic information about the facility, including the following:

- Identifiers such as a National Provider Identifier (NPI); Employer Identification Number (EIN); and Medicare, Medicaid, and the TRICARE provider numbers

- Healthcare organizations list (details a list of related healthcare organizations)

- Payer list (details a list of payers)

Figure 3.14   Facility Submenu

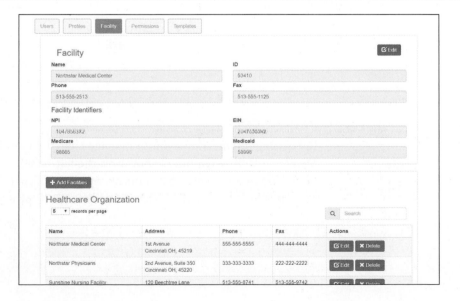

Figure 3.15 Facility Submenu (continued)

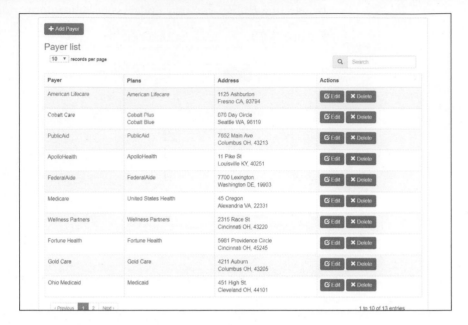

Permissions

The *Permissions* submenu in the EHR Navigator is where employee access to EHR functions is managed. Options to view, add, edit, and delete permissions are selected for each user. For example, all users are granted access to the *To Do* option on the *Users* menu, but only certain healthcare personnel that can order medications (such as physicians, physician assistants, nurse practitioners, and pharmacists) can override drug allergies. Figure 3.16 provides an example of how adjustments for permissions may be made to drug-drug and drug-allergy alerts.

Figure 3.16 Permissions for Drug Alerts

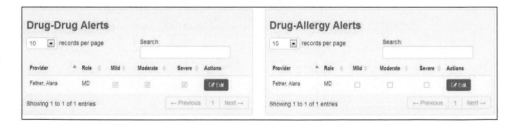

Templates

The *Settings* menu allows you to manage charting templates. When you select *Templates*, facility templates appear on the left panel, and a list of templates you may like to use in a patient's chart appears on the right panel. You may create custom templates by selecting *Add Templates*. Figure 3.17 provides a list of templates.

Figure 3.17 Facility and User Templates

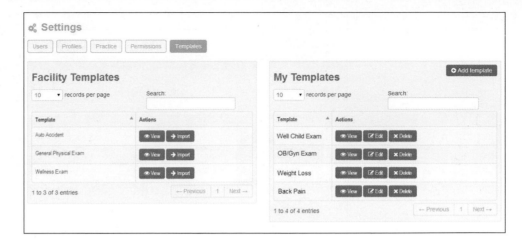

Tutorial 3.1   EHRNAVIGAT⊕R

Viewing Features in the EHR

Go to Navigator+ to launch Tutorial 3.1. As a physician, practice logging in, viewing permissions, examining the hibernation feature, and unlocking the system using the EHR Navigator.

Tutorial 3.2   EHRNAVIGAT⊕R

Adding a New Employee and Assigning Rights to the EHR

Go to Navigator+ to launch Tutorial 3.2. As an IT administrator, practice adding a new employee and assigning rights using the EHR Navigator.

Administrative Features

The administrative features in the EHR Navigator include reports, messages, scheduling, billing, some charting information, and documents.

Home

On the *Home* menu there are six submenus: *Calendar*, *To Do*, *Appointments*, *Patient Tracker*, and *Messages* (see Figure 3.18). The *Calendar* provides quick access to specific dates, and the *To Do* section allows you to create reminders, prioritize activities, and organize lists to be more efficient and effective on the job. *Appointments* displays appointments for the current week, and *Patient Tracker* identifies a patient's physical location while he or she is in the facility. *Messages* is an internal communication tool for all users of the EHR Navigator.

Figure 3.18 Home Menu

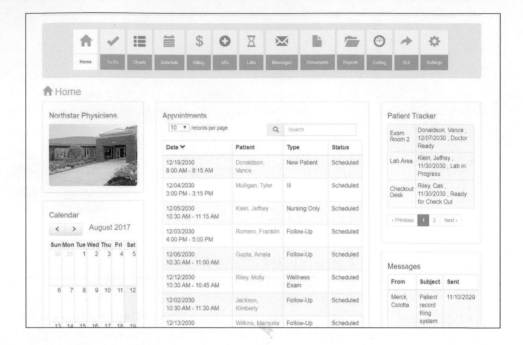

Patient Tracker

In the *Home* menu, a *Status* feature allows you to change the status of the patient. For instance, the patient status may change from *Scheduled* to *Arrived*, *No Show*, or *Canceled*. This allows the administrative staff to easily track patients. Once a patient's status is changed to *Arrived*, the patient is displayed in the *Patient Tracker*. Then the administrative staff or healthcare provider may change the status to *Arrived*, *Checked Out*, *Doctor Ready*, *Exam in Progress*, *Lab in Progress*, *Nurse Ready*, or *Ready for Checkout* in the system. Figure 3.19 shows the Patient Tracker status.

Figure 3.19 Patient Tracker Status

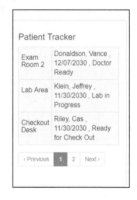

Reports

As you learned in Chapter 1, the Health Information Technology for Economic and Clinical Health Act (HITECH Act) provides incentives for implementing an EHR system based on meaningful use criteria, and many of these systems have a dashboard to track this use. Typically, an administrator of an EHR system monitors the progress the healthcare facility has made toward completing each criterion. In the EHR Navigator, the meaningful use information can be accessed under the *Reports* tab. Figure 3.20 illustrates an example of a typical *Meaningful Use* report. Criteria may be calculated based on provider, year, attestation duration, and start and end dates.

Figure 3.20 Meaningful Use Report

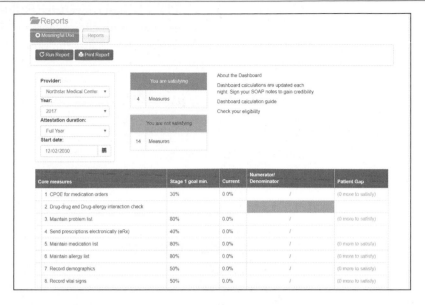

You can also access the Activity Feed feature on the Reports tab. The *User Activity Feed* feature in the EHR Navigator tracks your access to various components in the system. Each time you log in or out, or each time you make updates or add data to a patient's chart, the activity is tracked. If you create an appointment or submit a prescription to the pharmacy, that activity will also appear in the *User Activity Feed*. This feed, seen in Figure 3.21, enables the administrator to get a longitudinal view of actions occurring in the healthcare facility.

Figure 3.21 User Activity Feed

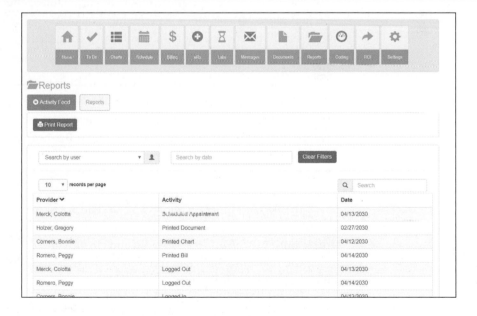

The *Reports* feature in the EHR Navigator allows users of Northstar Medical Center and Northstar Physicians to convert the facility's data into information that can be analyzed. Reports may be run on clinical data or administrative information, or by provider and date range. Figure 3.22 lists the various reports and descriptions available in the EHR Navigator.

Figure 3.22 List of Reports

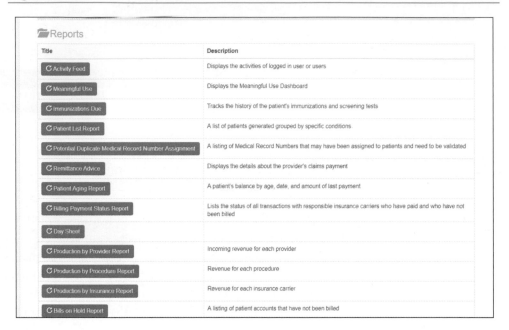

The EHR Navigator *Reports* feature queries special reports based on particular criteria. An example of a query report might include generating a list of women age 50 and older who have not yet scheduled mammography in the past year. Many of the reports will be covered more in depth in Chapter 9.

Messages

The EHR Navigator messaging system allows you to communicate with other system users in your organization. Some EHR systems contain a HIPAA-compliant messaging feature that permits physicians, nurses, and other healthcare providers to communicate with medical colleagues outside their healthcare facilities. This feature is similar to a social media type of messaging system used to improve the collaboration and continuity of patient care.

The *Message* function allows you to send messages to patients, providers, and employees of the healthcare facilities using the EHR Navigator. The menu provides three options: *Inbox, Sent Messages*, and *Archived Messages*.

The *Inbox* lists messages received by the user or healthcare facility. Figure 3.23 illustrates the EHR Navigator Inbox. You may reply, forward, save, or delete messages. You may also send a new message, as illustrated in Figure 3.24. As shown in Figure 3.25, messages may be archived to allow you to document communication among healthcare providers, facilities, pharmacies, and the patient.

Figure 3.23 Messages—Inbox

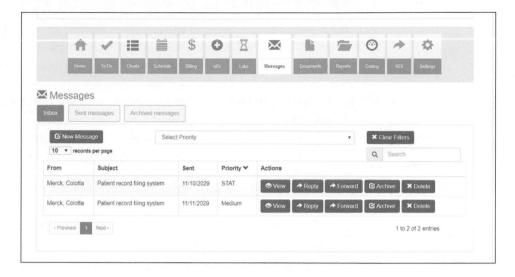

Figure 3.24 Messages—New Message

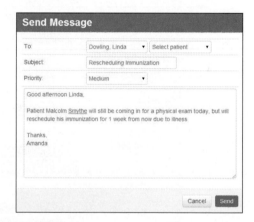

Figure 3.25 Messages—Archived Messages

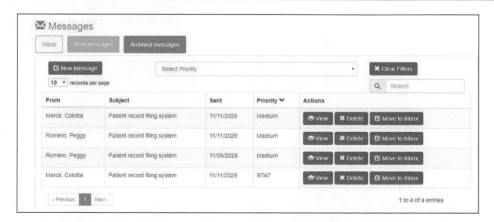

Schedules

The *Schedules* feature in the EHR Navigator gives you access to the calendar in daily and monthly views. The *Schedules* overview allows you to quickly view the available practice areas at the facility and see what patients have appointments there on any given day. For example, a front desk clerk at Northstar Physicians can view all of the the appointments in Exam Room 1 and potentially move a patient to Exam Room 2 by dragging and dropping the appointment (see Figure 3.26).

The view-only calendar overview allows you to quickly see all of the appointments for the entire month. The appointment types are color coded for easy viewing (see Figure 3.27).

In addition to the schedule and calendar overviews, Northstar Medical Center and Northstar Physicians can use the *Hours* feature to customize the availability of appointments by setting parameters for the days and times that Northstar is able to schedule patients. Figures 3.28 and 3.29 illustrate how Northstar may select days and hours, respectively, when appointments are available.

Figure 3.26   Schedules Overview—Northstar Physicians

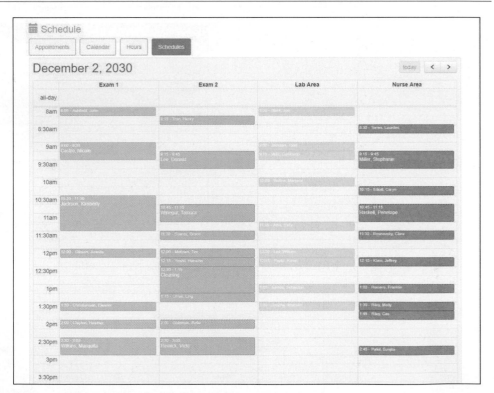

Figure 3.27 View Only Calendar—Northstar Physicians

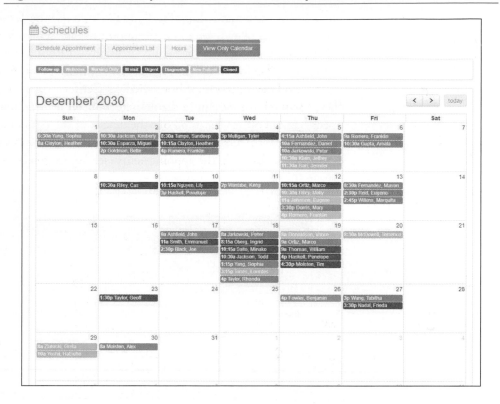

Figure 3.28 Facility Days and Hours

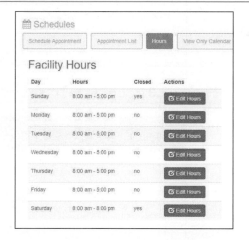

Figure 3.29 Customize Hours

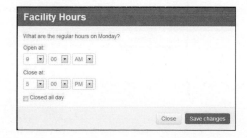

Schedules

The administrative and clinical staff are likely to use the *Schedules* feature in a variety of ways. *Schedules* allows you to see the appointments scheduled for the healthcare facility on a given day in each of the facility areas (Exam Room 1, Exam Room 2, Lab Area, and Nurse Area for Northstar Physicians; Clinic, Operating Room, Radiology, and Labor and Delivery for Northstar Medical Center). An appointment can be made by clicking an open time slot in the desired room. A *Schedule Appointment* dialog box opens, allowing the user to fill out the details of the patient appointment (see Figure 3.30). Appointments can also be dragged from one room to another, or they can be edited when you click the appointments (see Figure 3.31).

Figure 3.30   Schedule Appointment Dialog Box

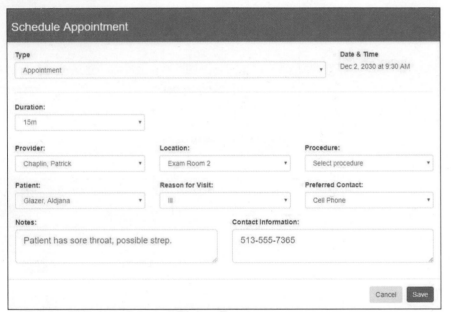

Figure 3.31   Edit Appointment Dialog Box

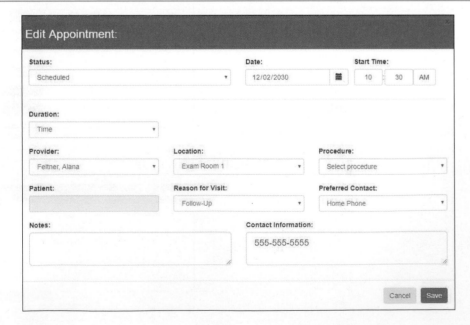

$ Billing

Billing for treatment and services rendered is a main function of any healthcare organization. Figure 3.32 shows the main billing screen found in the EHR Navigator.

Figure 3.32 Billing

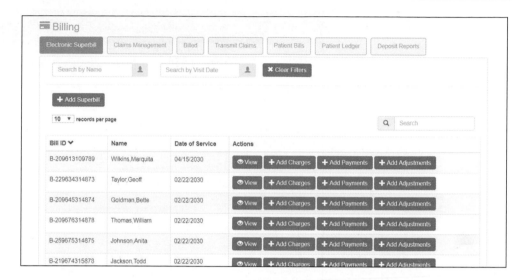

The main subsections of the *Billing* tab are *Electronic Superbill*, *Claims Management*, *Billed*, *Transmit Claims*, *Patient Bills*, *Patient Ledger*, and *Deposit Reports*.

On the *Electronic Superbill* subsection, a biller can view a superbill (a list of all charges relating to a patient visit) and can also add charges, add payments, and add adjustments using the buttons in the *Actions* section. Figure 3.33 shows the Add Superbill dialog box.

Figure 3.33 Add Superbill

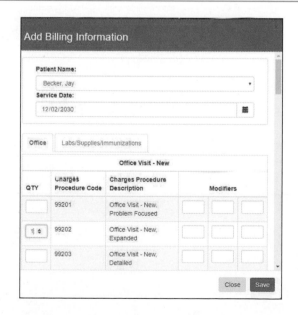

Under *Claims Management*, a biller can view, edit, and bill for patient visits. You can also access the CMS-1500 form on this screen in Northstar Physicians and CMS-1450/UB-04 form in Northstar Medical Center. These are specialized billing forms that will be covered in more detail in Chapter 9. See Figures 3.34 and 3.35.

Figure 3.34   CMS-1500 Form

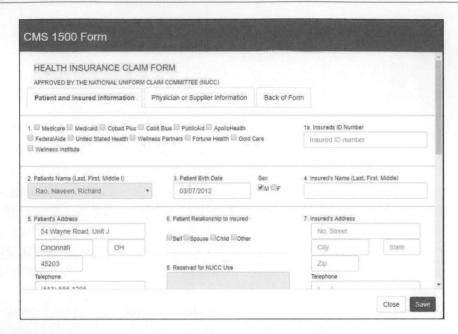

Figure 3.35   CMS-1450/UB-04 Form

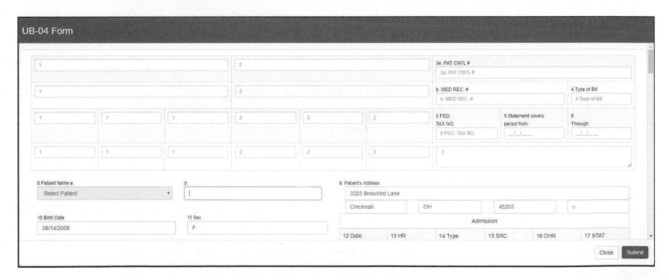

The *Billed* subsection shows the patient bills that have already been processed. *Transmit Claims* allows you to see the visits that are ready for review and transmit the claims (see Figure 3.36).

Figure 3.36 Transmit Claims

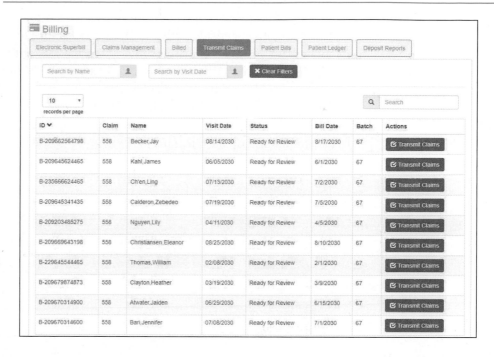

Patient Bills shows an archive of patient bills. The *Patient Ledger* allows you to see a history of services, payments, and adjustments for a patient (see Figure 3.37).

You will experience the billing functions of the EHR Navigator in Chapter 9.

Figure 3.37 Patient Ledger

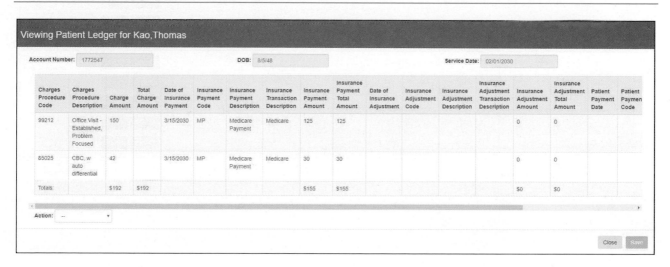

⊞ Charts

The *Charts* feature in the EHR Navigator contains both administrative *and* clinical information. This section addresses only the administrative information, and the clinical information will be discussed in the Clinical Features section on page 92. In the *Charts* feature, a list of patients treated at the healthcare facility appears. The user is able to find, filter, and add patients. The administrative features in the EHR Navigator contain patient demographics, insurance information, setting, clinical information, and a list of appointments. Within the patient chart, the healthcare facility can enroll a patient in a PHR, print a patient chart, send a referral or response letter, export a patient record, export an immunization registry, and provide public health surveillance information. Figures 3.38 and 3.39 provide examples of the patient list and patient chart found in the *Charts* feature.

Figure 3.38 Charts—List of Patients

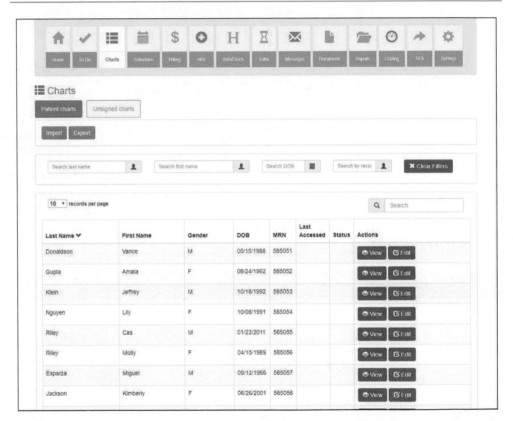

Figure 3.39 Charts—Patient Chart

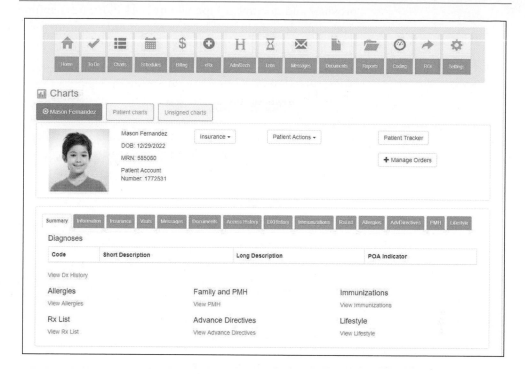

Documents

The EHR Navigator allows you to add documents from a predetermined list—Summary Report, Insurance Form, or a dictation—to a patient's chart. This action can be taken at the *Documents* tab or on the patient's chart. The system also allows you to make notations on a document before assigning the file to a patient's chart and to digitally sign documents. Figure 3.40 shows how to add a document.

Figure 3.40 Adding Documents

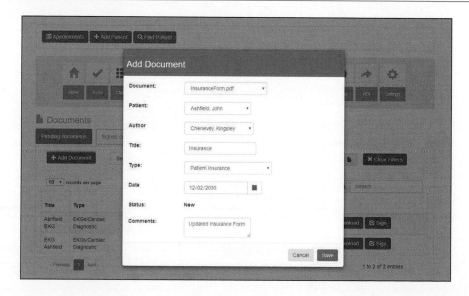

Documents can be viewed either as pending or signed, and they may be filtered by provider and document type. Figure 3.41 illustrates pending documents. For example, a pending document may be a physician order waiting for a doctor to authenticate.

Figure 3.41 Pending Documents

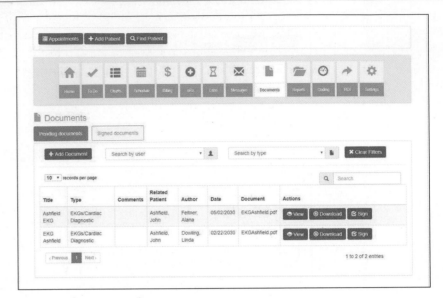

CHECKPOINT 3.2

1. Explain why *Messages* is an important feature in an EHR system.

   _____

   _____

   _____

2. Name two different ways to view appointments in the *Schedules* tab.

   a. _____

   b. _____

Tutorial 3.3

Scheduling an Appointment

Go to Navigator+ to launch Tutorial 3.3. As a physician, practice the administrative features using the EHR Navigator

Clinical Features

In addition to the administrative features, there are a number of clinical features available to an EHR user. The clinical features of the EHR Navigator include patient chart information, e-prescriptions (eRx), managing physician orders, and viewing laboratory and diagnostic test results.

Charts

The EHR Navigator *Charts* feature is the source for the patient's clinical data, including medical diagnoses, treatments, procedures, allergies, medical history, medications, test results, and reports. *Charts* provides you with a unique view of the entire record at a glance, without having to navigate to other areas of the EHR system to view patient information. The EHR Navigator allows multiple users to have access to a patient's chart. Figure 3.42 illustrates the past medical history component of the patient chart.

The EHR Navigator *Charts* feature also allows you to add a chart note, as shown in Figure 3.43.

Figure 3.42   Charts—Patient History

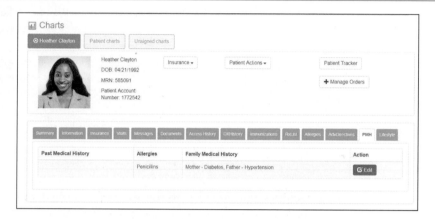

Figure 3.43   Add Chart Note

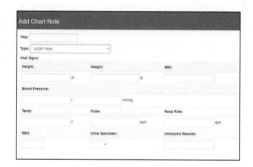

eRx

A typical EHR system has an eRx (electronic prescription) feature that enables the system to electronically submit prescriptions to pharmacies all across the United States. The use of e-prescribing helps to reduce medication errors, thus improving patient safety and increasing practice efficiency. An EHR system that integrates an e-prescribing function increases facility productivity and efficiency by allowing a healthcare provider to view the patient's medication history in the EHR rather than pulling a chart and writing a prescription by hand. Figure 3.44 shows the *eRx* screen in the EHR Navigator.

Figure 3.44 eRx

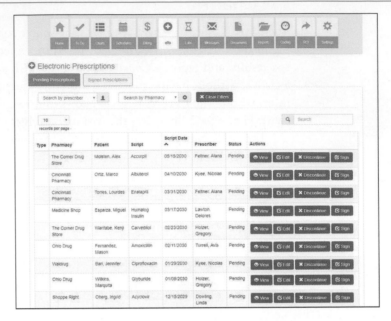

⧗ Labs

EHR systems include an integrated laboratory feature, which enables healthcare facilities and providers to connect with national and regional laboratories or maintain an existing laboratory partner. The EHR Navigator *Labs* feature allows you to view *Pending Labs* and *Signed Labs*. Pending labs are those awaiting test processing and results reporting. Signed labs are those that have been viewed and signed by a physician, physician assistant, or nurse practitioner. Integrating laboratories into an EHR system gives you the ability to create laboratory orders and view results from any computer at any time, with abnormal results flagged and organized for easy review. Figure 3.45 illustrates the *Labs* feature in the EHR Navigator.

Figure 3.45 Labs—Views

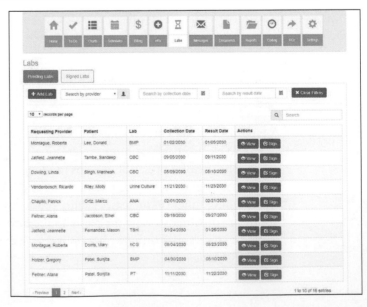

Manage Orders

Every EHR system contains a computerized physician order entry (CPOE) component. In the EHR Navigator, the CPOE component is located by clicking *Charts*, selecting the patient, and clicking *Manage Orders*. *Manage Orders* is a button located on the patient's chart. Depending on their level of access, users add, view, and cancel physician orders for treatment and care—for example, laboratory orders, dietary orders, and therapy orders—by using *Manage Orders*. Figure 3.46 illustrates the *Manage Orders* dialog box in EHR Navigator. You will learn about CPOE, in detail, in Chapter 8 of this text.

Figure 3.46 Manage Orders

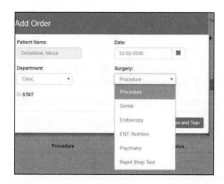

CHECKP✚INT 3.3

1. Name four types of clinical information found in a patient's chart.

   a. _____

   b. _____

   c. _____

   d. _____

2. Explain the importance of an integrated laboratory feature.

   _____

   _____

   _____

Tutorial 3.4

EHRNAVIGAT✚R

Reviewing a Patient's Chart and Locking and Unlocking the EHR

Go to Navigator+ to launch Tutorial 3.4. As a physician, practice reviewing patient clinical information using the EHR Navigator.

Backing Up and Accessing EHR Systems

EHR systems can be web-based or locally installed. Regardless, the EHR system data belongs to the healthcare facility. If the healthcare facility decides to switch from a web-based to a locally installed EHR system, the data may be exported from a cloud-based server into the local EHR system.

Backup System

No matter what type of server is used, the EHR system must have a secure backup plan. This contingency plan is critical in the event of a disaster that destroys the health records.

Web-based or locally installed EHR systems should have a secure backup system. A healthcare facility that has a locally installed EHR system should have its backup plan recorded in the facility's policy and procedure manual. The backup system must provide an exact copy of patient health records. Depending on the backup system—be it on-site, magnetic storage, cloud-based, or off-site—the same security measures must be followed to prevent the unauthorized access or release of patient PHI. Policies and procedures must include controlled access, password protection, and a secure location. A web-based EHR system is stored on a secure server utilizing the highest levels of encryption software.

Mobile Devices

An EHR system may be accessible through a mobile device such as a smartphone or tablet with computer capabilities. Mobile devices allow you to remotely access the EHR system, which will help improve your productivity and quality of patient care. Healthcare providers may choose to use a mobile device because they can bring the device with them when caring for patients. These easy-to-use devices help inform and show patients images such as the location of an injury. However, digital devices in a healthcare facility are not without their challenges; you must ensure that they comply with the security requirements of HIPAA. Integration with the EHR system can be difficult with some devices. Figure 3.47 illustrates the use of an EHR system, drchrono, on an iPad.

Figure 3.47   Drchrono for the iPad

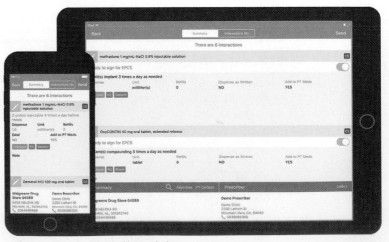

Source: drchrono. Used with permission.

EXPAND YOUR LEARNING

According to a study published in the US National Library of Medicine's online research journal, approximately 50% of healthcare providers use some type of mobile device for clinical decision-making. Review the study at http://EHR2 .ParadigmEducation .com/Smartphones to learn more about the advantages and challenges healthcare providers face while using mobile devices when caring for patients.

Chapter Summary

There are two primary healthcare settings—inpatient and outpatient—and each setting requires its own features within an electronic health record (EHR) system. Rather than learning one specific EHR system, mastering the knowledge behind an EHR system allows you the flexibility of working with a variety of EHR systems that you may encounter in the workplace. ONC-certified EHRs possess similar capabilities and functions as a result of standardized requirements for compliant EHRs.

With that in mind, the EHR Navigator provides you with the hands-on activities to help you master this basic knowledge. Assigning rights and permissions, managing and scheduling patients, reviewing medical documents, charting, reviewing laboratory results, filling e-prescriptions, and sending secure messages are all important features to understand, no matter what EHR system you use. The structure of an EHR system, such as the information processing cycle, is also crucial background knowledge to learn.

Data security and accessibility are important features of an EHR system. EHRs should always have a backup system and a secure server location. Accessing this server via mobile devices is becoming more commonplace as mobile technology becomes more affordable, secure, and adaptable to various EHR systems.

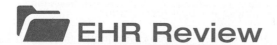 EHR Review

Navigator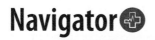

The following EHR Review, EHR Application, and EHR Evaluation activities are also available online in the Navigator+ learning management system. Your instructor may ask you to complete these activities online. Navigator+ also provides access to flash cards, study games, and practice quizzes to help strengthen your understanding of the chapter content.

Acronyms/Initialisms

Study the following acronyms discussed in this chapter. Go to Navigator+ for flash cards of the acronyms and other chapter key terms.

CCHIT: Certification Commission for Health Information Technology

CPOE: computerized physician order entry

EIN: Employer Identification Number

HIPAA: Health Insurance Portability and Accountability Act

HITECH Act: Health Information Technology for Economic and Clinical Health Act

HL7: Health Level Seven International

IT: information technology

LAN: local area network

NPI: National Provider Identifier

PHI: protected health information

PHR: personal health record

WAN: wide area network

Check Your Understanding

To check your understanding of this chapter's key concepts, answer the following questions.

1. Data storage in an electronic health record (EHR) may be handled by all of the following methods *except* a

   a. cloud server.

   b. vendor server.

   c. facility server.

   d. flash drive.

2. The four components of the information processing cycle are

   a. input, print, output, and save.

   b. input, output, print, and storage.

   c. input, processing, output, and storage.

   d. enter, print, save, and storage.

3. Which of the following is the organization that is responsible for certifying EHR vendors?

   a. Certified Commission for Health Information Technology

   b. American Medical Association

   c. Office of the National Coordinator for Health Information Technology

   d. Health Information Technology

4. Meaningful use provides

   a. incentives for a healthcare facility that meets established criteria for an EHR system.

   b. a report to the patient on his or her healthcare information.

   c. a measurement of the functionality of the EHR system.

   d. incentives for patients who use a personal health record.

5. Mobile devices include

   a. iPads.

   b. iPhones.

   c. Androids.

   d. all of the above.

6. True/False: Interoperability allows various healthcare facilities to communicate with each other.

7. True/False: A microphone is a type of input device.

8. True/False: A local area network is a computer connected to the Internet.

9. True/False: All users of an EHR system have the right to access all components of the EHR.

10. True/False: EHR systems may be customized to meet the needs of the facility.

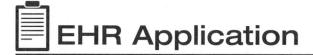 EHR Application

Go on the Record

To build on your understanding of the topics in this chapter, complete the following short-answer activities

1. Discuss the importance of assigning passwords and rights to users of an electronic health record (EHR) system.

2. Explain why it is important to lock an EHR system when not actively working with it.

3. Compare and contrast the advantages and challenges of using mobile devices with an EHR system.

4. Explain the advantage of using the e-prescribing feature of an EHR system.

Navigate the Field

To gain practice in handling challenging situations in the workplace, consider the following real-world scenarios and identify how you would respond to each.

1. You are the health information technology (HIT) training specialist at Northstar Medical Center, and you have been tasked with training new employees on the EHR Navigator. Prepare an outline you will follow for training employees.

2. After completing an overview of the EHR Navigator in this chapter, prepare a list of features that are most important to your job as the HIT training specialist at Northstar Medical Center. Explain why each feature is important and how each will help you complete your job more effectively and efficiently.

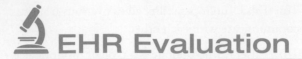

EHR Evaluation

Think Critically

Continue to think critically about challenging concepts and complete the following activities.

1. Tabitha Iris Wang calls to schedule an appointment with Dr. Alana Feltner. List the steps of an EHR system that you must take to schedule this patient.

2. You are the information technology (IT) manager for your healthcare facility. A new employee will begin in the Health Information Management (HIM) department. Prepare a list of the steps you would take to add a new user and assign permissions to this new HIM employee.

Make Your Case

Consider the scenario and then complete the following project.

You are chairing a committee on selecting the EHR system for Cincinnati Grace Medical Center. The committee has decided to select a web-based EHR system because the facility does not have a large IT staff. You are in charge of researching Practice Fusion, a free, web-based EHR system. Create a presentation based on the instructions provided to you by your instructor.

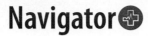

Explore the Technology

Complete the EHR Navigator practice assessments that align to each tutorial and the assessments that accompany Chapter 3 located on Navigator+.

> " Health care is becoming more digitized and consumer oriented. It's not an overnight change, but more like how summer turns into fall—gradual yet very perceptible. "

—Greg Scott, Principal, Deloitte Consulting

Are You Ready?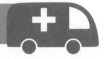

By choosing to pursue a career in health information technology (HIT), you are at the start of something monumental. The number of healthcare jobs is increasing, and it is estimated that 10 of the 20 fastest-growing occupations over the next 10 years will be in health care. Additionally, an estimated 50,000 new jobs will need to be filled to implement electronic health record (EHR) systems.

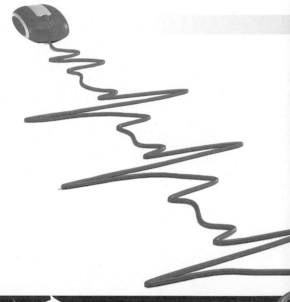

Beyond the Record

- 40% of consumers say information found on social media influences how they deal with healthcare issues.

- 19% of smartphone owners have at least one app on their phones.

- 41% of people say social media would affect their choice of a healthcare provider or facility.

- 26% of hospitals participate in social media.

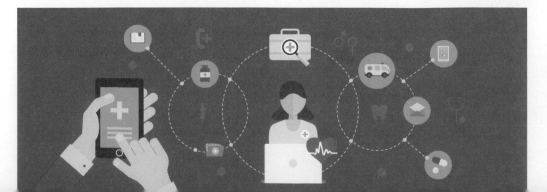

4

Administrative Management

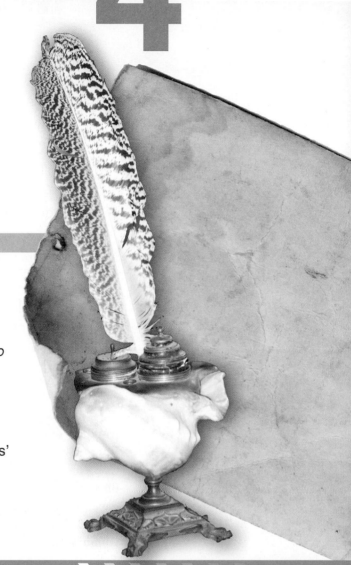

EHR Historical Context

Did you know that the roots of informed consent date back to the Middle Ages? Early medical practitioners would ask their patients to sign a *pro corpore mortuoto* ("hold harmless document"), absolving them of responsibility for any adverse effects from medical procedures or treatments. Ironically, the vast majority of patients at this time could not read or write and, consequently, had to place their trust in their caregivers' verbal communication about their treatment plans and possible complications.

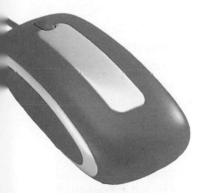

Advance Directives 〉〉〉

National Healthcare Decisions Day is April 16. This annual initiative, which started in 2007, was established to educate adults about the importance of advance care planning and to encourage them to document their wishes for end-of-life care. To find out more about this initiative, visit http://EHR2.ParadigmEducation.com/NHDD. This website provides a wealth of information on advance directives, including a list of sites that individuals can visit to download documents for completion.

4.1 Differentiate between the two main healthcare setting categories, and identify four types of healthcare settings.

4.2 Identify key elements of the patient entry process.

4.3 Identify the purpose, goals, and elements of the master patient index.

4.4 Explain the process for a patient requiring acute care.

4.5 Explain the registration process for a patient requiring ambulatory care.

4.6 Differentiate between a new and established patient.

4.7 Identify the importance of insurance information in the administrative management process.

4.8 Identify the purpose of the documents included in an acute or ambulatory care patient's health record.

Healthcare providers create and maintain an individual health record for every patient. Each health record contains the reason for the visit, the services rendered, diagnoses, and recommended treatments. Regardless of whether a patient is treated in a clinic, hospital, physical therapy facility, or imaging clinic, his or her health records require administrative management. As more healthcare facilities implement electronic health record (EHR) systems, more administrative functions will be electronically performed. This technology will change the daily tasks of healthcare personnel, streamline the workflow of health records, and improve the accuracy of documentation. For example, front desk personnel will input patient appointments into the EHR system rather than enter the data on a physical calendar, thus reducing the chance of error. Staff will directly input patient demographic data into the EHR instead of pulling it from a paper form. Billing specialists will enter insurance data into the system and update the electronic record if the patient's insurance changes, thus ensuring accurate billing. These administrative functions will also allow healthcare providers and other staff members easy access to a patient's medical record, providing them with a complete picture of the patient's health history.

Generally, the initial contact for a patient is the healthcare personnel at the admission or registration desk. This person, called a **registrar**, is often required to collect information before and at the time the patient is seen. Increasingly, healthcare facilities may refer to professionals performing the registration or admission process as *patient access specialists*.

At the initial visit, the patient provides **demographic information** that connects the registrar to the correct record. If no record exists for the patient, the registrar must create a new record and add it to the **master patient index (MPI)**. MPI will be discussed in more detail in Chapter 5.

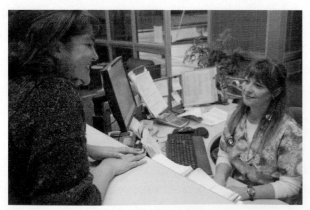

A registrar usually works at the front desk of a healthcare facility.

Depending on the nature of the appointment, patient information may be new or may require updating such information as insurance coverage, contact information, or demographic data. The Health Insurance Portability and Accountability Act (HIPAA) Notice of Privacy Practices for Protected Health Information and the advance directives notice are also given at registration. Copayments or coinsurance for acute care and for outpatient services at a hospital are collected at the time of service. Collecting accurate information from the patient is a critical job requirement for the registrar who completes the admission and registration process for the patient. Accurate data entry is also crucial to ensuring patient safety and preventing communication problems among providers.

Different Types of Healthcare Settings

As discussed in Chapter 2, patient care is divided into two main setting categories: acute care and ambulatory care.

An acute care facility's goal is to care for patients who have short-term illnesses and require an overnight stay in a hospital. Acute care facilities provide round-the-clock diagnostic, surgical, and therapeutic care to patients.

An ambulatory care facility provides care to patients who do not require an overnight stay. Ambulatory care centers have grown within the past 30 years as technology has improved and fewer medical procedures require patients to stay overnight. In addition, health insurance has changed how patients pay for services and procedures, and many policies will not cover extended overnight care in a hospital if it is not medically necessary. There are times when a patient may go to an ambulatory care facility for a procedure and complications occur, requiring the patient to be admitted to an acute care facility. The patient would then be an acute care patient rather than an ambulatory care patient.

Patient care in the acute and ambulatory settings is different. The following sections examine the differences in these two care setting categories and identify additional types of healthcare settings that are differentiated by length of stay or specialty of care.

Patient Care in an Acute Care Setting

Hospital personnel provide acute care to patients who experience sudden health issues or illnesses and cannot be treated in an outpatient care facility. Patients requiring acute care are either admitted to a hospital through the emergency department or sent from an outpatient clinic or a physician.

Acute care can range from a minimum stay of 24 hours to a maximum stay of 30 days, although exceptions to this guideline may occur. For example, if a patient dies before treatment, this patient is still considered as acute care because the physician planned for the patient to be admitted.

The day and time the patient is admitted to the acute care facility is the **admission date**. The admission registrar is the initial contact with the

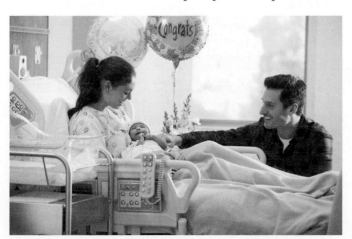

A hospital is an acute care facility.

patient, which is, in part, why this interaction is increasingly referred to as patient access. In the acute care setting, the patient will receive room, board, and care from the hospital. The day and time the patient leaves the facility are considered the **discharge date**. A patient is admitted to the hospital by the physician, who must document the admission order in the patient record. The physician must also document a discharge order to officially discharge the patient from the hospital.

Patient Care in an Ambulatory Care Setting

Ambulatory care includes services provided to the patient that do not require hospitalization or institutionalization. In most cases, the patient is discharged from the ambulatory care center in less than 24 hours. However, there are some exceptions to this rule, such as a patient who is placed on observation status.

Ambulatory care settings are numerous and include (but are not limited to):

- Birthing centers
- Cancer treatment centers
- Clinics
- Correctional facilities
- Dentist offices
- Dialysis clinics

- Emergency departments
- Home care
- Physician offices
- Surgery centers
- Therapeutic services
- Urgent care centers

Patient Data Management in Acute and Ambulatory Care Settings

Although gathering patient data is similar within an acute care or ambulatory care setting, there are some differences. Table 4.1 compares the types of patient data managed in the the two healthcare delivery settings.

Table 4.1   Patient Data Managed in Acute and Ambulatory Care Settings

Data Category	Acute Care	Ambulatory Care
Patient Contact	Admit a patient	Schedule an appointment
Health Record Content	History and physical exam, diagnostic records, treatment records, and discharge summary	SOAP, progress, or chart note
Patient Care	Admission	Visit
Length of Stay	More than 24 hours	Length of appointment, or less than 24 hours
List of Patients	Master patient index (MPI)	Patient list
Completion of Patient Care	Discharge	Check out
SOAP = subjective, objective, assessment, plan		

Other Healthcare Settings

Other types of healthcare settings are identified either by length of stay or by specialty of care:

- A **long-term care facility** typically has patients who reside more than 30 days.

- A **behavioral health setting** provides care to patients with psychiatric diagnoses. The facility may offer a combination of acute care and ambulatory care for patients.

- A **rehabilitation facility** may also offer acute care and ambulatory care, typically serving patients recovering from accidents, injuries, or surgeries.

- **Hospice care** is palliative, or short-term, care provided to terminally ill patients within acute care or home care settings. The purpose of hospice care is to make patients comfortable until death and to support their families during this difficult time.

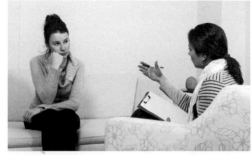
Behavioral health therapists may provide both acute care and ambulatory care.

CHECKPOINT 4.1

1. Name four types of healthcare settings.

   a. _____

   b. _____

   c. _____

   d. _____

2. When may a patient transition from an ambulatory care to an acute care setting?

   _____

   _____

   _____

Patient Entry into the Healthcare System

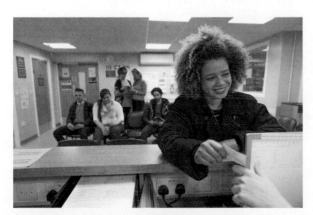
A patient provides insurance and copayments when checking in for an appointment.

Patients enter healthcare facilities for a number of reasons. For example, patients might be urgently admitted to a hospital via the emergency room, a nursing home, or an emergency from home. A patient may also be admitted electively for the delivery of a child or other medical or surgical treatment requiring an overnight stay in the hospital.

Patients might also be treated at a hospital as an outpatient. Outpatients treated at an acute care hospital might be treated in the emergency room and released to their homes without the need to be admitted to the hospital. Patients may also be treated as outpatients when they are seen in a clinic setting or testing area. Many hospitals also have outpatient surgical centers where patients have minor surgery and are sent home without the need to spend the night.

Patients may be treated in a variety of outpatient settings, including a physician's office, drug or alcohol treatment center, psychologist's office, or dialysis facility.

One thing that all of these patients have in common is that they need to be admitted or registered in the EHR prior to care and treatment. The next section will discuss admission and registration processes.

Admission and Registration

The admission or registration begins when the patient or healthcare provider contacts the acute care or ambulatory care facility to make an appointment or schedule an admission in person or by telephone, email, or secure patient portal. Some ambulatory care facilities provide an opportunity for patients to register by using a self-service kiosk, which is a computer station located in the patient waiting area that connects newly entered patient information to the registration system. If the healthcare facility uses a combination of electronic and paper forms for registration, a patient may download forms from a healthcare facility website, or the forms may be provided by mail, email, or in person when the patient arrives. Registration clerks might also telephone the patient to collect information over the phone. All of these methods of data collection help streamline the registration process and reduce the amount of face-to-face time needed upon arrival of the patient to the inpatient admission or outpatient appointment. In addition to demographic information, the data collected also includes payer information. This information is used to determine patient benefits and any required approvals from the third-party payer. Figure 4.1 shows a sample of a patient registration form.

Check-In Process

When the patient arrives at a healthcare facility, a staff member must verify the patient's identity by copying or scanning the patient's insurance card and checking a driver's license or other proof of identification. Verification of identify is necessary to ensure proper rendering of patient care and to lessen the opportunities for insurance fraud.

Following the proof of identification, a copy of the patient's insurance is scanned into the EHR, and consents for treatment, billing, notice of privacy practices acknowledgement, and release of patient information for billing and continuity of care are signed. The patient's insurance is verified, and the copayment is collected from the patient.

Tutorial 4.1   EHRNAVIGAT⊕R

Checking in a Patient

Go to Navigator+ to launch Tutorial 4.1. As an admission clerk, practice checking in a patient using the EHR Navigator. After completing the tutorial, apply your skills with the Checking in a Patient practice assessments.

EXPAND
YOUR LEARNING

The healthcare community is still debating the need to implement a unique patient identification system. To learn more on this controversy, visit:

http://EHR2.Paradigm Education.com/ PatientID.

Master Patient Index

Most acute care facilities that use an EHR system call their list of patients a **master patient index (MPI)** or a patient list. The MPI is a database created by a healthcare organization to assign a unique medical record number to each patient served, thus allowing easy retrieval and maintenance of patient information.

Figure 4.1 Patient Registration Form

For Office Use Only:

MRUN: _____

Registrar: _____

Northstar Physicians

Northstar Physicians

Patient Registration Form

PATIENT INFORMATION

Patient's Last Name		First	Middle Initial	Type of Care: ☐ Inpatient ☐ Same-Day Surgery ☐ Maternity ☐ Surgery ☐ Outpatient

Race	Marital Status	Religion	Primary Language	Date of Birth (mm/dd/yyyy)	Date of Scheduled Visit

Physician's Last Name   First Name   ☐ Female ☐ Male   Social Security No.

Patient's Street Address   Apt. No.   City   State   ZIP

Home Phone ( )   Work Phone ( )   Cell Phone ( )   Visit Reason or Diagnosis   Admission Date

Temporary Address   Apt. No.   City   State   ZIP

Patient's Current Employer Name   Employer Address   City   State   ZIP

Employer Phone ( )   Patient's Occupation   Employment Status: ☐ Not Employed ☐ Full Time ☐ Part Time ☐ Student ☐ Retired and Date:

Full Name of Emergency Contact   Relationship   Home Phone ( )   Work Phone ( )

Have you ever been a patient at EMC Medical Center? ☐ Yes ☐ No   If yes, when was your last visit?   Under what name?

Guarantor

Last Name   First   Middle Initial   Relationship   Date of Birth (mm/dd/yyyy)

Street Address   Apt. No.   ☐ Female ☐ Male   Marital Status   Social Security No.

City   State   ZIP   Home Phone ( )   Work Phone ( )   Cell Phone ( )

Employer Name   Employer Address   City   State   ZIP

Employer Phone ( )   Occupation   Employment Status: ☐ Not Employed ☐ Full Time ☐ Part Time ☐ Student ☐ Retired and Date:

Insurance Information

Primary Insurance Name   Name of Insured (exactly as it appears on card)

Insurance Billing Address   City   State   ZIP   Phone No. ( )

Policy No.   Group No.   Plan Code   State   Effective Date   Expiration Date

Subscriber's Full Name   Subscriber's Soc. Sec. No.   Subscriber's Date of Birth (mm/dd/yyyy)   ☐ Female ☐ Male

Subscriber's Employer Name (if self-employed, company name)   Relation to Insured   Subscriber's Employment Status: ☐ Not Employed ☐ Full Time ☐ Part Time ☐ Student ☐ Retired and Date:

Subscriber's Employer Address   City   State   ZIP   Phone No. ( )

Effective Date (mm/dd/yyyy) _____ ☐ Part A (Hospital Benefit) ☐ Part B (Medical Benefit)

Effective Date   State

Name of Insured (exactly as it appears on card)

State   ZIP   Phone No. ( )

State   Effective Date   Expiration Date

Subscriber's Date of Birth (mm/dd/yyyy)   ☐ Female ☐ Male

Subscriber's Employment Status: ☐ Not Employed ☐ Full Time ☐ Part Time ☐ Student ☐ Retired and Date:

State   ZIP   Phone No. ( )

Date of Accident: (mm/dd/yyyy)   Claim No.

Phone No. ( )   Insurance Name

State   ZIP   Phone No. ( )

Advance Directive

Do you have an Advance Directive, such as a Living Will or Durable Power of Attorney for Health Care? ☐ Yes ☐ No

Please specify the type: _____

*** If yes, please bring a copy at the time of your admission. ***

Self-Pay

* If insured but your procedure is not covered or verified by your plan, a deposit is required at the time of admission.

* If you do not have insurance, please call our *EMC Financial Services at (513)-555-1122* before your scheduled arrival date to discuss financial terms.

Additional Information

Do you need special accommodations, such as translation, visual aid, etc.? ☐ Yes ☐ No

*** If yes, please specify so that prior arrangements can be made for the day of your visit. ***

☐ Language Interpreter _____   ☐ Sign Language Interpreter   ☐ Visual Aid   ☐ Other: _____

Patient Identifiers

Typically, the EHR system automatically generates and assigns a unique patient or medical record number, also known as the **patient identification number**. Figure 4.2 illustrates the dialog box used to generate the patient's medical record number in the EHR Navigator.

HIPAA proposes the implementation of a unique patient identification system. In this system, a patient identifier is generated that has a purpose similar to a Social Security number. The patient identifier consists of a set of numeric or alpha characters that seamlessly connects a person to his or her healthcare information.

It is crucial that healthcare providers use the MPI to verify that a patient has only one patient identifier (i.e., medical record number). If a patient has multiple identifiers, then providers may not see the true picture of a patient's health status because important healthcare information may be misplaced, lost, or duplicated.

Figure 4.2   Generating a Patient Number

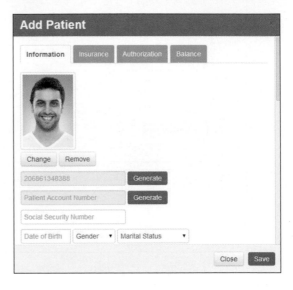

Purpose and Goals of the Master Patient Index

The EHR system stores the MPI permanently (see Figure 4.3). The following are goals of the MPI:

- Match the patient with his or her MPI record
- Minimize duplication
- Merge and enterprise the MPI
- Retain lifelong health records

An efficient and effective MPI system makes it possible to meet these goals.

The MPI contains the patient medical record number, with each information field containing data about a patient. These data fields produce a unique record. Healthcare providers use the MPI to determine whether a patient record exists in the EHR system. If such a record exists, that same patient identifier is used each time a healthcare provider or facility sees the patient. In doing so, the patient identifier can be used to track all of the patient's encounters at the healthcare facility.

Figure 4.3 Master Patient Index

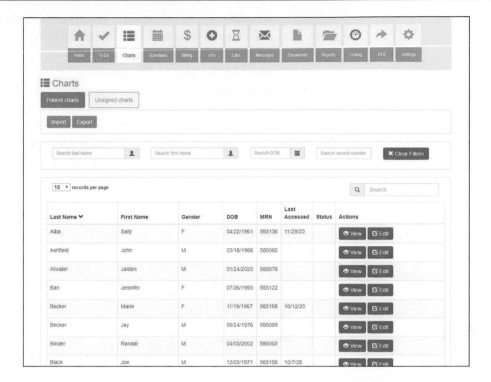

Core Data Elements

The American Health Information Management Association (AHIMA) recommends searching for a patient based on **core data elements** for indexing. In an MPI, the core data elements of a patient record include the following:

- Medical record number
- Name
- Date of birth
- Sex
- Race
- Ethnicity
- Address

- Previous name
- Social Security number
- Facility identifier
- Account number
- Admission date
- Discharge date
- Service type

Optional Data Elements

AHIMA has identified the following **optional data elements** for the MPI:

- Marital status
- Telephone number
- Mother's maiden name
- Place of birth
- Advance directive decision-making

- Organ donor status
- Emergency contact
- Allergies
- Problem list

Enterprise Master Patient Index

As health care continues to incorporate acute care and ambulatory care practices, there is a need to maintain patient identifier information across an EHR system for all healthcare settings. This systemwide database is called the **enterprise master patient index (EMPI)**. The EMPI allows the healthcare organization to compile the patient's information into one index using registration, scheduling, financial, and clinical information.

Two key data elements differentiate the MPI from the EMPI: the **enterprise identification number (EIN)** and the **facility identifier**. The EIN in the EMPI is an identifier used by the organization to identify the patient across the various healthcare settings, whereas the facility identifier is used to indicate the healthcare setting where the patient is seeking care. Healthcare providers have created a system in the EHRs that automates the data elements in the patient record. Recommended EMPI data elements include the following:

- EIN
- Facility identifier
- Internal patient identification
- Patient name
- Date of birth
- Sex

- Race
- Ethnicity
- Address
- Social Security number
- Telephone number

Tutorial 4.2   EHRNAVIGAT⊕R

Searching for a Patient's Chart

Go to Navigator+ to launch Tutorial 4.2. As an admission clerk, practice the various ways to search for a patient using the EHR Navigator.

Patient Registration and Admission

The patient registration and admission processes may be slightly different for acute care and ambulatory care settings, but personnel in both settings focus on collecting accurate patient information.

Acute Care Registration

As mentioned earlier, the registrar is typically the first person the patient approaches upon arrival at the care facility. The registrar collects demographic and administrative information from the patient. If the patient is already in the EHR system, then the registrar will verify the accuracy of that information. Although similar to the registration process for ambulatory care, acute care personnel must follow the **Uniform Hospital Discharge Data Set (UHDDS)** for inpatient care. Developed by a committee in 1969, the UHDDS outlined a set of patient-specific data elements. This protocol, revised by the National Committee on Vital and Health Statistics

(NCVHS) in 1984, was adopted by federal health programs in 1986. Since then, the UHDDS has been revised several times.

The recommended **UHDDS core data elements** include the following:

- Patient identifier
- Date of birth
- Sex
- Ethnicity
- Address
- Healthcare setting identification
- Admission date
- Type of admission
- Discharge date
- Attending physician identification

- Surgeon identification
- Principal diagnosis
- Other diagnoses
- Qualifier for other diagnoses
- External cause of injury code
- Birth weight of neonate
- Significant procedures and dates
- Disposition of patient
- Expected source of payment
- Total charges

Ambulatory Care Registration

In an outpatient or a physician office setting, the front office staff usually handles the registration process. The information gathered in the outpatient setting should follow the **Uniform Ambulatory Care Data Set (UACDS)** for outpatient services. The primary purpose of using this data set is to ensure that all healthcare settings and providers are gathering identical types of information on each patient and that the data collected is defined consistently across all healthcare settings.

The NCVHS approved this data set in 1989. The UACDS is used in surgery centers, physician offices, outpatient clinics, and emergency departments. The UACDS is not required but highly recommended.

Some of the recommended UACDS data elements include:

- Patient identification
- Address
- Date of birth
- Sex
- Ethnicity
- Provider identification
- Provider address
- Provider specialty
- Place of encounter
- Reason for encounter
- Diagnostic services
- Problem, diagnosis, and assessment
- Therapeutic services

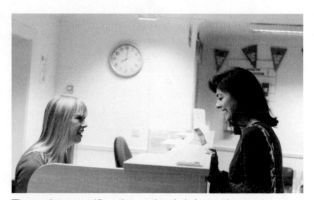
The registrar verifies the patient's information.

- Preventive services
- Disposition
- Source of payment
- Total charges

New versus Established Patients

After identifying the patient, you must determine if he or she is an established patient or a new patient. To make this determination, it is important to understand the differences between these types of patients.

New Patient

For the purposes of admission and registration, a **new patient** is defined as a patient who has not received any services from a provider or a provider in the group in the same specialty and subspecialty within the past three years. For instance, if the patient was seen two years and eleven months ago, then he or she is considered an established patient; however, if the patient was seen three years and one day ago, then he or she is considered a new patient.

To add a new patient to the system, the registrar must collect administrative information, including demographics used to identify the patient, report statistics, conduct research, and allocate resources. The demographic information gathered includes the following:

- First, middle, and last names
- Medical record number (if known by the patient)
- Address
- Telephone numbers: home, work, and cell
- Sex
- Date of birth
- Place of birth

- Marital status
- Ethnicity
- Social Security number
- Emergency contact
- Date of service
- Physician
- Dentist

Consider This

When a patient arrives at an emergency department (ED), he or she is neither a new patient nor an established patient. The patient may have a record in the EHR system, but patients in the ED are not identified as being new or established. The terms *new* and *established* are primarily used for patients in an ambulatory care setting. Patients may have been to the ED for previous visits, but they would not be classified as *established*.

How would you handle a situation in which a patient states that he has been to Shoreview Emergency Department before and, consequently, should not have to provide his information again?

Tutorial 4.3

EHRNAVIGATOR

Adding a New Patient

Go to Navigator+ to launch Tutorial 4.3. As an admission clerk, practice preadmitting a patient using the EHR Navigator.

Established Patient

An **established patient** has received professional services from a healthcare provider or a provider in the same group and same specialty and subspecialty within the past three years.

The process begins by searching for the patient to determine whether the patient record is entered in the EHR Navigator. There are multiple ways to search for a patient using a variety of criteria, such as the following:

- The patient's full or partial name in the *Last Name* and *First Name* fields

- The patient's medical record or patient number in the *Patient Record* field

- The patient's date of birth in the *Date of Birth (DOB)* field

Healthcare staff members can also use a combination of these criteria to find an established patient.

When searching for an established patient, search by different core data elements, such as patient name, patient record number, DOB, Social Security number, or admission date, to ensure the patient record exists in the EHR system.

Figure 4.4 shows the Find Patient dialog box. Use this dialog box to determine if the patient is registered in the EHR Navigator.

If the patient is registered in the EHR system, the existing information needs to be confirmed with the patient. If the patient needs to edit or update any demographic information, select the patient record and click the Edit Patient button to display the Edit Patient dialog box, as shown in Figure 4.5, and then update any patient demographic information required. To edit patient information, select the field and key in the appropriate data.

Figure 4.4 Dialog Box to Search for a Patient

Figure 4.5 Dialog Box to Update Patient Demographic Information

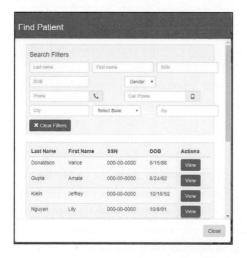

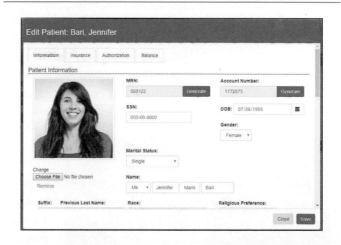

Tutorial 4.4

EHRNAVIGAT⊕R

Editing a Record for an Established Patient

Go to Navigator+ to launch Tutorial 4.4. As a front desk clerk, practice updating a record for an existing patient using the EHR Navigator.

Figure 4.6 Insurance Card

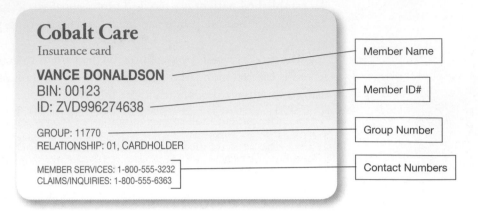

Insurance Information

Insurance information includes details about the patient's insurance coverage, such as the insurance company, copay, and identification numbers, to assist with processing claims. Some patients may not have insurance or may not wish to use insurance and are considered cash payers. Figure 4.6 is an example of a typical insurance card a patient may provide to the healthcare facility. The insurance card contains the member name, member identification number, group number, and contact numbers for member services and claims and inquiries. A staff member will scan the insurance card and enter the scanned image and insurance coverage information into the EHR system.

Insurance Subscriber and Guarantor

Two other key components of health insurance coverage are the subscriber and the guarantor. The **subscriber** is the person whose insurance coverage is used for acute or ambulatory care. The **guarantor** is the person or financial entity that guarantees payment on any unpaid balances on the account. Further explanation of health insurance is covered in Chapter 9.

When entering the patient's insurance and financial information into the EHR, you must also enter the patient's guarantor and guarantor account information. Subsequently, if an acute or ambulatory healthcare facility sends a bill for a balance of a service or services not covered by insurance, the bill will go to the patient's guarantor.

A guarantor is the person or financial entity financially responsible for the patient. The guarantor may be the patient, another person, or a financial entity. Most patients older than 18 years are their own guarantors. Minors usually have their parents or legal guardians as their guarantors. Any patient with decreased mental capacity typically has a guarantor.

Every patient must have at least one guarantor account prior to being admitted or checked in to a healthcare facility. The **guarantor account** is a record that saves the information about the guarantor, including the guarantor's name and address.

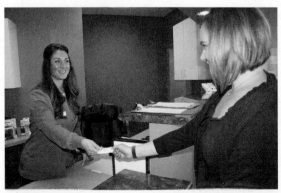

A patient provides insurance and copayments when he or she checks in for an appointment.

There are several types of guarantor accounts, as shown in Table 4.2.

Table 4.2   Guarantor Types

Type	Description
Personal/Family	For general healthcare services, the guarantor is typically the subscriber of the primary insurance.
Workers' Compensation	The employer's workers' compensation insurance carrier is billed, and then if there are remaining charges, or injuries are deemed not work-related, the patient is responsible for the charges.
Third-Party Liability	A third party, such as an insurance company, is responsible for payment.
Corporate	A company requires the patient to receive services from a healthcare facility or provider.
Research	The patient is involved in research or is a provider at the healthcare facility.

Tutorial 4.5   **EHR**NAVIGAT✚R

Adding Insurance

Go to Navigator+ to launch Tutorial 4.5. As a biller, practice adding insurance information using the EHR Navigator.

Updating Insurance Information in the EHR

If a patient's current health insurance information is missing or does not match what is in the EHR, then the EHR will need to be updated, which is done by finding the patient's EHR and selecting the Insurance menu option on the left panel. You can make changes to existing coverage or add new coverage. If changing existing coverage, it is important to enter the end date of the old insurance coverage to ensure that claims are submitted to the correct insurance provider.

The patient's current and previous health insurance coverages will appear on the Insurance tab of the Edit Patient dialog box, as shown in Figure 4.7.

In most cases, a patient may be scheduled for appointments and receive care only after the EHR is updated with current patient insurance information.

Figure 4.7   Dialog Box to Review Patient's Insurance Information

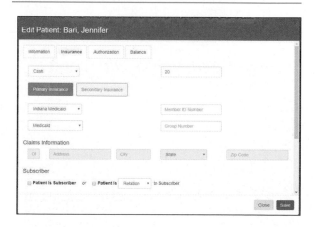

Coverage of Treatment

How insurance covers a patient's healthcare costs is based on the primary reason for the visit and a list of established insurance rules.

- If a patient is injured, the healthcare setting must determine how the injury occurred. If there was an accident, primary coverage may be provided by the company, property insurance, or accident insurance.

- If a service at an acute care or ambulatory care setting is not accident-related, and each adult on the policy has his or her own insurance, then the patient's own insurance is primary.

- If a child is seen at an acute care or ambulatory care setting, and there are two insurance plans that cover the child, then the **birthday rule** is applied. The birthday rule specifies that the insurance of the parent whose birthday falls first in a calendar year will be the primary insurance. The ages of the separate cardholders have no bearing on this rule.

- If a patient has Medicare coverage and the services meet Medicare coverage guidelines, primary coverage is provided by Medicare.

- If a patient older than 65 years is being seen for something other than an injury, has two insurances (Medicare and a supplemental plan), is unemployed, and is not covered by a spouse's insurance, the primary insurance would be Medicare and the supplemental plan would be the secondary insurance. Typically, a supplemental plan pays the deductible, copay, and any other charges not paid by Medicare.

- If a patient has Medicaid and a private insurance plan, the private insurance would be primary and Medicaid would be secondary.

For patients with insurance coverage through more than one provider, the primary coverage is determined by industry rules adopted by state insurance commissioners. The patient or the insured is responsible for informing the healthcare facility whether he or she has more than one insurance coverage.

CHECKPOINT 4.2

1. Name the five different types of guarantors.

a. _____

b. _____

c. _____

d. _____

e. _____

2. Explain the birthday rule. Why is it important?

_____

_____

_____

Adding Documents to a Patient Record

The EHR system gives you the ability to add scanned or uploaded documents to the patient's chart. The types of documents depend on the type of facility but may include privacy notices, financial agreements, consent forms, and advance directives.

Privacy Notices

An ambulatory care facility may scan or upload a Notice of Privacy Practices for Protected Health Information, which is a rule based on a US Department of Health and Human Services (HHS) rule that informs patients about the use and disclosure of information by the healthcare facility. The document informs patients of their rights and responsibilities and provides contact information for any questions they may have.

The patient or the patient's representative must review and approve the Notice of Privacy Practices (NPP). An example of an NPP is shown in Figure 4.8. Each patient must receive a copy of the NPP at his or her first contact with the healthcare organization—for example, the first visit to a physician's office or first admission to a hospital.

Figure 4.8 Notice of Privacy Practices

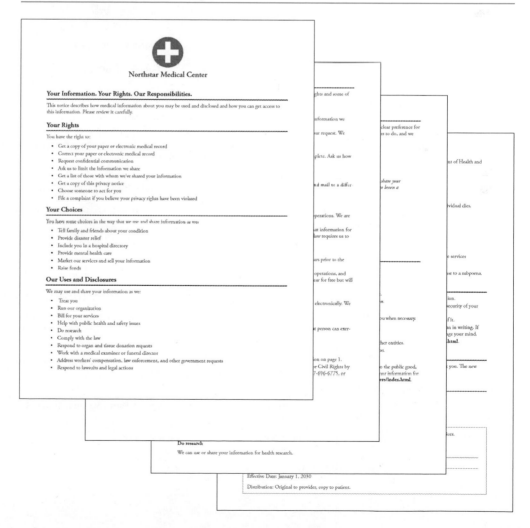

Either the patient or the patient's legal representative must sign the NPP. Some facilities use electronic patient signatures for these documents, while other facilities use paper copies, which need to be scanned after they are signed. A digital copy of the signed document must be saved in the patient's EHR.

Financial Agreements

An example of a financial agreement that may be attached to a patient's EHR is the Assignment of Benefits form. The **Assignment of Benefits** form is an authorization by the patient to allow his or her health insurance or third-party provider to reimburse the healthcare provider or facility directly. A sample financial agreement is shown in Figure 4.9. If a healthcare facility requires patients to have a financial agreement on file, a staff member may ask for the patient's signature and then upload the signed document into the patient's EHR.

Figure 4.9 Assignment of Benefits

Northstar Physicians

Assignment of Benefits

In consideration of the patient receiving services from Northstar Physicians, I agree that:

- I am responsible for all expenses for treating the patient.
- Payment of charges is due at the time of the appointment.
- If Northstar Physicians files my insurance for me, I agree to pay for noncovered insurance benefits, coinsurance, copays, and deductibles.

Patient Signature	Responsible Party's Signature (Parent/Guardian of Minor)
Printed Name	Printed Name
Date	Date

AUTHORIZATION TO RELEASE INFORMATION AND TO PAY BENEFITS

I authorize Northstar Physicians to release any of my medical information, including drug, alcohol, and HIV-positive test results, to my insurance company(s) as needed to process my insurance claim.

I authorize my insurance company to make payments directly to Northstar Physicians for covered medical and/or surgical services.

Patient's Signature	Responsible Party's Signature (Parent/Guardian of Minor)
Printed Name	Printed Name
Date	Date

Consent Forms

A **general consent for treatment** form is used in acute care facilities. The patient or the patient's legal representative signs the general consent for treatment, giving the healthcare provider the right to treat him or her. The provider may require an informed consent form if the patient is having a specialty procedure. A sample consent form is provided in Figure 4.10. This consent may also request permission to bill the patient and/or the patient's insurance for services rendered.

Figure 4.10 Consent Form

Northstar Medical Center

Informed Consent for Invasive, Diagnostic, Medical, and Surgical Procedures

Patient's Name_____

Date of Birth_____

Medical Record #_____

I hereby authorize _____ and/or _____ and/or such assistants and associates as may be select-ed by him/her/they to perform the following procedure(s)/treatment(s) upon myself/the patient.

Procedure(s)/Treatment(s) _____

The procedure has been explained to me, and I have been told the reasons why I need the procedure. The risks of the procedure have also been explained to me. In addition, I have been told that the procedure may not have the results that I expect. I have also been told about other possible treatments for my condition and what might happen if no treatment is received.

I understand that, in addition to the risks described to me about this procedure, there are risks that may occur with any surgical or medical procedure. I am aware that the practice of medicine and surgery is not an exact science and that I have not been given any guarantees about the results of this procedure.

I have had enough time to discuss my condition and treatment with my healthcare providers, and all of my questions have been answered to my satisfaction. I believe I have enough information to make an informed decision, and I agree to have the procedure performed. If something unexpected happens and I require additional or different treatment(s) from the treatment I expect, I agree to accept any treatment necessary.

I agree to have transfusion of blood and other blood products that may be necessary in addition to the procedure I am having. The risks, benefits, and alternatives have been explained to me, and all of my questions have been answered to my satisfaction. If I refuse to have transfusions, I will cross out and initial this section and sign a Refusal of Treatment form.

I agree to allow this facility to keep, use, or properly dispose of tissue and parts of organs removed during this procedure.

_____   _____
Signature of Patient or Parent/Legal Guardian of Minor Patient   Date

If the patient cannot consent for himself or herself, the signature of either the healthcare agent or legal guardian acting on behalf of the patient, or the patient's next of kin who is asserting to the treatment for the patient, must be obtained.

_____   _____
Signature of Patient or Parent/Legal Guardian of Minor Patient   Date

_____   _____
Signature and Relationship of Next of Kin   Date

Witness:

I, _____, am a facility employee who is not the patient's physician or authorized healthcare provider named above, and I have witnessed the patient or other appropriate person voluntarily sign this form.

_____
Signature and Title of Witness

Interpreter/Translator (to be signed by the interpreter/translator if the patient required such assistance)

To the best of my knowledge, the patient understood what was interpreted/translated and voluntarily signed this form.

_____
Signature of Interpreter/Translator

Advance Directives

An **advance directive** is a document that provides information about how the patient would like to be treated if he or she is no longer able to make his or her own medical decisions. There are several types of advance directives. Figure 4.11 provides a sample of one type of document that may be attached to a patient's chart in the EHR system.

Figure 4.11   Advance Directive

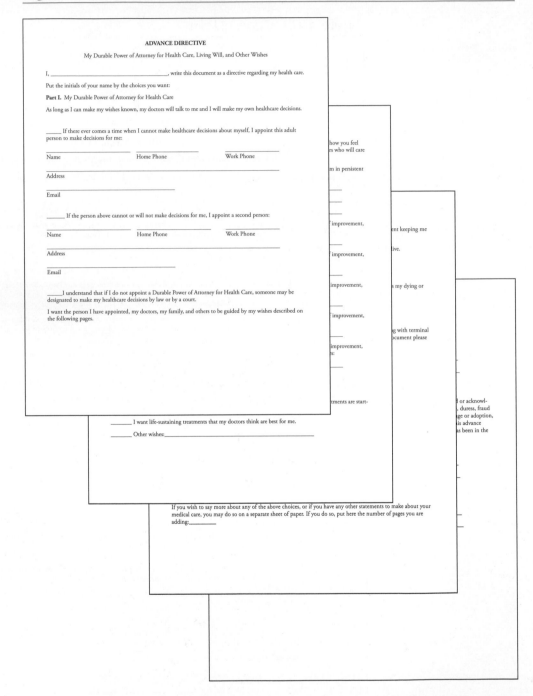

Figure 4.12 shows the documents that have been uploaded in the EHR system.

Figure 4.12 Patient Documents in the EHR Navigator

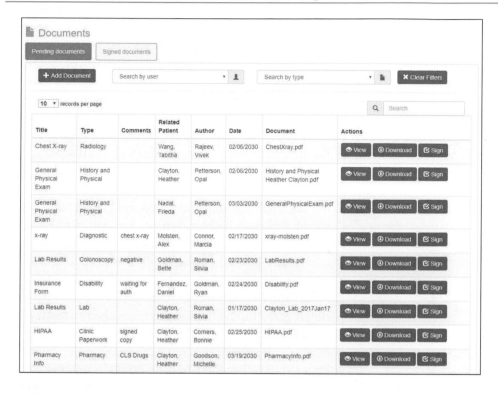

Tutorial 4.6

EHRNAVIGAT✛R

Attaching Documents to a Patient's Chart

Go to Navigator+ to launch Tutorial 4.6. As an admission clerk, practice attaching documents to a patient's chart using the EHR Navigator.

Consider This

The Documents feature of an EHR system offers many benefits for healthcare personnel. For providers, this feature allows them to scan or upload documents, such as test results or handwritten notes, and attach them to a patient's chart. This feature also allows providers to sign the notes. For all healthcare staff members, the Documents feature allows them access to view the documents and helps prevent misplaced or misfiled paperwork. In short, the ability to attach documents in an EHR system increases efficiency, productivity, and quality of patient care. With all these benefits, do you think there are still opportunities for documentation errors? What types of errors may occur?

Patients seek health care at acute care and ambulatory care facilities. Acute care services are provided by hospitals, long-term care facilities, inpatient behavioral units, inpatient rehabilitation units, and hospice care facilities. Ambulatory care services are delivered by clinics, group practices, home care, dentist offices, and many other types of facilities. In fact, ambulatory care facilities represent a growing segment of health care as more procedures and services are completed on an outpatient basis.

Depending on the type of care facility, patient visits are managed differently. An important factor of the patient visit in an acute care facility is the master patient index (MPI), which keeps track of the patient encounters and services at the facility. The design of the MPI is based on the core data elements proposed by the National Committee on Vital and Health Statistics (NCVHS). The American Health Information Management Association (AHIMA) recommends using the core data elements when searching the database. The data collected by an acute care facility is based on the Uniform Hospital Discharge Data Set (UHDDS), whereas the data collected by an ambulatory care facility is based on the Uniform Ambulatory Care Data Set (UACDS). Care for a patient in the ambulatory setting is based on the "new versus established" patient rule.

No matter the healthcare setting or whether the patient is new or established, healthcare staff members must collect insurance information. They also are required to gather and complete many documents during the patient's initial visit, including the Notice of Privacy Practices, Assignment of Benefits, Consents, and Advance Directives. In an EHR system, these documents may be electronically signed and attached to the patient's record.

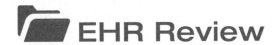

EHR Review

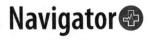 **Navigator**

The following EHR Review, EHR Application, and EHR Evaluation activities are also available online in the Navigator+ learning management system. Your instructor may ask you to complete these activities online. Navigator+ also provides access to flash cards, study games, and practice quizzes to help strengthen your understanding of the chapter content.

Acronyms/Initialisms

Study the following acronyms discussed in this chapter. Go to Navigator+ for flash cards of the acronyms and other chapter key terms.

AHIMA: American Health Information Management Association

EIN: enterprise identification number

EMPI: enterprise master patient index

HIPAA: Health Insurance Portability and Accountability Act of 1996

MPI: master patient index

NCVHS: National Committee on Vital and Health Statistics

UACDS: Uniform Ambulatory Care Data Set

UHDDS: Uniform Hospital Discharge Data Set

UPI: universal patient identifier

Check Your Understanding

To check your understanding of this chapter's key concepts, answer the following questions.

1. Demographic information includes

   a. date of birth.

   b. laboratory results.

   c. diagnostic history.

   d. immunizations.

2. The master patient index is a/an

   a. spreadsheet of patient invoices.

   b. database of patients seen at the healthcare facility.

   c. index of patient telephone numbers.

   d. index of patient insurance coverage.

3. AHIMA recommends using which core data element when searching for a patient record in an EHR?

   a. Marital status

   b. Mother's maiden name

   c. Telephone number

   d. Patient identification number

4. The Uniform Hospital Discharge Data Set includes all of the following *except*

   a. date of birth.

   b. sex.

   c. reason for encounter.

   d. admission date.

5. If a child is covered by two insurance plans, the primary coverage is the insurance of the

   a. parent who is older.

   b. parent who is younger.

   c. parent whose birth date occurs first in a calendar year.

   d. parent who has the best coverage.

6. True/False: Long-term care facilities have patients who reside more than 30 days.

7. True/False: There is only one type of ambulatory care facility.

8. True/False: Workers' Compensation is a type of guarantor account.

9. True/False: Most EHR systems allow documents to be uploaded to a patient's chart.

10. True/False: EHR systems do not have the capability for a healthcare provider to electronically sign documents.

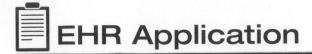

EHR Application

Go on the Record

To build on your understanding of the topics in this chapter, complete the following short-answer activities.

1. Compare the registration processes in acute care versus ambulatory care settings.

2. Describe the different types of ambulatory care settings.

3. Explain the differences between the Uniform Hospital Discharge Data Set (UHDDS) and the Uniform Ambulatory Care Data Set (UACDS).

4. Review the image of Vance Donaldson's Cobalt Care insurance card. Identify the different parts of the insurance card.

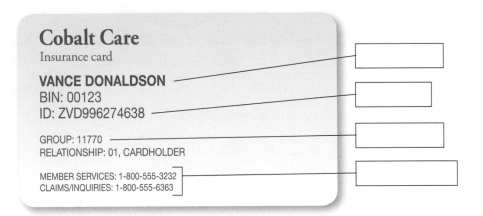

5. Discuss how a patient is identified as either a new patient or an established patient.

Navigate the Field

To gain practice in handling challenging situations in the workplace, consider the following real-world scenarios and identify how you would respond to each.

1. You are part of the team from Lincoln County Hospital working with the EHR Savvy company on the design of the master patient index (MPI). What elements are required for the MPI? Create a table with the elements that must be included in the MPI.

2. You are the EHR training specialist with Lincoln County Hospital. You are meeting with the registration staff to review the appropriate procedures for searching for patients. What steps should those procedures contain? Create a checklist for the registrars to follow when determining whether a patient is new or established.

 # EHR Evaluation

Think Critically

Continue to think critically about challenging concepts and complete the following activities.

1. A new patient calls the admissions desk at Northstar Medical Center to preregister for a surgery. Prepare a list of steps that you would take to add the new patient to the EHR system.

2. Identify common errors made in the registration process. How could these errors be avoided or minimized? What is the impact of these errors on patient care?

Make Your Case

Consider the scenario and then complete the following project.

You are a member of the Medical Records Department at Lincoln County Hospital. You are training the registration staff on the admission process. Prepare a presentation for your class that provides detailed guidelines to follow when collecting patient information.

Explore the Technology

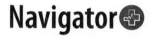

Complete the EHR Navigator practice assessments that align to each tutorial and the assessments that accompany Chapter 4 located on Navigator+.

Are You Ready?

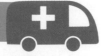

Not sure where to begin your career in health information management (HIM)? Volunteering and job shadowing are worthwhile ways to learn about different HIM disciplines. Choose a hospital, physician's office, or other type of facility where you might like to work to get a good idea of the profession's day-to-day responsibilities and gain insight into the type of atmosphere that will be a good fit for your personality and skill set. Plus, you will be able to add valuable experience to your résumé!

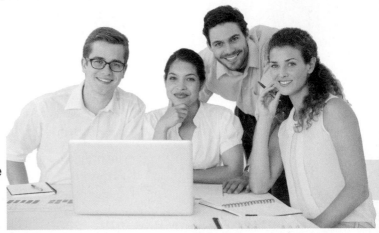

Beyond the Record

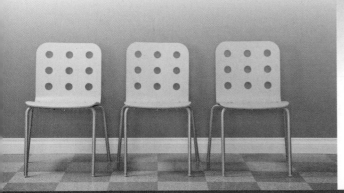

- The average wait time in a doctor's office is 19 minutes and 19 seconds.

- The average wait time in an emergency department is 30 minutes, and the treatment wait time is 90 minutes.

- Electronic health records can reduce wait time by streamlining the registration process.

Room for Improvement

No-shows affect a healthcare organization through lost revenue, jumbled employee work schedules, and increased expenses. A missed appointment on average costs the healthcare organization $120 per no-show. Due to the cost, many healthcare organizations charge patients for missed appointments. For a healthcare facility that has an average of 160 appointments with a 5% no-show rate, the cost for no-shows is $11,520. Healthcare organizations are using different technologies to reach patients to remind them of their appointments. In the past, healthcare organizations sent postcards that often went into the trash, made telephone calls that went unanswered, and sent emails that went to a patient's spam file. However, 90% of all text messages are viewed within three minutes, making them an effective mode of communication. Text messages can create more engagement between patients and healthcare facilities, and they also save staff time.

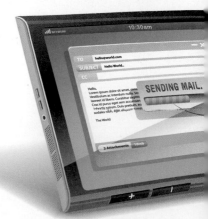

Chapter

5

Scheduling and Patient Management

EHRs in the News

In February 2017, the US Department of Defense (DoD) launched an inpatient and outpatient EHR called MHS Genesis. The EHR connects medical and dental information. MHS Genesis supports 9.4 million DoD beneficiaries and approximately 205,000 military personnel globally.

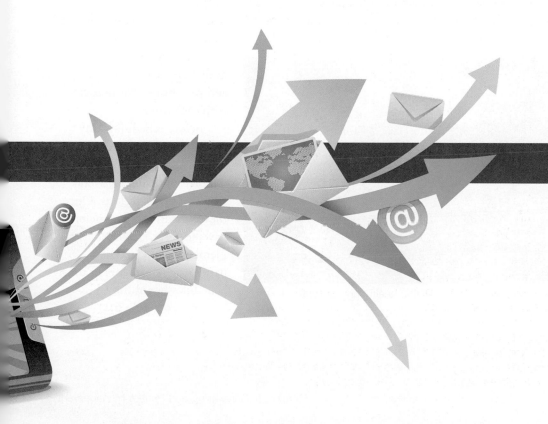

5.1 Explain the importance of using the scheduling feature in an EHR.

5.2 Customize a healthcare facility's schedule.

5.3 Describe the five types of scheduling methods.

5.4 Describe the benefits of allowing patients to schedule appointments using a patient portal.

5.5 List the information required to schedule an appointment.

5.6 Schedule, cancel, and reschedule an appointment in the EHR.

5.7 Generate a provider schedule from the EHR.

5.8 Transfer a patient in the EHR.

5.9 Check out or discharge a patient in the EHR.

5.10 Explain how the patient tracker can improve workflow.

Scheduling appointments is a common task among healthcare staff members, particularly in an ambulatory care setting. An electronic health record (EHR) system that includes a scheduling feature helps simplify the scheduling and billing processes in a healthcare facility. Using the EHR scheduling feature will decrease the administrative responsibilities of the admissions and front desk staff. The use of the EHR schedule features will help to streamline the scheduling process. An EHR system should provide the healthcare facility with a way to schedule patient appointments directly in the system, as you will learn how to do within the EHR Navigator. Some systems will use a separate electronic program to handle scheduling and communicate with the EHR system via a Health Level Seven International (HL7) interface. The system's scheduling component also includes a messaging system for the healthcare facility, provider, and patient to communicate with each other.

Before scheduling any patient visits, however, the facility must set up a facility template showing its overall schedule of operations. Once these scheduling parameters have been set, healthcare staff members can schedule patient appointments in the Schedules tab of the EHR system (see Figure 5.1).

Patients make contact with a healthcare facility to make an appointment.

Figure 5.1 Scheduling Tab on the EHR Navigator

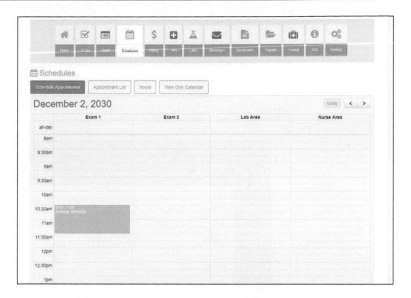

Healthcare Facility Schedule

A healthcare facility should create a matrix that shows available and unavailable appointment times. Unavailable times may include meetings, holidays, lunch hours, surgical schedules, physician rounds, or emergencies. The schedule may be viewed as daily, weekly, or monthly calendars, and it may be viewed by patient, provider, or facility. The scheduling tools are used to insert, edit, cancel, or clear an appointment from the schedule. When setting up the EHR system, the acute care or ambulatory care facility enters the parameters for scheduling patients. Typically, a practice administrator or a representative from the healthcare facility works with the EHR vendor to create available days, times, and types of appointments. Such parameters typically include available providers, available scheduling days and hours, and types of visits. A typical EHR schedule for an ambulatory care facility displays a calendar; lists of available providers such as physicians, nurse practitioners, and physician assistants; and a list of open appointments, currently scheduled patients, contact information, types of appointments, and notes (see Figure 5.2).

Figure 5.2 EHR Schedule for an Ambulatory Care Facility

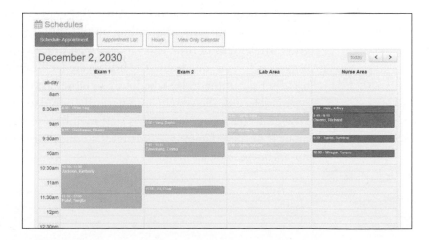

As mentioned earlier, the EHR scheduling system must block off time for holidays, lunch hours, vacations, personal time, and meetings, as necessary. These unavailable hours should be blocked off as soon as possible so patients are not scheduled during those times (see Figure 5.3). This can be accomplished by using the Schedules feature and adding the blocked off time directly to the calendar, or by clicking Hours and adjusting the times or days the facility is open.

Figure 5.3 Blocked-Off Time in a Facility Schedule

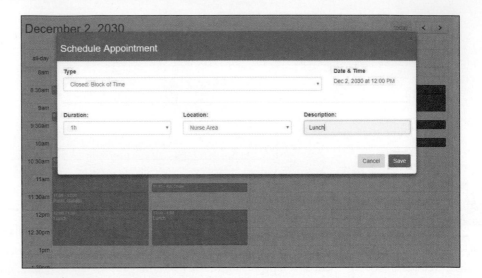

Tutorial 5.1

Blocking Time in the EHR Schedule

Go to Navigator+ to launch Tutorial 5.1. As an office manager, practice closing the office and adjusting the hours for Northstar Physicians using the EHR Navigator.

Appointment Scheduling Process

Patients who want to be seen by a healthcare provider or receive care at a facility typically make an appointment for a specific date and time. Most healthcare facilities use a fixed schedule, whereas others, such as urgent care clinics or after-hours clinics, take walk-in appointments. Depending on the appointment type (e.g., office visit, surgery), the length of time will vary, with an office visit usually ranging from 10 minutes to as long as one hour. The healthcare facility typically has each type of appointment set up in the EHR scheduling parameters; therefore, when an appointment type is selected, the system automatically populates the length of the appointment. However, the system also allows staff members to customize the length of an appointment if needed. Figure 5.4 illustrates a typical process for scheduling an appointment for an outpatient.

Figure 5.4 Scheduling an Outpatient Appointment

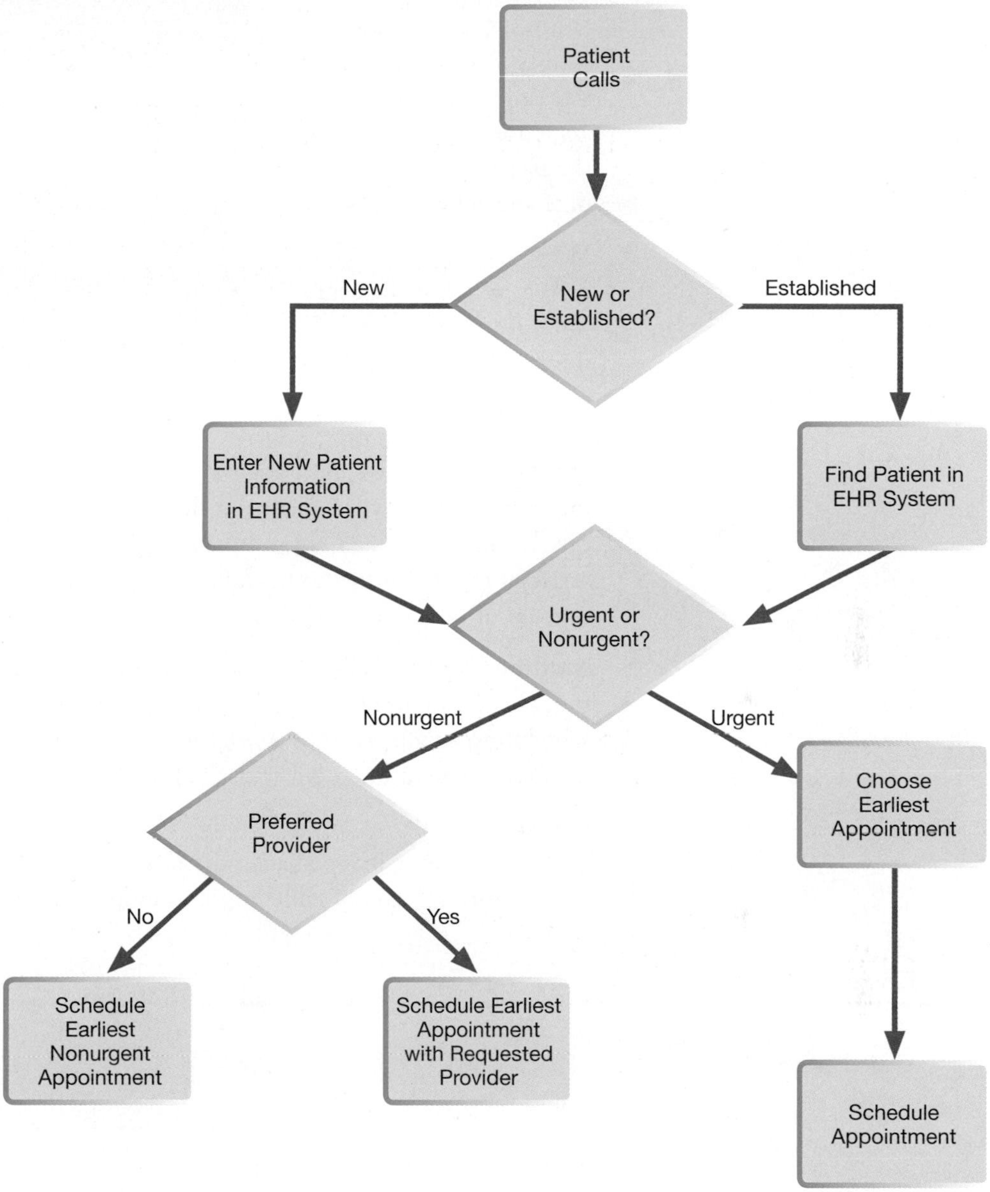

Scheduling Methods

There are several ways healthcare facilities choose to schedule appointments. No matter the type of scheduling method selected by the healthcare facility, the schedule must meet the needs of the facility's providers and patients. The types of scheduling methods that may be implemented include: open hours, time-specified, wave, modified wave, and cluster.

- **Open Hours** Patients are seen throughout certain time frames or on a first-come, first-served basis. This type of scheduling is typically used in an urgent care setting.

- **Time-Specified** Patients are given a specific date and time to arrive at a facility. A time-specified schedule may be used in an acute care setting where the patient has a specific date and time for surgery.

- **Wave** Patients are scheduled to arrive at the beginning of the hour (hence, the term *wave*), and the number of appointments is determined by dividing the hour by the length of an average visit or procedure. The expectation is that patient visits will average out the time usage during that hour. This type of scheduling may be used in a primary care office where a group of patients arrive at the top of the hour, and then no appointments are scheduled at the bottom of the hour.

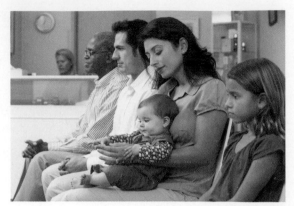

In wave scheduling, all patients arrive at the beginning of the hour.

- **Modified Wave** Patients arrive at planned intervals in the first half hour, then, in the second half hour, the healthcare provider catches up. This type of scheduling may be used in an internal medicine office where the provider does not have to be in the room with the patient for the entire appointment.

- **Cluster** Similar appointments are scheduled together at specific times of the day. For example, in a pediatrician's office, well-child visits may be scheduled in the morning, and ill-child appointments may be scheduled after lunch.

CHECKP⊕INT 5.1

1. What types of events are placed on the schedule as blocked-off time?

_____

_____

_____

2. List the five types of scheduling methods.

a. _____

b. _____

c. _____

d. _____

e. _____

Patient Appointment Scheduling

Once the facility schedule includes the necessary parameters, patient appointments may be scheduled. There are a few ways to schedule an appointment in the EHR scheduling system. A patient can schedule an appointment through a secure patient portal, which gives the patient the opportunity to request his or her preferred appointment. Or more traditionally, patients contact the healthcare facility to schedule their appointments.

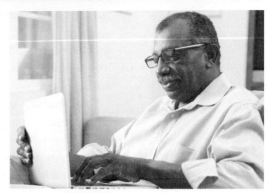

A patient can make an appointment from a home computer using a patient portal.

Information Needed to Schedule an Appointment

When a patient, whether inpatient or outpatient, initiates an admission or appointment, specific patient information must be collected. For a new patient, this information includes the following:

- Patient's full name
- Telephone number
- Date of birth
- Chief complaint or reason for appointment
- Type of insurance
- Insurance identification number

- Referring physician
- Social Security number
- Sex
- Address
- Emergency contact
- Responsible party information
- Employer information

Using the master patient index (MPI), the healthcare facility may populate the admission or appointment for an established patient by collecting the following information to schedule an appointment:

- Patient's full name
- Date of birth
- Telephone number
- Chief complaint or reason for appointment

The patient information that already exists in the EHR must be verified and updated at the time of scheduling.

Using the Patient Portal to Schedule an Appointment

Many EHR systems contain either a patient portal or a personal health record (PHR) component. The **patient portal** provides a secure communication tool between patients and healthcare providers that complies with the Health Insurance Portability and Accountability Act of 1996 (HIPAA). Patient portals can also provide patients

MAKE AN
IMPACT!

The number of digital devices has increased to more than 5 billion worldwide, making it easy for healthcare organizations to communicate with patients. Health Services Research found that text message reminders increased appointment attendance by nearly 50%. A Kaiser Permanente study showed that a text message pilot program saved $275,000.

with information for their PHRs. Some patient portals are web-based and provide 24-hour, self-service components for patients to use. The patient portal links to the facility's EHR system and thus allows the patient to view a provider's calendar of available dates and times and to schedule an appointment. This type of portal also allows the patient to update demographic, insurance, medical history, and current health information prior to an appointment. Patients who use the patient portal reduce the resources necessary from the healthcare facility.

The patient portal scheduling component is used only by established patients of an acute care or ambulatory care facility. The healthcare provider gives an established patient an access code that allows him or her to schedule an appointment, send a message, update information, view laboratory appointments, request prescription refills, and view his or her health record. See Figures 5.5 and 5.6 for examples of a patient portal. Chapter 12 will cover the personal health record and the patient portal in more detail.

The patient accesses the patient portal by entering a username and password. Once logged in, the patient can view upcoming appointments, schedule appointments, view past appointments, and request referrals.

To begin, the patient would select *Schedule an Appointment*. The patient is able to select a provider and appointment type. The patient is then able to see the available appointments based on the criteria he or she has selected. Once a patient selects an appointment, the information is sent to the healthcare facility, and then the healthcare facility sends an email message to the patient with a confirmation. Figure 5.7 shows an example of the Inbox area on the Messages tab of a patient portal.

Figure 5.5   Log-In Screen of a Patient Portal

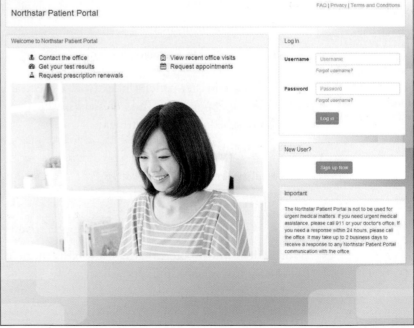

Figure 5.6   Dialog Box to Schedule an Appointment in a Patient Portal

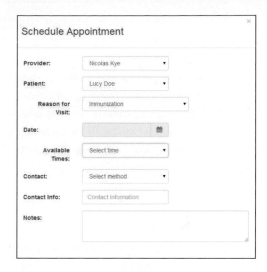

Figure 5.7   Messages in a Patient Portal

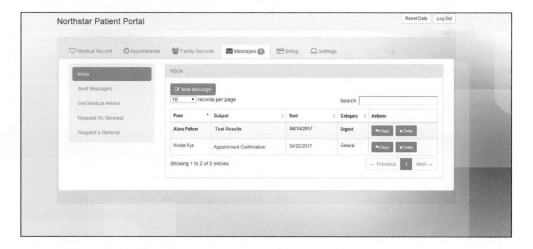

The patient portal makes scheduling convenient for the patient and the health-care facility. Practices that implement a patient portal provide value to the patient by increasing patient access, enhancing the relationships between patients and providers, improving quality of care, and securing information. The patient portal also meets these four meaningful use criteria:

- Patient engagement criteria 1: electronic copy of health information

- Patient engagement criteria 2: clinical summaries

- Patient engagement criteria 3: appointment recalls

- Patient engagement criteria 4: timely access to health information

Initiating an Appointment in the EHR System

When a patient telephones the healthcare facility or is present to schedule an appointment, there are two ways to initiate an appointment within the EHR Navigator scheduling feature.

- Select Schedules: This method is the easiest way to schedule an appointment, as it allows the user to see all the available time slots and facility areas at a glance (see Figure 5.8). Users click in an open time slot and can add the appointment details in the dialog box.

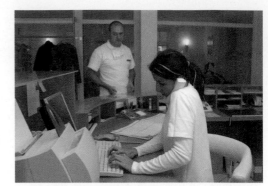

The healthcare worker searches for available appointments when a patient calls the facility.

- Select Appointment List and then Add Appointment: This method allows the user to modify the traditional appointment times. Figure 5.9 shows the Add Appointment dialog box.

Both methods produce the same result: an appointment. The difference in the various ways to schedule appointments depends on user needs and preferences. The scheduling feature shows various colors that define the visit type or scheduled department.

Figure 5.8 Schedule an Appointment

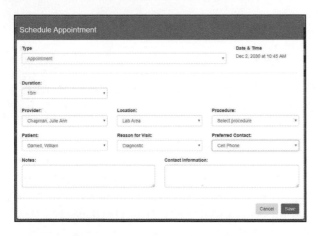

Figure 5.9 Add Appointment Dialog Box

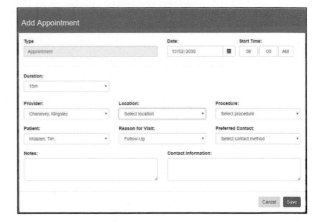

CHECKPOINT 5.2

1. Describe the benefits of scheduling using a patient portal.

_____

_____

2. What are two methods for scheduling an appointment in the EHR?

a. _____

b. _____

Tutorial 5.2

EHRNAVIGAT⊕R

Scheduling an Inpatient Procedure

Go to Navigator+ to launch Tutorial 5.2. As a unit clerk, practice scheduling an inpatient procedure using the EHR Navigator.

Tutorial 5.3

EHRNAVIGAT⊕R

Scheduling an Outpatient Appointment

Go to Navigator+ to launch Tutorial 5.3. As a front desk clerk, practice scheduling an outpatient appointment using the EHR Navigator.

EXPAND YOUR LEARNING

Most healthcare practices begin each day with the thought that all patients will show up and there will not be any no-shows. This is often not the case. Read the article on how practice workflow can be improved by examining the patient schedule.

http://EHR2
.ParadigmEducation
.com/
PatientScheduling

Canceling and Rescheduling Appointments

Many facilities struggle with patients who cancel appointments or those who do not show for their scheduled appointments (called **no-shows**). Patients cancel their appointments for a variety of reasons, including scheduling conflicts, emotional issues, financial concerns, and—for no-shows—forgetfulness. Regardless of the reason, each facility must set its own policy on cancellation fees, and each canceled appointment or no-show should be documented in the EHR system. Tracking these types of appointments will enable the healthcare facility to run reports and determine its rate of no-shows. See Figure 5.10 for a sample No-Show Report.

Confirming appointments decreases the incidences of no-shows, which in turn increases practice productivity and revenue. Healthcare staff can decrease the number of no-shows by setting up automated confirmation of appointments in the EHR system. To maximize the results of confirming appointments, patients can be given an option to receive a phone call, text message, or secure email reminder based on personal preference. Rescheduling may be the outcome of a canceled or no-show appointment.

Figure 5.10 No-Show Report

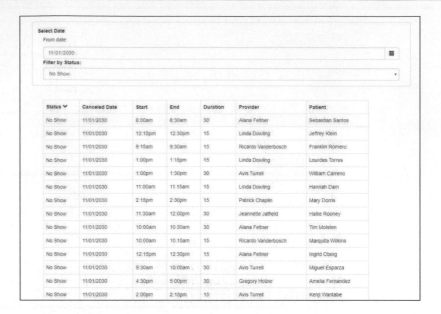

Select Date						
From date:						
11/01/2030						
Filter by Status:						
No Show						

Status ∨	Canceled Date	Start	End	Duration	Provider	Patient
No Show	11/01/2030	8:00am	8:30am	30	Alana Feltner	Sebastian Santos
No Show	11/01/2030	12:15pm	12:30pm	15	Linda Dowling	Jeffrey Klein
No Show	11/01/2030	9:15am	9:30am	15	Ricardo Vanderbosch	Franklin Romero
No Show	11/01/2030	1:00pm	1:15pm	15	Linda Dowling	Lourdes Torres
No Show	11/01/2030	1:00pm	1:30pm	30	Avis Turrell	William Carreno
No Show	11/01/2030	11:00am	11:15am	15	Linda Dowling	Hannah Dam
No Show	11/01/2030	2:15pm	2:30pm	15	Patrick Chaplin	Mary Dorris
No Show	11/01/2030	11:30am	12:00pm	30	Jeannette Jatfeld	Hallie Rooney
No Show	11/01/2030	10:00am	10:30am	30	Alana Feltner	Tim Molsten
No Show	11/01/2030	10:00am	10:15am	15	Ricardo Vanderbosch	Marquita Wilkins
No Show	11/01/2030	12:15pm	12:30pm	15	Alana Feltner	Ingrid Oberg
No Show	11/01/2030	9:30am	10:00am	30	Avis Turrell	Miguel Esparza
No Show	11/01/2030	4:30pm	5:00pm	30	Gregory Holzer	Amelia Fernandez
No Show	11/01/2030	2:00pm	2:15pm	15	Avis Turrell	Kenji Wantabe

Tutorial 5.4   **EHR**NAVIGAT✛R

Pulling a No-Show Report

Go to Navigator+ to launch tutorial 5.4. As a front desk clerk, practice pulling a report of no-show patients using the EHR Navigator.

Tutorial 5.5   **EHR**NAVIGAT✛R

Canceling and Rescheduling an Appointment

Go to Navigator+ to launch Tutorial 5.5. As a medical assistant, practice canceling and rescheduling an appointment using the EHR Navigator.

Printing a Provider's Schedule

The EHR must generate reports of clinical or administrative information. One example is to print the provider's schedule.

Tutorial 5.6   **EHR**NAVIGAT✛R

Printing a Provider's Schedule

Go to Navigator+ to launch Tutorial 5.6. As a medical assistant, practice printing a provider's schedule using the EHR Navigator.

Patient Transfers in the EHR System

While receiving care in a hospital, a patient may need to be transferred from one unit or room to another. Some of the reasons for a patient transfer include a change in patient condition, change in isolation status, or patient preference. All intrafacility transfers must be documented within the EHR system to ensure accuracy in patients' locations and hospital census data.

Change in Patient Condition

During an inpatient stay, a patient's condition may improve or deteriorate to the point that he or she must be transferred to a nursing unit in the hospital that can more adequately address his or her needs. For example, a patient in a room on a postoperative hospital unit who experiences cardiac arrest will likely be transferred to a more intensive nursing unit such as a cardiac intensive care unit. As the patient stabilizes and improves, he or she may be moved to a less intensive care unit.

Change in Isolation Status

Isolation status refers to the precautions that must be taken by healthcare staff and visitors to prevent the spread of bacterial or viral infections. Many hospital rooms are semiprivate, meaning there are two patients occupying a room. Patients can be admitted to the same room only if they have the same isolation status. For example, a patient infected with methicillin-resistant *Staphylococcus aureus* (MRSA) cannot be admitted to the room of a patient without the same infection, as there is a substantial risk that the other patient may also become infected with MRSA.

Patient Preference

Patients may ask to be transferred to another hospital room for many reasons, such as noise levels or roommate issues.

All EHR systems should have a transfer patient function. In the EHR Navigator, this function is accessed through the Admission/Discharge tab.

Tutorial 5.7   **EHR**NAVIGAT✛R

> Transferring a Patient
>
> Go to Navigator+ to launch Tutorial 5.7. As a unit clerk, practice transferring a patient using the EHR Navigator.

Checkout/Discharge Procedures

The procedure for a patient leaving a medical facility varies depending on whether the patient is **checking out** at an outpatient facility or being **discharged** from an inpatient facility.

Outpatient Checkout

Following an outpatient visit, the patient will check out. The checkout procedure may include collecting payments, ordering tests, making referrals, or scheduling a future appointment for the patient. During the checkout process, all the necessary prescriptions and completed forms must be verified.

Inpatient Discharge

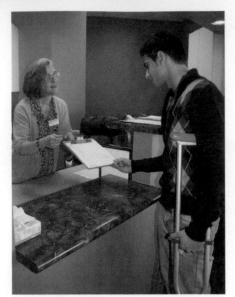

Before checking out of an outpatient facility, a patient may be asked to schedule a follow-up appointment.

The discharge of an inpatient from an acute care hospital is entered into the EHR Navigator via the Admission/Discharge tab. The date and time of the patient's discharge are automatically captured when the nurse or staff member enters the discharge into the EHR system. The **discharge disposition**, or the patient's destination following a stay in the hospital, is also entered. Examples of discharge dispositions include home, skilled nursing facility, rehabilitation hospital, and long-term acute care hospital. If an inpatient dies, the discharge disposition entered is "expired." Discharge documents may be generated from the EHR system. These documents may include discharge instructions specific to the patient's diagnoses and the procedures performed. Discharge documents may also include information regarding recommended follow-up with the patient's surgeon or primary care physician. In addition, to comply with accreditation requirements, a current medication list should be provided from the EHR system to the patient at the time of discharge. At time of discharge, the patient or patient representative should acknowledge and sign receipt of discharge summary and instructions.

Tutorial 5.8   EHRNAVIGAT⊕R

Discharging a Patient
Go to Navigator+ to launch Tutorial 5.8. As a unit clerk, practice discharging a patient using the EHR Navigator.

Electronic Patient Tracker

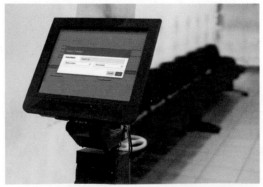

Workstations in the waiting room can be used to check in a patient and begin tracking his or her location.

An EHR system has the ability to track a patient's location from admission to discharge (for inpatients) or from check-in to checkout (for outpatients). This feature offers a real-time, at-a-glance view of a patient's current status and location. For example, when a patient checks in at Northstar Physicians, the patient tracking feature would be activated and would follow the patient until checkout.

Electronic patient tracking (EPT) is an important function of an EHR system. EPT tracks a patient's location from the time of his or her arrival at the healthcare organization to discharge (for inpatients) or checkout (for outpatients). The EPT function offers a real-time, at-a-glance view of a patient's current status and location. The electronic patient tracking replaces the traditional use of a whiteboard.

Benefits of Electronic Patient Tracking

Knowing the location and status of all patients at all times is the obvious benefit of an electronic patient tracking system. Other benefits of EPT include real-time monitoring of patient wait times and bottlenecks in the flow of patient care, room and provider utilization statistics for analysis, and identification of opportunities for improvement in patient flow and care. Improving the flow of patients with the use of EPT results in operational cost savings for the healthcare organization and increased patient satisfaction because of a reduction in wait times. Busy hospital emergency departments (EDs) benefit greatly from the use of EPT, because patients in the most serious conditions can be identified, located, and triaged much faster. Patient families may also benefit from EPT. Have you ever waited for news about a family member undergoing a surgical procedure? Many hospitals and surgical centers have HIPAA-friendly electronic displays that update as a patient is moved from preop, surgery, postop, and recovery room.

Simple or Complex?

The functionality of EPT can be simple or complex. Electronic patient tracking at its simplest is an outpatient checking in for a scheduled appointment. The staff member indicates the patient's arrival in the EPT, the medical assistant enters the patient's location as the patient is taken back to an exam room, and then a staff member enters the patient's departure at the time of check-out. To locate a patient, a staff member has to access one of the office's computers.

A more complex EPT functionality might have patients check in via a kiosk. The kiosk prints a wristband that contains a computer chip that tracks the patient via the organization's secure wireless Internet. Authorized users of the healthcare organization can determine a patient's location via the organization's computers and their authorized mobile devices. Consider the time savings for providers and staff who are able to quickly determine whether a patient is in his or her hospital room, CT scanning room, surgery, or somewhere else. The EHR Navigator's Patient Tracker feature is illustrated in Figures 5.11 and 5.12.

Figure 5.11 Dialog Box to Update the Patient's Location

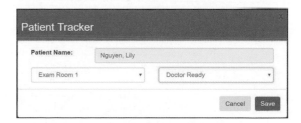

Figure 5.12   Patient Status Summary

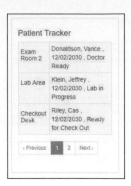

CHECKP⊕INT 5.3

1. List three reasons a patient might be transferred.

   a. _____

   b. _____

   c. _____

2. Describe the purpose of a patient tracker system.

   _____

   _____

   _____

Tutorial 5.9   **EHR**NAVIGAT⊕R

Using the Patient Tracker

Go to Navigator+ to launch Tutorial 5.9. In this activity, practice using the EHR Navigator Patient Tracker to follow the patient from arrival to checkout. You will log in as several different staff members of Northstar Physicians.

Chapter Summary

Scheduling patients in an acute care or ambulatory care facility is a key factor in the delivery of health care. Scheduling depends on the type of facility and type of appointment. In an acute care facility, the appointment depends on resources, such as the availability of the healthcare provider and/or the equipment and the type of procedure ordered. Ambulatory care patients are typically labeled as new or established. When scheduling a new patient, healthcare staff must gather demographic and financial information.

There are five scheduling methods, each designed to meet the specific needs of the facility. The scheduling methods include open hours, time-specified, wave, modified wave, and cluster. The electronic health record (EHR) system provides features for scheduling, canceling, and rescheduling appointments.

An EHR system must display a schedule of patient appointments and generate reports of clinical or administrative information.

Transferring patients may be necessary because the patient's condition or isolation status changes or because he or she is dissatisfied with the room.

Tracking patients allows facilities to know immediately the location and status of a patient, increasing workflow efficiency and patient satisfaction.

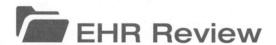 EHR Review

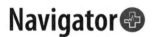

The following EHR Review, EHR Application, and EHR Evaluation activities are also available online in the Navigator+ learning management system. Your instructor may ask you to complete these activities online. Navigator+ also provides access to flash cards, study games, and practice quizzes to help strengthen your understanding of the chapter content.

Acronyms/Initialisms

Study the following acronyms discussed in this chapter. Go to Navigator+ for flash cards of the acronyms and other chapter key terms.

EPT: Electronic Patient Tracker

PHR: personal health record

Check Your Understanding

To check your understanding of this chapter's key concepts, answer the following questions.

1. Scheduling an appointment requires that the scheduler collect all of the following pieces of information *except*

   a. health insurance information.

   b. patient demographics.

   c. reason for the visit.

   d. means of arrival.

2. An electronic health record (EHR) contains unavailable times for scheduling appointments. Unavailable times may include all of the following *except*

   a. holidays.

   b. hospital rounds.

   c. lunch.

   d. pharmaceutical sales visits.

3. A healthcare facility may choose one of the following scheduling methods to create its appointment schedule.

   a. modified cluster

   b. wave

   c. open wave

   d. cluster time

4. A patient portal is

   a. owned and controlled by a patient, may contain additional information not in the medical record, and is used for managing health information.

   b. generated by a healthcare provider to document a patient's medical and health information and is not directly accessed by a patient.

   c. a secure website that allows patients to access a personal health record (PHR) to communicate with healthcare providers, request prescription refills, review laboratory test results, or schedule appointments.

   d. a nonsecure website that allows patients to access a PHR to communicate with healthcare providers, request prescription refills, review laboratory test results, or schedule appointments.

5. Which of the following is *not* an appropriate reason for a patient transfer?

   a. The patient's condition has changed.

   b. The patient does not like his or her roommate.

   c. The patient is in isolation status.

   d. A nurse does not like the patient.

6. True/False: Scheduling is used to insert, edit, delete, or remove an appointment.

7. True/False: The patient tracker feature in an EHR follows the patient from admission or check-in to discharge or checkout.

8. True/False: Time-specified appointment scheduling requires the patient to be seen on a first-come, first-served basis.

9. True/False: A patient may request a transfer because he or she finds the room too noisy.

10. True/False: A patient portal provides the patient with an opportunity to schedule his or her own appointments.

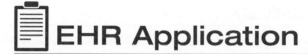

EHR Application

Go on the Record

To build on your understanding of the topics in this chapter, complete the following short-answer activities.

1. Why would a healthcare facility choose to use a specific type of scheduling?

2. There are times when a schedule should be blocked from appointments. Explain the different types of activities of a healthcare facility or provider that would necessitate blocked schedule time.

3. What are the different reasons that a patient's appointment may need to be adjusted?

4. Why is it important to track a patient during his or her stay at a healthcare facility?

5. Describe how the patient tracker feature may improve the healthcare facility's work flow and patient satisfaction.

Navigate the Field

To gain practice in handling challenging situations in the workplace, consider the following real-world scenarios and identify how you would respond to each.

1. You receive an appointment request from Ms. Ying through the patient portal. She is requesting an appointment time already filled by another patient. You contact Ms. Ying, and she informs you that when she requested the appointment, the time was available and she needs to be seen right away. How should you handle this situation?

2. You are preparing the 2030 calendar for Northstar Physicians. You are working with the physicians, staff, and IT manager to create the schedule in the EHR Navigator. What are the steps you would take to prepare the calendar to be customized for the EHR Navigator? What would be the best way to communicate this to the IT manager so that the EHR Navigator calendar may be customized?

 # EHR Evaluation

Think Critically

Continue to think critically about challenging concepts and complete the following activities.

1. A new patient calls to schedule an appointment. Describe the process you would follow to schedule the initial appointment.

2. Dr. Nelson's office contacts the Scheduling Department at St. Francis Hospital to schedule Mr. Yadav's double bypass surgery. Mr. Yadav will have to stay a minimum of three days in the hospital. Prepare a list of steps you would follow to schedule the surgery for Dr. Nelson's patient.

Make Your Case

Consider the scenario and then complete the following project.

You work for Pleasant Valley Urgent Care, which is implementing a new electronic health record (EHR) system. You are responsible for working with the EHR vendor to determine the scheduling parameters of the system and must provide the vendor with a presentation on the type of scheduling Pleasant Valley Urgent Care will use. Include in the presentation the urgent care days, times, a list of healthcare providers, number of examination rooms, necessary equipment, any nonpatient times, and any additional resources that will be used for scheduling. You will be presenting to the vendor and the director of Pleasant Valley Urgent Care.

Explore the Technology

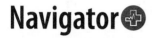

Complete the EHR Navigator practice assessments that align to each tutorial and the assessments that accompany Chapter 5 located on Navigator+.

Are You Ready?

Have you found a job that sounds perfect for you? If so, you will want to spend some time perfecting your résumé and cover letter to make a good first impression on a potential employer. Research how to craft an interesting and effective cover letter, and consider meeting with your school's career services office for tips on writing an effective résumé.

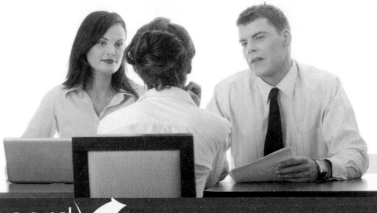

Beyond the Record

- The penalties for criminal violations of the Health Insurance Portability and Accountability Act of 1996 (HIPAA) are steep.

- Knowingly obtaining or disclosing identifiable patient information can result in one year of imprisonment and a $50,000 fine per violation.

- Obtaining patient information for personal or commercial gain or with malicious intent can result in 10 years of imprisonment and a $250,000 fine.

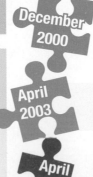

HIPAA Time Line

1996 — HIPAA signed into law.

1999 — US Department of Health & Human Services (HHS) becomes responsible for developing privacy standards.

1999 — HHS proposes privacy standards and receives more than 50,000 comments on the proposed standards.

December 2000 — HHS publishes the Final Rule for Standards for Privacy of Individually Identifiable Health Information, or the Final HIPAA Privacy Rule.

April 2003 — Deadline for covered entities to comply with the Privacy Rule.

April 2005 — Deadline for covered entities to comply with the Security Rule.

Chapter 6

Privacy, Security, and Legal Aspects of the EHR

Case Study

In August 2016, Advocate Health Care, one of the largest healthcare providers in Illinois, agreed to pay $5.5 million to settle multiple patient data breaches that involved 4 million patients. These data breaches primarily involved stolen laptops. This is one of the largest HIPAA–related settlements.

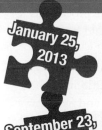

January 25, 2013

HHS publishes modifications to the HIPAA Privacy, Security, and Enforcement Rules to comply with the provisions of the Health Information Technology for Economic and Clinical Health (HITECH) Act. This is known as the HIPAA Omnibus Final Rule.

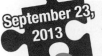

September 23, 2013

HIPAA Omnibus Final Rule compliance is mandatory for covered entities, business associates, and subcontractors.

October 1, 2015

HIPAA Code Set Rule: Effective this date, the use of ICD-10 (International Classification of Diseases) codes is mandatory.

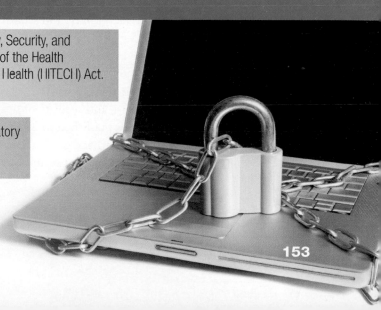

6.1 Define Health Insurance Portability and Accountability Act of 1996 (HIPAA), specifically the Administrative Simplification provisions and the date enacted.

6.2 Identify who is and who is not considered to be a covered entity under HIPAA.

6.3 Identify the basic principles of the Privacy Rule and differentiate between when disclosure of protected health information is permitted and when it is not permitted.

6.4 Demonstrate release of information (ROI) functions carried out by health information management (HIM) staff in the electronic health record (EHR) environment.

6.5 Demonstrate how to produce an accounting of disclosures log.

6.6 Discuss the concept of "minimum necessary" as it relates to the release of health information.

6.7 Explain the enforcement and penalty process for violations of HIPAA privacy and security regulations.

6.8 Demonstrate competency in the use of EHR software as it relates to the release of health information.

6.9 Discuss the HIPAA Breach Notification Rule.

6.10 State the two primary purposes for the development of the security standards of HIPAA.

6.11 List the major sections of the standards of the HIPAA Security Rule and provide safeguard examples that apply to each section.

6.12 Discuss the difference between required and addressable implementation specifications.

As you have already learned, privacy and confidentiality of health information is a major focus when implementing an electronic health record (EHR) system. As a user of an EHR system, you must understand and follow the laws and regulations regarding privacy, safety, and security of health information. In addition, there are procedures for safeguarding health information that are not mandated by law but should be considered when implementing and using EHRs.

A challenging topic to address is patients' access to their health information and their rights regarding its release to others. Federal legislation that revolutionized the release and security of health information includes the HIPAA Privacy and Security Rules published in 2000, which were subsequently updated in 2010 and 2013. These rules provide guidance about the release and security of paper health records, as well as the release and security of EHR data.

HIPAA

The **Health Insurance Portability and Accountability Act of 1996 (HIPAA)** was enacted on August 21, 1996. HIPAA includes many provisions that affect all healthcare facilities. For example, HIPAA allowed for health insurance to be "portable"—in other words, the insurance could be moved from one employer to another without denial or restrictions. HIPAA mainly addresses the confidentiality of patients' medical records, including the safeguards that need to be implemented by a healthcare facility to protect the privacy and security of its patients. In addition to setting standards for health information privacy and security, HIPAA also addresses standards to improve the efficiency and effectiveness of healthcare systems. For example, Sections 261–264, known as the Administrative Simplification Provisions, required the US Department of Health and Human Services (HHS) to adopt national standards for electronic healthcare transactions and code sets, unique health identifiers, and security. To gain a broad picture of the tenets of HIPAA, see Figure 6.1. This chapter will specifically focus on the provisions for the electronic exchange, privacy, and security of health information.

Figure 6.1 HIPAA Administrative Simplification Provisions

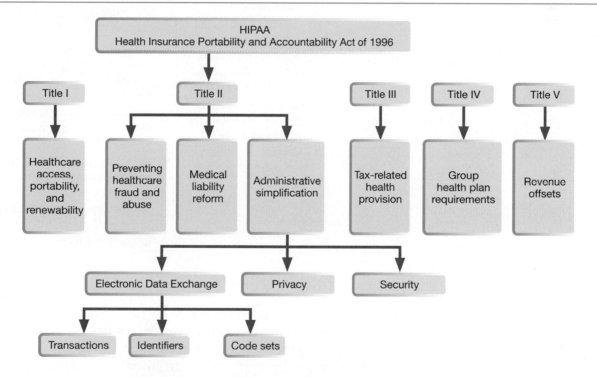

HIPAA Privacy Rule

In response to the US Department of Health and Human Services (HHS) legislation, the HHS secretary published the Privacy Rule on December 28, 2000, and later modified the HIPAA Privacy, Security, and Enforcement Rules on January 25, 2013, to comply with the provisions of the Health Information Technology for Economic and Clinical Health (HITECH) Act, particularly with regard to EHRs.

Covered Entities

The Privacy and Security Rules apply to healthcare providers, health plans, and healthcare clearinghouses transmitting health information in an electronic format. These entities are called **covered entities** (see Table 6.1). Individuals, organizations, and agencies meeting the definition of a covered entity under HIPAA must comply with the rules' requirements to protect the privacy and security of health information, and they must provide individuals with certain access rights with respect to their health information.

Business associates of a covered entity must also follow Privacy and Security Rules if they perform services for the covered entity involving the use or disclosure of individually identifiable health information.

Table 6.1 Covered Entities

Healthcare Provider	Health Plan	Healthcare Clearinghouse
The term *healthcare provider* refers to a provider who transmits health information in an electronic format, such as the following: • Doctors • Clinics • Psychologists • Dentists • Chiropractors • Nursing homes • Pharmacies • Hospitals	The term *health plan* refers to the following entities: • Health insurance companies • Health maintenance organizations • Company health plans (some self-administered company health plans with fewer than 50 participants are not covered) • Government programs that pay for health care, such as Medicare, Medicaid, and military and veterans' health care programs	The term *healthcare clearinghouse* refers to public or private entities, including billing services, repricing companies, community health management information systems, community health information systems, or value-added networks and switches, that do either of the following functions: • Processes, or facilitates the processing of, health information received from another entity in a nonstandard format or containing nonstandard data content into standard data elements or a standard transaction • Receives a standard transaction from another entity and processes or facilitates the processing of health information into nonstandard format or nonstandard data content for the receiving entity

Noncovered Entities

If an entity is not considered a covered entity, it does not have to comply with HIPAA Privacy and Security Rules. Some examples of **noncovered entities** include workers' compensation carriers, employers, marketing firms, life insurance companies, pharmaceutical manufacturers, casualty insurance carriers, pharmacy benefit management companies, and crime victim compensation programs.

Health Information and the Privacy Rule

Certain types of health information are classified under the HIPAA Privacy Rule. These types include protected health information, individually identifiable health information, and deidentified health information.

Protected Health Information

The Privacy Rule defines **protected health information (PHI)** as all individually identifiable health information held or transmitted by a covered entity or its business associate, in any form or media, whether electronic, paper, or oral.

Individually Identifiable Health Information

Individually identifiable health information is information, including demographic data, that identifies the individual, or for which there is a reasonable basis to believe that the information can be used to identify the individual, and that it relates to at least one of the following:

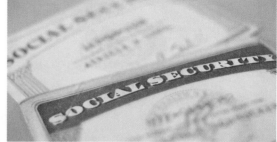

Your Social Security number is a type of common identifier.

- The individual's past, present, or future physical or mental health condition

- The provision of health care to the individual

- The past, present, or future payment for the provision of health care to the individual

Individually identifiable health information includes many common identifiers, such as name, address, birth date, and Social Security number.

Deidentified Health Information

The term **deidentified health information** was coined by the Privacy Rule and is health information that neither identifies an individual nor provides a reasonable basis to identify an individual. Therefore, the Privacy Rule does not restrict the use of deidentified health information. Healthcare staff primarily use deidentified health information for summary purposes, as illustrated by the following scenarios:

- The marketing department of a healthcare provider wants to know how many patients are from each zip code.

- A dentist's office wants to know the number of patients who recently had a cavity filled to determine if the office's use of dental supplies is appropriate.

- A home care agency wants to know the number of physical therapy home care visits made last year to determine whether additional physical therapists should be hired.

Basic Principles of the Privacy Rule

A major purpose of the Privacy Rule is to define and limit the circumstances in which an individual's protected health information may be used or disclosed by covered entities. A covered entity may not use or disclose PHI except either (1) as the Privacy Rule permits or requires, or (2) as the individual who is the subject of the information (or the individual's personal representative) authorizes in writing.

Required Disclosures

A covered entity *must* disclose PHI in only two situations:

1. To an individual (or his or her personal representative), specifically when he or she requests access to, or an accounting of disclosures of, his or her PHI

2. To HHS, specifically during a compliance investigation, review, or enforcement action

Permitted Disclosures

HIPAA regulations permit health information to be used and/or disclosed in the following scenarios without a prior authorization signed by the patient:

- To the individual patient

- For treatment purposes

- For payment purposes

- For healthcare operations

- Incidental to an otherwise permitted use or disclosure

- For public interest and benefit activities

- As a limited data set for purposes of research, public health, or healthcare operations

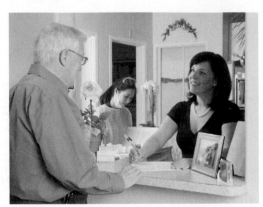

A patient is often asked to sign a HIPAA disclosure asking if it is acceptable to release his or her health information in certain situations.

To learn more about these specific provisions for the disclosure of health information, refer to the following sections.

Individual Patient A patient has the right to view and receive a copy of his or her health information. The covered entity must release the health information in the format requested by the patient (e.g., paper or on an electronic storage medium). As a result of the HIPAA Omnibus Final Rule, patients also now have the right to download and transmit their health information electronically.

TPO Clause Three types of permitted disclosures are commonly known in the healthcare industry collectively as **treatment, payment, healthcare operations (TPO)**. When health information managers, compliance officers, or administrators are asked questions related to the appropriate release of healthcare information and reply with, "Yes, you can release the health information under the TPO clause," they are referring to these permitted disclosures.

The treatment provision of the TPO clause applies to the application, coordination, or management of health care and related services for an individual by one or more healthcare providers, including consultation among providers regarding a patient and referral of a patient by one provider to another.

HIPAA has made it easier and faster for providers to release information for patient care purposes because written patient authorization is not necessary. This HIPAA provision is particularly important for EHRs, allowing healthcare practitioners to obtain health information within minutes or seconds. In comparison, a written authorization could take hours or days.

Consider This

A teenage patient brought to the emergency department (ED) of a hospital drifts in and out of consciousness. The ED physician suspects an adverse event from a medication the patient is taking or a possible drug overdose. The physician learns that the patient takes medications that have been prescribed by the patient's primary care physician. Because the patient's EHR is interoperable with the hospital's EHR, the ED physician is able to access the medications prescribed for the patient. How does permitted disclosure of health information in HIPAA's Privacy Rule allow the patient to receive the necessary care? What could happen if the patient needs to wait while the hospital seeks authorization to release her information?

The payment provision of the TPO clause allows the health plan to review healthcare information to determine premiums, to identify coverage responsibilities and benefits, and to furnish or obtain reimbursement for health care delivered to an individual. Under this provision, healthcare providers are allowed to release health information to receive payment for services rendered. In addition, health insurance companies can obtain health information to identify a subscriber's coverage and provision of benefits, as well as to offer reimbursement for healthcare services provided. For example, a nursing home is allowed to provide health information to an ambulance transportation company so that the ambulance company can be reimbursed for the transfer of a nursing home resident to the hospital.

The healthcare operations provision of the TPO clause applies to any of the following activities:

- Quality assessment and improvement, including case management and care coordination

- Competency assurance activities, including providers of health plan performance evaluation, credentialing, and accreditation

- Conducting or arranging for medical reviews, audits, and legal services, including fraud and abuse detection and compliance programs

- Specified insurance functions, such as underwriting, risk rating, and reinsuring risk

- Business planning, development, management, and administration

- Business management and general administrative activities of the entity, including—but not limited to—deidentifying PHI, creating a limited data set, and certain fundraising for the benefit of the covered entity

A covered entity is allowed to use health information for its own facility or the company's internal operations. The specific activities allowed by HIPAA are listed in the previous definition of healthcare operations. Some specific examples of permitted use and disclosures of health information under this provision are as follows:

- Health insurance companies want to contract for healthcare services from only the best providers, which are those providing the highest quality of care and services for the lowest cost. To select these high-quality, low-cost providers, the insurance company reviews specific health information, and HIPAA permits the use and disclosure of health information for this purpose.

- Healthcare providers conduct internal quality assessments to identify policies and procedures to be changed to provide higher-quality care. The HIPAA healthcare operations clause allows providers to use health information for these assessments.

It is important to note that covered entities may choose to require a signed patient authorization for any and all disclosures of patient health information, even in circumstances in which HIPAA does not require a patient's written authorization. For example, most healthcare providers request that patients sign an authorization to release healthcare information to insurance companies or other payers prior to rendering healthcare services. A good rule for a healthcare provider to follow is to obtain a written patient authorization prior to the release, disclosure, or use of an individual's health information. The authorization form should be HIPAA compliant and depict certain elements required by law.

Incidental to a Permitted Use or Disclosure The Privacy Rule does not require that every risk of an incidental use or disclosure of PHI be eliminated. A use or disclosure of this information that occurs as a result of, or as "incident to," an otherwise permitted use or disclosure is permitted as long as the covered entity has adopted reasonable safeguards as required by the Privacy Rule. For example, a hospital visitor may overhear a provider's confidential conversation with another provider, or a patient may glimpse another patient's information on a sign-in sheet or nurses' station whiteboard.

Public Interest and Benefit Activities The Privacy Rule permits the use and disclosure of PHI without an individual's authorization or permission for 12 national priority purposes, including subpoenas and court orders, certain law enforcement purposes, approved research purposes, public health purposes, organ donations, use by coroners or funeral homes, or compliance with workers' compensation laws.

Limited Data Set Use A **limited data set** is PHI from which certain specified direct identifiers of individuals and their relatives, household members, and employers have been removed. A limited data set may be used and disclosed for research, healthcare operations, and public health purposes, provided the recipient enters into a data use agreement promising specified safeguards for the PHI within the limited data set.

When patient authorization is required or optionally used, specific core elements and required statements must be included in the authorization, including the date the authorization expires and a statement that the authorization is revocable. Covered entities should use a standard patient authorization form drawn up by legal counsel that includes all of the elements required by law.

Release of Information

Typically, HIM professionals, in conjunction with compliance and information technology professionals, ensure that all healthcare staff members are educated in the organization's release of information (ROI) policies and procedures.

Rules and regulations related to the release of PHI are the same whether you are releasing information from a paper record or an EHR. However, the ROI process is significantly more streamlined in an EHR environment for many reasons, including the following:

- Physical records do not need to be located, resulting in significant time savings for HIM staff.

- Records can be printed to paper, saved to a digital storage medium, or emailed directly from the EHR rather than being copied or scanned by hand, resulting in significant time savings for HIM staff.

- Records can be released faster because the process takes less time.

The ROI workflow process follows these steps:

1. A requester submits a written ROI request.

2. For verbal requests, the HIM staff completes a Verbal Request for Information.

3. The HIM staff logs the request into the EHR system or other designated ROI software.

4. A staff member scans the request, along with other pertinent documents such as patient authorization, into the patient's EHR or ROI software.

5. A staff member reviews the request to verify the legitimacy for release of information. He or she looks at items such as identification of the patient whose information is being requested, types of documents requested, and service dates.

6. The HIM staff produces the records in the format requested (paper or electronic).

7. An HIM staff member generates a correspondence letter to accompany the records.

8. The HIM staff mails or sends the records.

Tutorial 6.1   **EHR**NAVIGAT⊕R

Releasing Patient Information
Go to Navigator+ to launch Tutorial 6.1. As an RHIT, practice releasing patient information using the EHR Navigator.

Accounting of Disclosures

As you learned earlier in this chapter, the Privacy Rule states that a patient has the right to receive an accounting of disclosures of his or her PHI made by the covered entity. These accountings of disclosure are provided by the covered entity. ROI software that is either part of the EHR system or interfaces with the EHR system makes the release of an accounting of disclosures relatively simple because the ROI software automatically produces these documents on paper or electronically.

A sample accounting of disclosures log is found in Figure 6.2.

Figure 6.2 Accounting of Disclosures Log

Northstar Medical Center

NORTHSTAR MEDICAL CENTER

Accounting of Disclosures Log

Patient Name:______________________________

Medical Record Number: ______________________

Date Requested	Name of Requestor	Address	Authorization or Written Request (Y/N)	Purpose	PHI Disclosed	Date Disclosed	Disclosed By

Tutorial 6.2

EHRNAVIGATOR

Printing an Accounting of Disclosures Log

Go to Navigator+ to launch Tutorial 6.2. As an RHIT, practice printing an accounting of disclosures log using the EHR Navigator.

Privacy Rule and State Laws

State laws that contradict the Privacy Rule are overruled by the federal requirements, unless an exception applies. Examples of exceptions are when the state law:

- provides greater privacy protections or rights with respect to individually identifiable health information;
- allows for the reporting of injury, illness, child abuse, birth, death, or for public health surveillance, investigation, or intervention; and
- requires health plan reporting—for example, for management or financial audits.

In these examples, a covered entity is not required to comply with a contrary provision of the Privacy Rule.

CHECKPOINT 6.1

1. True/False: A healthcare provider may not release patient health information without a specific authorization or consent signed by the patient.

2. True/False: HIPAA regulations cover only health information documented on paper.

3. The HIPAA Privacy and Security Rules apply only to health plans, healthcare clearinghouses, and healthcare providers who transmit health information in electronic format. What term is used for these plans, clearinghouses, and providers?

Minimum Necessary Concept

Covered entities must make reasonable efforts to limit the use of, disclosure of, and requests for the minimum amount of PHI necessary to accomplish the intended purpose. This concept is called **minimum necessary** and is required by the Privacy Rule.

An example of a covered entity *not* following the minimum necessary concept is as follows. An insurance company needs to determine whether physical therapy services were necessary for a patient residing in a nursing home. So one of its representatives requests a copy of the patient's entire medical record, including physician progress notes, laboratory and radiology results, medical history and physical examination findings, physical therapy progress notes, nutrition progress notes, and case management reports. This is more information than is needed. The insurance company representative should be able to determine whether physical therapy was necessary based on the history and physical examination, physician's orders, and physical therapy progress notes.

An example of a covered entity that *adheres to* the minimum necessary concept is as follows. A new patient is scheduled for a hemodialysis run tomorrow at an outpatient dialysis clinic. The hospital where the patient had hemodialysis discharged the patient yesterday. The outpatient dialysis clinic needs a copy of the last hemodialysis run sheet to plan the patient's hemodialysis run for tomorrow. The dialysis clinic requests only the last dialysis run sheet from the hospital.

Privacy Rule Enforcement

As with any law, there are consequences when the HIPAA Privacy and Security Rules are not followed. Within HHS is the **Office for Civil Rights (OCR)**, which is responsible for enforcing the HIPAA Privacy and Security Rules. The enforcement process begins with a complaint and follows through to a resolution with the Department of Justice when violations are criminal or the OCR when violations are civil, as illustrated in Figure 6.3.

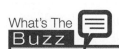

What's The
Buzz

Researchers at Binghamton University, State University of New York have devised a new way to protect personal electronic health records using a patient's own heartbeat. Read more about this at the following website:

http://CHR2.ParadigmEducation.com/Heartbeat.

Figure 6.3 HIPAA Privacy and Security Rules Complaint Process

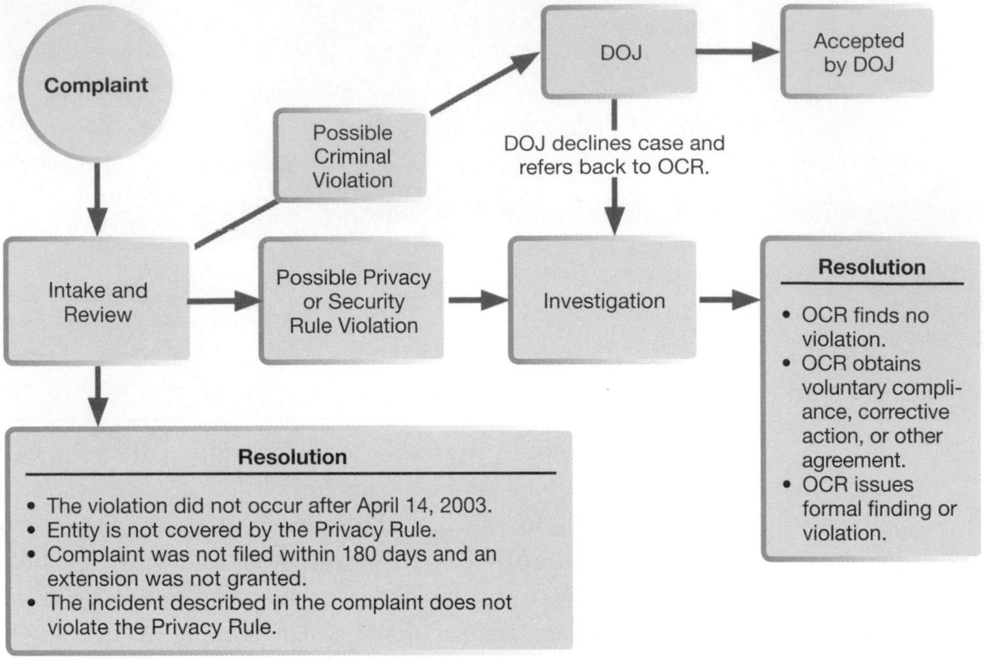

Complaint

Possible Criminal Violation

DOJ

Accepted by DOJ

DOJ declines case and refers back to OCR.

Intake and Review

Possible Privacy or Security Rule Violation

Investigation

Resolution
- OCR finds no violation.
- OCR obtains voluntary compliance, corrective action, or other agreement.
- OCR issues formal finding or violation.

Resolution
- The violation did not occur after April 14, 2003.
- Entity is not covered by the Privacy Rule.
- Complaint was not filed within 180 days and an extension was not granted.
- The incident described in the complaint does not violate the Privacy Rule.

Violations of the Privacy Rule fall into one of two categories: civil or criminal violations. The major difference between civil and criminal violations involves the intent behind the violation.

Civil Violations

If a person *mistakenly* obtained or disclosed individually identifiable health information in violation of HIPAA, and the covered entity corrected the violation within 30 days of when it knew or should have known of the violation, then a penalty is not imposed, as per the HITECH Act. Since the HITECH Act, civil monetary penalties of $100 to $50,000 per failure may be imposed on a covered entity failing to comply with a Privacy Rule requirement. The cumulative penalties may not exceed $1.5 million per year.

Criminal Violations

If a person *knowingly* obtains or discloses individually identifiable health information in violation of HIPAA, this is considered a criminal violation, and the person can be penalized with a fine of $50,000 and one year of imprisonment. Criminal penalties increase to $100,000 and up to five years of imprisonment if the wrongful conduct involves false pretenses. The penalties increase up to $250,000 and up to 10 years of imprisonment if the wrongful conduct involves the intent to sell, transfer, or use PHI for commercial advantage, personal gain, or malicious harm.

© Mike Baldwin / Cornered

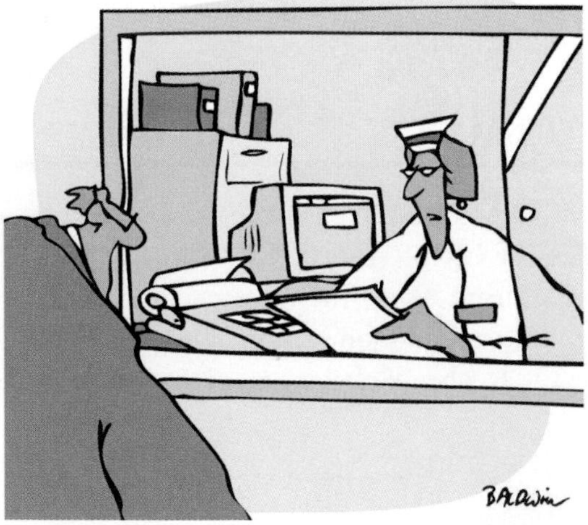

"Somehow your medical records got emailed to a complete stranger. He has no idea what's wrong with you either."

In addition to monetary penalties and imprisonment, the federal government can also require a **Resolution Agreement** with a covered entity, which is a contract signed by the federal government and a covered entity in which the covered entity agrees to perform certain obligations (e.g., staff training regarding privacy and confidentiality, audits of all releases of health information to ensure compliance) and to send reports to the federal government for a certain time period (typically three years). During this period, the federal government monitors the compliance of the covered entity with the obligations it has agreed to perform.

Cases of Privacy Rule Breaches

EXPAND YOUR LEARNING

Describe two recent breaches of the Privacy or Security Rules. A list can be found at the following website:

http://EHR2 .ParadigmEducation .com/Breaches.

In recent years, many high-profile cases of enforcement have included significant monetary penalties and resolution agreements.

In March 2008, Massachusetts General Hospital lost documents for 192 patients and was fined $1 million by the US government. A Massachusetts General Hospital employee left a patient schedule containing patient names and medical records on the subway. The employee also left billing encounter forms for 66 patients, containing names, birth dates, insurance policy numbers, and patient diagnoses. The violation was inadvertent on the part of the employee; however, because Massachusetts General Hospital did not have policies and procedures in place to ensure that PHI was protected when removed from the hospital, and because employees were not adequately trained, the hospital was fined.

On July 16, 2008, the federal government entered into a Resolution Agreement with Seattle-based Providence Health & Services to settle potential violations of HIPAA Privacy and Security Rules. The incidents giving rise to the agreement involved two entities within the Providence Health System, namely Providence Home and Community Services and Providence Hospice and Home Care. On several occasions between September 2005 and March 2006, backup tapes, optical disks, and laptops, all containing unencrypted electronic PHI, were removed from Providence premises and left unattended. The media and laptops were subsequently lost or stolen, compromising the PHI of more than 386,000 patients. The investigation focused on the failure of Providence to implement policies and procedures to safeguard this information. The healthcare facility agreed to pay $100,000 and implement a detailed corrective action plan to ensure that it would appropriately safeguard identifiable electronic patient information against theft or loss. It also agreed to revise its policies and procedures regarding physical and technical safeguards (e.g., encryption) and off-site transport and storage of electronic media containing patient information.

In April 2010, Cignet Health of Prince George's County, MD, violated the rights of 41 patients by denying them access to their medical records when requested. This violation cost Cignet Health $1.3 million. Because Cignet refused to cooperate with the investigation, it was fined an additional $3 million by the federal government.

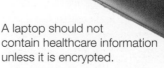

A laptop should not contain healthcare information unless it is encrypted.

In July 2013, the managed care company WellPoint Inc. agreed to pay HHS $1.7 million to settle potential violations of the HIPAA Privacy and Security Rules. OCR's investigation indicated that WellPoint did not implement appropriate administrative and technical safeguards as required under the HIPAA Security Rule. The investigation indicated WellPoint did not adequately implement policies and procedures for authorizing access to the online application database, perform an appropriate technical evaluation in response to a software upgrade to its information systems, or have technical safeguards in place to verify the person or entity seeking access to electronic PHI maintained in its application database. As a result, the investigation indicated that WellPoint impermissibly disclosed the PHI of 612,402 individuals via access over the Internet.

Although major cases with high-dollar penalties such as those described receive considerable media attention, they are the exception rather than the rule.

From the HIPAA compliance date in April 2003 through August 31, 2017, the federal government received 163,277 HIPAA privacy complaints. Of these complaints, 25,373 (16%) went through the investigative and enforcement phases, whereas 138,004 (85%) complaints were either not violations or were determined not to be eligible for the HIPAA enforcement process, and 3,644 (2%) were complaints that had not yet been resolved. Many different types of entities, including national pharmacy chains, major medical centers, group health plans, hospital chains, and small provider offices, were part of the cases investigated.

The most often investigated compliance issues are listed below in order of frequency:

1. Impermissible uses and disclosures of PHI

2. Lack of safeguards of PHI

3. Lack of patient access to his or her PHI

4. Uses or disclosures of more than the minimum necessary PHI

5. Lack of administrative safeguards of electronic PHI

The most common types of covered entities required to take corrective action are listed below in order of frequency:

1. Private practices

2. General hospitals

3. Outpatient facilities

4. Health plans (group health plans and health insurance issuers)

5. Pharmacies

As patients and the public at large have become more familiar with HIPAA privacy rights, there has been a steady increase in the number of complaints made to OCR.

CHECKPOINT 6.2

1. What is the difference between a civil violation and a criminal violation?

   _____

   _____

   _____

2. Name three of the top five investigated compliance issues.

   a. _____

   b. _____

   c. _____

Breach Notification Rule

Implemented in August 2009, breach notification regulations require HIPAA-covered entities and their business associates to provide notification to affected individuals following a breach of unsecured PHI.

Generally speaking, a **breach** is an impermissible use or disclosure under the Privacy Rule that compromises the security or privacy of PHI such that the use or disclosure poses a significant risk of financial, reputational, or other harm to the affected individual.

Following a breach of unsecured PHI, covered entities are required to provide notification of the breach to affected individuals, to the federal government (specifically HHS), and, in certain circumstances, to the media. In addition, business associates must notify covered entities that a breach has occurred.

Notice to Individuals Requirement

Covered entities must notify affected individuals following the discovery of a breach of unsecured PHI and must provide individual written notifications within 60 days following the discovery of a breach. These notifications must include the following items:

1. A description of the breach

2. A description of the types of information involved in the breach

3. The steps affected individuals should take to protect themselves from potential harm

4. A brief description of what the covered entity is doing to investigate the breach, mitigate the harm, and prevent further breaches

5. Contact information for the covered entity

Notice to the Media Requirement

Covered entities experiencing a breach affecting more than 500 residents of a state or jurisdiction are required to notify the affected individuals and provide notice to prominent media outlets serving the state or jurisdiction. Covered entities will likely provide this notification in the form of a press release to appropriate media outlets serving the affected area. Like individual notices, they must provide this media notification within 60 days following the discovery of a breach and must include the same information required for the individual notice.

HIPAA Security Rule

Privacy of health information is one of the main subjects addressed by HIPAA. Another important component of HIPAA is the security of health information. Just as the Privacy Rule was developed to address the privacy provisions of HIPAA, the **Security Standards for the Protection of Electronic Protected Health Information** were developed to address the security provisions of HIPAA and are commonly known as the **Security Rule**. Security Rule provisions pertain exclusively to electronic health information. The Security Rule required all HIPAA-covered entities (the same covered entities discussed earlier in this chapter) to reach compliance no later than April 20, 2005, with the exception of small health plans, which had until April 20, 2006, to comply with the rule.

Prior to HIPAA, no national security standards or general requirements existed to protect health information. With healthcare delivery systems moving away from paper records and toward electronic systems to process claims, manage health information, and document clinical and administrative activities, it became clear that federal guidance was necessary to protect patient information. Covered entities are using web-based applications and other portals that give physicians, clinical staff, administrative staff, health plan employees, and pharmaceutical companies greater access to electronic health information. In addition to web-based products, an increasing number of healthcare providers use internal EHR software to varying degrees. As the United States moves toward its goal of a **Nationwide Health Information Network (NwHIN)** and a greater use of EHRs, protecting the confidentiality, integrity, and availability of **electronic protected health information (ePHI)** becomes even more critical. The security standards in HIPAA were developed for two primary purposes: (1) to protect certain electronic healthcare information that may be at risk, and (2) to promote the use of electronic health information in the healthcare industry.

Protecting an individual's health information, while permitting appropriate access and use of that information, ultimately promotes the use of electronic health information in the healthcare industry.

Objectives of the Security Rule

Although HIPAA established the two broad purposes of health information security standards as just noted, the Security Rule was adopted to more specifically define the objectives that covered entities would need to attain to be in compliance with HIPAA. In the General Rules section of the Security Rule, the four major objectives include the following:

1. Each covered entity must ensure the confidentiality, integrity, and availability of ePHI that it creates, receives, maintains, or transmits.

2. Each covered entity must protect against any reasonably anticipated threats and hazards to the security or integrity of ePHI.

3. Each covered entity must protect against reasonably anticipated uses or disclosures of such information that are not permitted by the Privacy Rule.

4. Each covered entity must ensure compliance by the workforce.

Major Differences between the Privacy and Security Rules

When HHS developed the Security Rule, it chose to closely align it with the provisions in the Privacy Rule. Because both rules were developed in response to HIPAA, it made sense to ensure that the two rules were in sync. Therefore, it is easier for covered entities to implement the provisions of both rules and achieve the goals of HIPAA. However, although the two rules are closely aligned, there are two areas of distinction:

1. The Privacy Rule applies to all forms of patient PHI, whether that information is in electronic, written, or oral format. In contrast, the Security Rule covers only PHI in electronic form, including ePHI that is created, received, maintained, or transmitted. For example, ePHI may be transmitted over the Internet or stored on a server, computer, disc, flash drive, magnetic tape, or electronic storage media. The Security Rule does not cover PHI transmitted or stored on paper or provided in oral form.

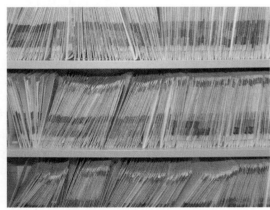

2. The Privacy Rule contains minimum security requirements for the protection of PHI, whereas the Security Rule provides comprehensive security requirements.

The Privacy Rule applies to all forms of patients' PHI, including paper records. The Security Rule covers PHI that is in electronic form.

Sections of the Security Rule

The standards of the Security Rule are divided into six main sections: General Rules, Administrative Safeguards, Physical Safeguards, Technical Safeguards, Organizational Requirements, and Policies and Procedures and Documentation Requirements.

General Rules

The General Rules section includes general requirements that all covered entities must meet. This section establishes the flexibility of approach that covered entities have when implementing and identifying the standards required and those addressable. Information in this section also addresses the required maintenance of security measures to continue reasonable and appropriate protection of ePHI.

Administrative Safeguards

Generally speaking, the Administrative Safeguards section includes the assignment or delegation of security responsibility to an individual and the need for security training for employees and users. Employees must be trained in security, and covered entities must have appropriate policies and procedures for security (e.g., a disaster backup plan, incident reporting of security breaches).

Physical Safeguards

The Physical Safeguards section includes mechanisms necessary to protect electronic systems and the data they store from threats, environmental hazards, and unauthorized intrusion. These safeguards include restricting access to ePHI and retaining off-site computer backups.

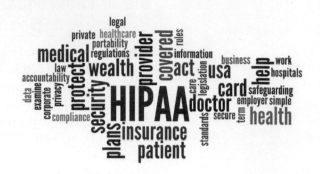

Technical Safeguards

The Technical Safeguards section primarily covers the automated processes used to protect data and control access to data. These processes include the use of authentication control to verify that the person signing onto a computer is authorized to access that ePHI or encryption and decryption of data as it is being stored, transmitted, or both.

Organizational Requirements

The fifth major section of the Security Rule, the Organizational Requirements, includes standards for business associate contracts and other arrangements and the requirements for group health plans.

Policies and Procedures and Documentation Requirements

The section titled Policies and Procedures and Documentation Requirements addresses the implementation of reasonable and appropriate policies and procedures to comply with the Security Rule standards. The covered entity must maintain written documentation and records that include policies, procedures, actions, activities, or assessments required by the Security Rule.

CHECKP⊕INT 6.3

1. List the six main sections of the Security Rule.

   a. _____

   b. _____

   c. _____

   d. _____

   e. _____

   f. _____

2. Encryption of healthcare data before transmission is an example of which type of security safeguard?

   _____

3. Security training of employees is an example of which type of security safeguard?

   _____

Security Standards Matrix

The Centers for Medicare & Medicaid Services (CMS) created a Security Standards Matrix, which is Appendix A of the Security Rule, to assist covered entities in the assessment of their compliance with the Security Rule (see Figure 6.4).

Note that the first column is a description of the Security Standard. The second column lists the section of the Security Rule published within the *Federal Register*. The third and fourth columns list a more specific reference to a portion of the security standards along with a designation of *R* (required) or *A* (addressable). A **required standard** must be met, while an **addressable standard** should be met if it is a reasonable and appropriate safeguard in the entity's environment. Addressable standards should not be considered merely optional.

Figure 6.4   The Security Standards Matrix

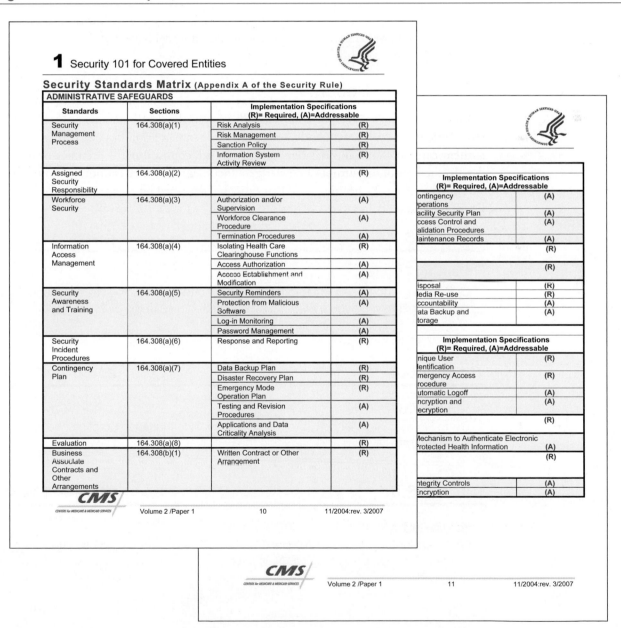

EXPAND YOUR LEARNING •))

Conduct an Internet search and identify a certification for a healthcare privacy or security specialty. Who offers the certification? What are the qualifications or requirements for the certification?

Because HIPAA is applicable to a variety of organizations classified as covered entities, HIPAA includes flexibility that allows covered entities to tailor security measures to their own situations while still keeping health information secure. Determining whether an addressable portion of the standard is applicable to a particular covered entity can be challenging. It involves analyzing the standard in reference to the likelihood of protecting the entity's ePHI from reasonably anticipated threats and hazards.

If the covered entity does not implement an addressable standard based on its assessment, the covered entity must document the reason why the implementation of the standard is not appropriate or reasonable. For example, a solo practitioner without any employees would likely not need to implement the Administrative Safeguards of the Security Rule. This specification states that employees should be sent security reminders about potential security threats via email, newsletters, and so on. Because there are no employees to be notified, this safeguard is not applicable.

Every covered entity is responsible for complying with the required and addressable standards or documenting why it does not need to comply with certain addressable elements. Covered entities should conduct an internal review of their compliance with the security standards.

EHR System Security

Because electronic data can be changed with a keystroke, EHR systems can track and record user activity. Consequently, once clinical documentation has been entered and authenticated (i.e., the author's signature is applied, confirming the accuracy of the data to the best of the author's knowledge), documented entries cannot be modified. Attempts to change a health record can easily be identified by an administrator by viewing the activity log.

Tutorial 6.3   **EHR**NAVIGAT⊕R

Denying Access

Go to Navigator+ to launch Tutorial 6.3. As a lab technician, you will experience what happens when you try to access a restricted area in the EHR Navigator.

Tutorial 6.4   **EHR**NAVIGAT⊕R

Changing an Email

Go to Navigator+ to launch Tutorial 6.4. As an office manager, practice changing a staff member's email address using the EHR Navigator.

Tutorial 6.5   **EHR**NAVIGAT⊕R

Reviewing a User Activity Log

Go to Navigator+ to launch Tutorial 6.5. As an IT administrator, practice reviewing a user activity log using the EHR Navigator.

HIPAA Security Rule Enforcement

Enforcement of the Security Rule follows the same process as enforcement of the Privacy Rule. The OCR has the responsibility for the enforcement, and the enforcement process starts with a complaint and follows through to a resolution with the Department of Justice when violations are criminal or the OCR when violations are civil.

From October 2009 through May 2014, more than 880 complaints of violations of the Security Rule were made, about 25% of which were breaches of the Security Rule. Theft and loss of data contributed to 67% of these breaches, with unauthorized access/disclosure at 21%, hacking at 6%, improper disposal at 5%, and other breaches at 1%.

Just as there were many high-profile examples of breaches of the Privacy Rule, there have been many large breaches of the Security Rule in recent history.

In January 2015, Anthem, a major health insurance company, experienced one of the largest security breaches in history when hackers broke into its database containing 80 million records. The information that the hackers stole included names, birthdays, medical IDs, Social Security numbers, street addresses, email addresses, and employment information, including income data. Another large security breach occurred in September 2011, when backup tapes storing PHI for 4.9 million people from a military EHR system were stolen from the car of a Science Applications International Corporation (SAIC) employee. At the time, SAIC was under contract with TRICARE, a US military insurance carrier, to provide off-site data storage and backup data security.

In September 2013, data thieves hacked into a physician office EHR. The hackers not only gained access to the healthcare information of more than 7,000 patients but also made the data completely inaccessible for the physician practice. The thieves then posted an electronic ransom note demanding that the physicians pay to get access to their data.

Organizations can learn many lessons from these reported breaches, such as the following:

- The opportunity to reduce risk through network or enterprise data storage as an alternative to local devices. **Enterprise data storage** is a centralized system (online or offline) that businesses use for managing and protecting data.

- The importance of encryption of ePHI on any desktop or portable device

- The need for clear and well-documented administrative and physical safeguards on the storage devices and media that handle ePHI

- The need to raise employee awareness of security and to promote good data stewardship. **Data stewardship** can be defined as the authority and responsibility associated with collecting, using, and disclosing health information in its identifiable and aggregate forms. The principles of data stewardship apply to all the personnel, systems, and processes engaging in health information storage and exchange within and across organizations.

EXPAND YOUR LEARNING

For more information about enterprise data storage, visit:

http://EHR2
.ParadigmEducation
.com/
EnterpriseStorage.

EXPAND YOUR LEARNING

For more information about data stewardship, refer to the article found at:

http://EHR2
.ParadigmEducation
.com/
DataStewardship.

Consider This

An employee of the State Department of Health and Social Services left a portable electronic storage device (USB drive) in a car that was later stolen. The USB drive contained ePHI, so the State Department of Health and Social Services submitted a report to the OCR, as all covered entities are required to do when a breach of health information security has occurred. When the OCR investigated, it found evidence that the department did not have adequate policies and procedures in place to safeguard ePHI. In addition, the department had not completed a risk analysis,

implemented sufficient risk management measures, completed security training for its workforce members, implemented device and media controls, or addressed device and media controls or encryption, as required by the HIPAA Security Rule.

Does the State Department of Health and Social Services have to follow the HIPAA Security Rule? Why? Is there a possibility that the department would be fined in this scenario? What do you think the findings of the OCR should be in this scenario?

Chapter Summary

Privacy and security of health information is a major focus of healthcare entities implementing and using electronic health records (EHRs). As a user of an EHR system, you must understand and follow the laws and regulations regarding privacy, safety, and security of health information. Federal legislation that revolutionized the release and security of health information includes the HIPAA Privacy and Security Rules published in 2000, which were subsequently updated in 2010 and 2013. These rules provide guidance about the release and security of paper health records, as well as the release and security of EHR data.

Healthcare entities must carefully follow all of the Privacy and Security Rules of the Health Insurance Portability and Accountability Act of 1996 (HIPAA) when selecting and installing EHRs, and they must remain vigilant in monitoring the use of protected health information (PHI) and electronic PHI (ePHI) in their organizations. In addition to setting standards for health information privacy and security, HIPAA also addresses standards to improve the efficiency and effectiveness of healthcare systems.

The Privacy Rule was published on December 28, 2000. It was later modified to yield the HIPAA Privacy, Security, and Enforcement Rules on January 25, 2013, to comply with the provisions of the Health Information Technology for Economic and Clinical Health (HITECH) Act, particularly with regard to EHRs. The Privacy and Security Rules apply to healthcare providers, health plans, and healthcare clearinghouses transmitting health information in an electronic format. These entities are called covered entities.

Certain types of health information are classified under the HIPAA Privacy Rule. These types include protected health information, individually identifiable health information, and deidentified health information. The Privacy Rule defines protected health information (PHI) as all individually identifiable health information held or transmitted by a covered entity or its business associate, in any form or media, whether electronic, paper, or oral. The term deidentified health information was coined by the Privacy Rule. It is health information that neither identifies an individual nor provides a reasonable basis to identify an individual.

A major purpose of the Privacy Rule is to define and limit the circumstances in which an individual's protected health information may be used or disclosed by covered entities. The Privacy Rule generally requires covered entities to take reasonable steps to limit the use or disclosure of, and requests for, protected health information to the minimum necessary to accomplish the intended purpose. This concept is called *minimum necessary* and is required by the Privacy Rule.

Workers must receive initial and ongoing training in the proper use and release of PHI and ePHI, as well as the importance of keeping healthcare data safe and secure.

Violations of the Privacy Rule fall into one of two categories: civil or criminal violations. The major difference between civil and criminal violations involves the intent behind the violation. A breach is an impermissible use or disclosure under the Privacy Rule that compromises the security or privacy of PHI such that the use or disclosure poses a significant risk of financial, reputational, or other harm to the affected individual.

Another important component of HIPAA is the security of health information. The Security Standards for the Protection of Electronic Protected Health Information were developed to address the security provisions of HIPAA and are commonly known as the Security Rule. The standards of the Security Rule are divided into six main sections: General Rules, Administrative Safeguards, Physical Safeguards, Technical Safeguards, Organizational Requirements, and Policies and Procedures and Documentation Requirements.

The privacy and security of health information is the responsibility of all healthcare providers.

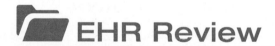# EHR Review

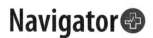**Navigator** The following EHR Review, EHR Application, and EHR Evaluation activities are also available online in the Navigator+ learning management system. Your instructor may ask you to complete these activities online. Navigator+ also provides access to flash cards, study games, and practice quizzes to help strengthen your understanding of the chapter content.

Acronyms/Initialisms

Study the following acronyms discussed in this chapter. Go to Navigator+ for flash cards of the acronyms and other chapter key terms.

CMS: Centers for Medicare & Medicaid Services

ePHI: electronic protected health information

HHS: US Department of Health & Human Services

HIPAA: Health Insurance Portability and Accountability Act of 1996

HITECH Act: Health Information Technology for Economic and Clinical Health Act

NwHIN: Nationwide Health Information Network

OCR: Office for Civil Rights

PHI: protected health information

ROI: release of information

TPO: treatment, payment, healthcare operations

Check Your Understanding

To check your understanding of this chapter's key concepts, answer the following questions.

1. What is an example of a *noncovered entity*?

    a. nursing home

    b. workers' compensation carrier

    c. military healthcare program

    d. healthcare clearinghouse

2. The acronym *TPO* stands for

    a. treatment, protection, organization.

    b. transmission, privacy, operations.

    c. treatment, payment, healthcare operations.

    d. type, patient, officials.

3. A breach is

    a. the transmission of health information in an electronic format.

    b. an impermissible use or disclosure under the Privacy or Security Rules.

    c. a data set used for healthcare research.

    d. a punishment enforced by the OCR.

4. After a Privacy Rule breach, _____ must be notified.

    a. the individual, the federal government, and in certain circumstances, the media

    b. the individual, the healthcare organization, and the insurance company

    c. the healthcare organization and the federal and state governments

    d. the federal and state governments and the media

5. Deidentified health information

   a. can never be used in marketing or research.

   b. neither identifies an individual nor provides a reasonable basis to identify an individual.

   c. does not directly identify an individual, but it may provide information that could be used to identify an individual.

   d. cannot be electronically transmitted.

6. True/False: Users of electronic health records are not required to follow the laws and regulations of the Health Insurance Portability and Accountability Act of 1996 (HIPAA).

7. True/False: If an entity does not meet the definition of *covered entity*, then it does not have to comply with the Privacy or Security Rule.

8. True/False: The Office for Civil Rights (OCR) has the responsibility for the enforcement of the HIPAA Privacy and Security Rules.

9. True/False: The major difference between criminal and civil punishments and penalties involves the intent behind the violation.

10. True/False: As patients and the public at large have become more familiar with HIPAA privacy rights, the number of complaints made to the OCR has steadily increased.

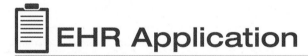 # EHR Application

Go on the Record

To build on your understanding of the topics in this chapter, complete the following short-answer activities.

1. What is the major purpose of the Privacy Rule?

2. What are the two situations in which disclosure of protected health information is required?

3. Describe a *limited data set* for purposes of research, public health, or healthcare operations.

4. Describe the differences between civil and criminal acts in violation of the Health Insurance Portability and Accountability Act of 1996 (HIPAA).

5. List the top five compliance issues that have been investigated by the federal government since HIPAA went into effect.

Navigate the Field

To gain practice in handling challenging situations in the workplace, consider the following real-world scenarios and identify how you would respond to each.

1. Hans Frank, office manager of Mountainview Surgical Clinic, was working on year-end reports at his home over the weekend. He spent several hours on Sunday compiling reports related to the 3,000 surgical patients who received treatment from Mountainview Surgical Clinic during the previous year. Unfortunately, while on his way to work on the subway on Monday, he inadvertently left his work laptop under his seat. In a panic, Mr. Frank tried to locate his laptop but was unsuccessful. Because this is clearly a breach of unsecured protected health information (PHI), what notification processes must Mountainview Surgical Clinic initiate?

2. Green Hills Valley Hospital has hired you to be the *Electronic Health Records Security Officer*. As you tour the hospital during your first week of employment, you notice that many of the nurses and other staff members are sharing user IDs and passwords to log onto the EHR system. As the security officer, what actions should you take to resolve this situation?

 # EHR Evaluation

Think Critically

Continue to think critically about challenging concepts and complete the following activities.

1. Interview a privacy or security officer at an acute care hospital to learn about the challenges of complying with the Health Insurance Portability and Accountability Act of 1996 (HIPAA) in a hospital that uses an EHR system.

2. Nearly everyone has seen news reports of cyberattacks against nationwide utility infrastructures or the information networks of the Pentagon. Healthcare providers may believe that if they are small and low profile, they will escape the attention of the criminals running these attacks. Yet, every day, new attacks are specifically aimed at small- to mid-size organizations, because they are low profile and less likely to have fully protected themselves. Criminals have been highly successful at penetrating these smaller organizations, carrying out their activities while their victims remain unaware until it is too late. Review the Office of the National Coordinator for Health Information Technology's cybersecurity checklist and discuss five best practices for a small healthcare environment to protect an EHR system. The checklist can be found at the following website:
http://EHR2.ParadigmEducation.com/SecurityChecklist.

Make Your Case

Consider the scenario and then complete the following project.

Describe the main components of the Privacy Rule and create a presentation with your findings.

Explore the Technology

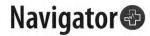

Complete the EHR Navigator practice assessments that align to each tutorial and the assessments that accompany Chapter 6 located on Navigator+.

Are You Ready?

A successful job search in the allied health field requires diligence and preparation. One area in which preparation is particularly critical is the job interview. The interview allows you to make a good first impression, emphasize your personal strengths and skills, and explain why you are the best candidate for the available position. With that in mind, do your homework before your interview by completing the following tasks:

- Research the company so that you are knowledgeable about the organization's history, structure, philosophy, and mission.

- Take time to practice your answers to typical interview questions regarding your personal characteristics, strengths and weaknesses, valuable work experiences, and professional goals.

- Prepare samples of your work and have them available to share with the interviewer.

- Plan your attire for the interview and ensure your clothing is appropriate for the position you are seeking.

The more prepared that you are, the easier the interview may be.

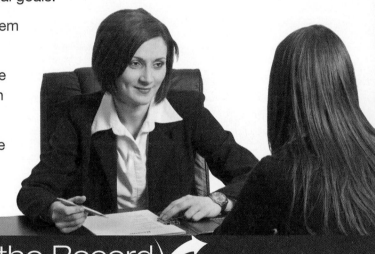

Beyond the Record

- 96% of US hospitals had adopted certified electronic health records (EHRs) by 2015.
- 87% of US physicians had adopted at least some form of EHRs by 2015.

- A survey conducted by the Centers for Disease Control and Prevention found that 75% of physicians said their organizations' EHR systems enhanced patient care.

7

Clinical Documentation and Reporting

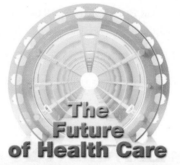

The Future of Health Care

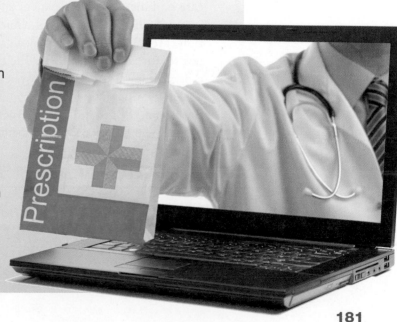

According to the US government's official website for health information technology, future technologies may offer many different ways for patients and their doctors to monitor and manage health care. These new practices could include the following:

- Use of global positioning system technology and real-time reminders and alerts to prevent and treat health conditions
- The ability to send health data to clinics from personal devices such as tablets and smartphones
- More virtual doctor visits and health coaching tailored to issues based on clinical data in a patient's EHR

7.1   Differentiate between *structured* and *unstructured* data and identify examples of each.

7.2   Explain manual and automated methods of data collection.

7.3   Identify the elements of a history and physical examination.

7.4   Understand how to enter progress notes into an EHR, as well the role of assessments, orders, test results, and other clinical documentation in the EHR system.

7.5   Identify the concerns related to cloned notes.

7.6   Define *e-prescribing* and its benefits and challenges.

7.7   Modify an e-prescription and override a drug allergy notification in the EHR.

7.8   Define *data mining* and its relationship to structured and unstructured data.

7.9   Understand clinical results reporting and discuss manual and automatic methods of results entry into the EHR.

7.10   Understand how EHR systems support public health initiatives.

7.11   Create a meaningful use report via the EHR Navigator.

7.12   Report an immunization in the EHR.

In 2008, only 41% of hospitals had a basic EHR system. By 2015, more than 80% of hospitals met meaningful use requirements for an EHR. The implementation of the EHR has streamlined data entry and encouraged interoperability of data and information. Depending on compatibility of the clinical system interface with other systems such as radiology, laboratory, pharmacy, and transcription services, healthcare staff members enter patient and clinical data either automatically or manually to create the EHR. Examples of clinical data include the history and physical examination (H&P), progress notes by all clinicians, immunization information, laboratory test results, and medications. The clinical input of medication information via the e-prescribing feature of EHR systems has improved the safety and efficiency of drug administration. While this textbook has explored many of the scheduling, administrative, and health information management data activities in an EHR system, this chapter will focus on clinical documentation and reporting.

Clinical Documentation in the EHR

Clinical documentation, also known as **clinical inputs**, contains data related to the patient's clinical status that is entered into the patient's EHR or paper record. Data entered into an EHR can be classified as either structured or unstructured.

Structured data is stored in a specific, organized fashion within a database. Examples of structured data include date of birth, sex, race, lab results, and International Classification of Diseases (ICD) codes. **Unstructured data** is information that is stored in a free-form format. Examples of unstructured data include primarily the narrative portions of the EHR such as progress notes, test interpretations, and operative reports. Data will be explored more indepth in Chapter 10.

Data Collection

EXPAND YOUR LEARNING

The Standards and Interoperability Framework within the Office of the National Coordinator for Health Information Technology (ONC) was formed to gather input from both public and private sectors regarding the creation of standardized health information technology specifications for use throughout the United States. In January 2013, the Standards and Interoperability Framework launched the Structured Data Capture initiative. Read about this initiative at the following website. Why is this initiative important to the interoperability of EHRs?

http://EHR2
.ParadigmEducation
.com/DataCapture

Data collection for the EHR occurs through a combination of manual and automated methods. **Manual data collection** of demographic and insurance information is often initiated by a staff member upon initial patient contact with a healthcare facility. The data is typically obtained from a preprinted form the patient has completed or during an in-person interview; however, at times, the information is collected over the telephone. A staff member subsequently enters this information into the EHR system. Some healthcare organizations ask patients to enter their own demographic data through a secure, personal Internet link that a staff member sends to the patient to begin developing the EHR.

Automated data collection occurs when the data from the initial patient encounter is automatically copied over to each new patient encounter using an automated data capture. Automated data

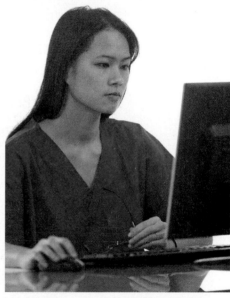

Healthcare workers manually enter demographic and insurance information into the EHR. On subsequent visits, this information is automatically copied over to the next patient encounter.

collection is the preferred method of data capture because it requires less personnel time, avoids repetitive requests of information from patients, and may allow for more consistent data capture. The era of patients entering EHR data highlights the importance of frontline review for errors and duplication of data. The success of patient-initiated entry of demographic data relies on a healthcare facility's structured auditing and correction procedures to reconcile data errors and/or duplications. As EHR technology has evolved, more data collection has been automated, and healthcare professionals enter less information manually.

History and Physical Examination

A **history and physical examination (H&P)** is a part of most patient encounters with healthcare providers and is a valuable tool for the healthcare provider in the identification of diagnoses. The H&P consists of two main elements: a subjective element and an objective element.

Subjective Element

The **history** is the subjective element of the H&P because it is obtained from the patient or a family member as well as a review of previous medical records. **Subjective element** is based on personal reporting and opinions. The history begins with the **chief complaint**, which is the patient's stated reason for seeking health services. The chief complaint is then followed by one or more of the following components:

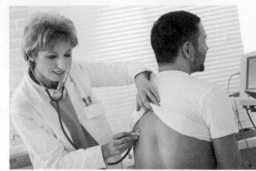

The physical examination is the objective portion of the history and physical.

- History of present illness

- Past medical issues

- Allergies

- Medications currently prescribed to the patient

- Family and social histories

Objective Element

The **physical examination** is the objective element of the H&P. **Objective information** is based on facts and not subject to the interpretation required for subjective information. This procedure is conducted by the nursing or medical staff and consists of an investigation of the patient's body systems, an assessment of his or her condition, and a treatment plan. The inventory of each body system is called the **review of systems (ROS)**. The ROS consists of the following system assessments:

1. General (documents the general appearance of the patient, such as, "A 66-year-old Caucasian woman in no acute distress. Patient is alert and able to discuss medical history.")

2. Vital signs (includes the patient's blood pressure, pulse, respiratory rate, pulse oximetry, and body temperature)

3. Head, ears, eyes, nose, and throat (HEENT)

4. Respiratory

5. Cardiovascular

6. Abdominal

7. Gastrointestinal

8. Genitourinary

9. Musculoskeletal

10. Neurologic

Depending on the reason for the patient's visit, the physician may conduct a complete ROS or a selective ROS that focuses on the body systems involved with the patient's chief complaint(s). For example, a high school student whose chief complaint is that he or she wishes to participate in sports will likely need a complete ROS to ensure his or her health status is appropriate for participation in the sport. However, a 10-year-old whose chief complaint is throat pain will likely receive only a general examination along with a check of vital signs and a review of the HEENT system.

Once the healthcare provider has reviewed the history of the patient, physically examined the patient, and evaluated all recent laboratory and diagnostic test results, the provider assesses the patient's diagnoses and decides on a **treatment plan** to alleviate the patient's condition.

Depending on the preference of the healthcare provider, the provider may type the H&P directly into the EHR or dictate a report and have a transcriptionist type and upload the report into the patient's EHR. **Uploading** is the process of transmitting a file from one computer to another computer or portal.

Tutorial 7.1   **EHR**NAVIGAT✚R

Viewing a History and Physical Report

Go to Navigator+ to launch Tutorial 7.1. As an occupational therapist, practice reviewing a patient's history and physical report using the EHR Navigator.

Electronic Health Record Templates

Many of the clinical inputs to an EHR system are accomplished using a **template**, which is a preformatted file that provides prompts to obtain specific, consistent information. For healthcare providers, the use of a template does the following:

- Indicates required fields that must be completed during the documentation process

- Ensures consistent data-gathering techniques among users

- Allows for efficient data entry through the use of structured input options such as drop-down menus and check boxes

- Provides immediate data population of the EHR system

- Avoids the added expense of hiring a transcriptionist to document patient information

- Facilitates easy access to data because of its consistent format, thus avoiding time-consuming searches

- Enables faster and more precise reporting and analysis of data because of its format and consistent elements

Clearly, EHR templates offer several advantages. However, their use should never hinder thorough documentation by a healthcare provider. For any selections not available in drop-down menus, a provider will need to input patient information to ensure accuracy and completeness of the patient record.

Certain patient diagnoses or conditions may dictate the creation of specialized templates that offer information fields tailored to specific documentation needs. Specialized healthcare providers may also need specialized templates. For example, a detailed eye examination template like the one shown in Figure 7.1 would be a useful tool for an ophthalmologist. Depending on the policies of a healthcare organization, staff members may conduct special assessments to determine these special needs.

Figure 7.1 Eye Examination Template

Choose an item. Visual Acuity OD	Choose an item. Visual Acuity OS
Choose an item. Pinhole OD	Choose an item. Pinhole OS
Yes ☐No ☐Afferent Pupillary Defect OD	Yes ☐No ☐Afferent Pupillary Defect OS
Yes ☐No ☐Dilated OD	Yes ☐No ☐Dilated OS
[ ] IOP OD	[ ] IOP OS
[ ] CVF OD	[ ] CVF OS
Yes ☐No ☐Lid OD WNL	Yes ☐No ☐Lid OS WNL
Choose an item. Lid OD	Choose an item. Lid OS
Yes ☐No ☐Conjunctiva/Sclera OD WNL?	Yes ☐No ☐Conjunctiva/Sclera OS WNL?
Choose an item. Conjunctiva/Sclera OD	Choose an item. Conjunctiva/Sclera OS

CHECKPOINT 7.1

1. Provide two reasons why automated data collection is the preferred method of data capture.

   _____

   _____

2. Define history and physical examination and identify the two main elements of an H&P.

   _____

   _____

Nursing Documentation

In an inpatient environment, such as an acute care hospital, rehabilitation hospital, or psychiatric hospital, nurses spend a considerable amount of their shifts documenting the care and treatment of the patients under their care. There are many patient assessments that nurses conduct and document upon admission and throughout a patient's stay. Nurses conduct an admission assessment shortly after the patient's arrival to the hospital room. This admission assessment is similar to the history and physical examination that was previously discussed but is completed from a nursing perspective. Major assessment areas on the nursing admission assessment typically include general admission data, patient history, physical assessments of all major body systems, and spiritual, cultural, and social histories and perspectives. Table 7.1 provides more detail of the major assessment areas.

Table 7.1 Nursing Admission Assessment

Major Assessment Area	Data Items Included
General Admission Data	• Patient demographics (name, address, date of birth, marital status, etc.) • Admission source (where was the patient admitted from, e.g., home, nursing home, emergency room) • Reason for admission • Vital signs (temperature, pulse, and blood pressure) • Height and weight • Communication needs (hard of hearing, needs interpreter, etc.) • Advance directives (living will, durable power of attorney for health care, code status) • Patient belongings (what the patient brought to the hospital, including clothes, glasses, cell phone, and money) • Physicians (including the admitting physician, attending physician, consulting physicians, and primary care physician)
Patient History	• Allergies • Medications • Diagnoses • Past diagnoses • Past surgical procedures
Physical Assessments	• Pain assessment • Neurological assessment • Fall risk assessment • Cardiac assessment • Respiratory assessment • Gastrointestinal assessment • Nutrition assessment • Genitourinary assessment • Skin assessment • Musculoskeletal assessment • Peripheral vascular assessment
Spiritual/Cultural/Social Assessments	• Spiritual needs • Cultural needs • Social situation (lives alone, with spouse, with children, etc.) • Discharge plans (where patient wants to live after discharge)

Progress Notes

Progress notes are the portion of the health record in which healthcare providers of all disciplines document the patient's progress, or lack thereof, in relation to the established goals of the care plan. Healthcare providers may choose to write or transcribe progress notes in any format. For healthcare organizations that have adopted an EHR system, this task can be easily completed through the use of customized templates.

Progress Note Templates

These templates provide information fields that cater to certain disciplines and specialties. For example, a template for a physical therapy progress note may include checkboxes to indicate whether the patient can bear weight on the right side and on the left side and drop-down menus with options for indicating the patient's range of motion and pain level. A progress note template for a cardiologist may allow healthcare providers to select different causes of syncope (i.e., cardiac, metabolic, neurologic). Use of a progress note template lessens data entry time and ensures the inclusion of all pertinent data elements.

Tutorial 7.2

EHRNAVIGAT⊕R

Entering a Progress Note

Go to Navigator+ to launch Tutorial 7.2. As a nurse, practice entering a progress note into a patient's chart using the EHR Navigator.

Cloned Progress Notes

One area of concern related to EHR progress notes has been the increased use of cloned progress notes. A **cloned progress note** is a note that has been partially or totally copied from an existing progress note. The copied note is then updated by the healthcare provider to include any new information. This shortcut may save time, but it can also result in inaccurate or outdated documentation regarding a patient's health status and progress if the healthcare provider forgets to make the necessary updates to the existing note. Consequently, other healthcare providers may make inappropriate medical decisions based on incorrect patient information, which could have dire consequences for the patient.

What's The **Buzz**

If you see this Blue Button on the website of a hospital, provider, insurance company, pharmacy, lab, clinic, or immunization registry, it signifies that patients are able to access their health information electronically. Widespread use of the Blue Button is encouraged by the Office of the National Coordinator for Health Information Technology (ONC) so that patients and their families can identify and access their health information and more fully participate in their health care.

Consider This

Dr. Sebold's progress note for 9/12/2030, 6:20 a.m.:
Patient examined and found in no acute distress. Patient has no complaints at this time. Lab values reviewed and all within normal limits. Continue current plan of treatment.

Nurse Akin's nurse's note for 9/13/2030, 4:50 a.m.:
Patient complains of nausea and headache. Vital signs: BP 180/101, T 101.8°, P 87, R 12. Resident telephoned and ordered CBC. Abnormal WBC of 9000. Resident telephoned and ordered urine culture. Awaiting results.

Dr. Sebold's progress note for 9/12/2030, 7:10 a.m.:
Patient examined and found in no acute distress. Patient has no complaints at this time. Lab values reviewed and all within normal limits. Continue current plan of treatment.

How does Dr. Sebold's progress note conflict with Nurse Akin's progress note? If you compare Dr. Sebold's progress notes on two different days, you will note that the documentation is identical, indicating the use of a cloned progress note.

Cloned progress notes may also affect the process of coding diagnoses and procedures for reimbursement purposes. Coding classification systems, such as the International Classification of Diseases (ICD) and Current Procedural Terminology® (CPT®), require detailed documentation for accurate coding. Coding classification systems will be covered in detail in Chapter 8. Cloned progress notes that do not accurately reflect patient diagnoses and treatment may result in inaccurate code assignment, which in turn could lead to reduced reimbursement and increased focus and monitoring from payer sources.

The Office of Inspector General (OIG) in the US Department of Health and Human Services is responsible for combating healthcare fraud, waste, and abuse and for working to improve healthcare efficiency. To that end, the OIG routinely audits the billing and coding practices of healthcare organizations. Health record documentation must support code assignment and bills submitted for Medicare and Medicaid reimbursement. The OIG establishes an annual **Work Plan** of areas of healthcare documentation and billing practices to be addressed and audited during the year. The goals of the OIG are to ensure that healthcare organizations maintain accurate coding and billing records and that documentation is accurate and consistent throughout health records. Because of initial problems with cloned documentation in the early years of EHR implementation, the OIG included cloned documentation as a focus area in the 2012, 2013, and 2014 Work Plans. The use of cloned documentation was sufficiently reduced so that the OIG removed it from the Work Plans subsequent to 2014.

Consider This

The Emergency Care Research Institute (ECRI) conducted a study looking at the frequency of cloning/copying and pasting in a random sample of 239 EHR notes. The study indicated that 10.8% of notes contained cloned material, and the frequency varied by specialty. Endocrinology notes were the highest, at 19.5% of notes containing cloned materials, and cardiology was the lowest, at 1.9% containing copied material. Obviously, cloning is a time-saving activity. However, what problems could arise from cloned progress note documentation?

E-Prescribing

Another documentation feature available to users of EHR systems is electronic prescribing, commonly known as **e-prescribing**. This feature allows a physician, nurse practitioner, or physician assistant to electronically transmit a new prescription or renewal authorization to a pharmacy. The healthcare provider enters the medication order along with the location of the patient's pharmacy into the patient's EHR, and the e-prescription is automatically transmitted to the pharmacy, where it is filled for patient pickup. All EHR systems must have the e-prescribing feature, because meaningful use requires that more than 50% of all permissible prescriptions written by an eligible healthcare provider are electronically transmitted using certified EHR technology.

Benefits of E-Prescribing

For healthcare providers, the benefits of e-prescribing include improved prescribing accuracy and efficiency, a decreased potential for medication errors and prescription forgeries, and more accurate and timely billing. Using e-prescriptions lessens the risk for potential medication errors due to unclear handwriting, illegible faxes, or misinterpreted prescription abbreviations. EHR systems also have the ability to alert a healthcare provider if he or she prescribes a drug to which the patient is allergic, resulting in improved medication safety. Many studies indicate that the use of the e-prescribing feature of EHR systems has reduced medication errors by 12% to 15%, which translates to 17.4 million medication errors averted per year. E-prescriptions also benefit patients in terms of improved accuracy in medication administration, more effective and efficient communication between patients and prescribers, and timely notifications for refills. Overall, e-prescription functionality improves patient care quality and reduces healthcare costs. Figure 7.2 illustrates an e-prescription.

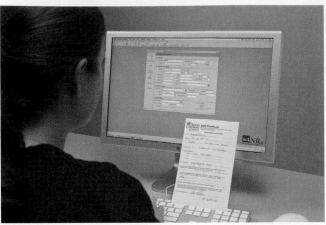

Practitioners enter orders for medications along with the patient's pharmacy location into the patient's EHR, and the prescription is automatically transmitted to the pharmacy.

The e-prescribing component of an EHR includes an alert function that notifies the prescribing healthcare provider of drug-to-drug interactions, drug-to-food interactions, and the patient's allergies to medications. These alerts are grouped into a hierarchy of potential risk and seriousness of the interactions or allergies, and healthcare prescribers

Figure 7.2   E-Prescription

```
---------------------------------------------------------------
!!! -- START SECURED ELECTRONIC PRESCRIPTION TRANSMISSION -- !!!
---------------------------------------------------------------
FROM THE OFFICES OF PHIL JACKSON, MD; ETHEL JACOBSON, MD;
                    PETER JARKOWSKI, PA; EUGENE JOHNSON, DO

OFFICE ADDRESS:          67 EAST ELM
                         CEDAR RAPIDS, IA 52411
OFFICE TELEPHONE:        (319) 555-1212    TRANSMIT DATE: FEB 20, 2030
OFFICE FAX:              (319) 555-1313    WRITTEN DATE:  FEB 20, 2030
---------------------------------------------------------------
TRANSMITTED TO           THE CORNER DRUG STORE
PHARMACY ADDRESS:        875 PARADIGM WAY
                         CEDAR RAPIDS, IA 52410
PHARMACY TELEPHONE:      (319) 555-1414
---------------------------------------------------------------
PATIENT NAME:            JEFFREY KLEIN     D.O.B.: OCT 18, 1994
PATIENT ADDRESS:         1157 NORTH PLAZA AVE
                         CEDAR RAPIDS, IA 52411
---------------------------------------------------------------
PRESCRIBED MEDICATION:   FLUOXETINE 20 MG
SIGNA:                   i PO QD
DISPENSE QUANTITY:       30
REFILL(S):               PRN
---------------------------------------------------------------
PHYSICIAN SIGNATURE:     [[ ELECTRONIC SIGNATURE ON FILE ]]
                         [[ FOR DR. ETHEL JACOBSON ]]
---------------------------------------------------------------
!!! -- END SECURED ELECTRONIC PRESCRIPTION TRANSMISSION -- !!!
---------------------------------------------------------------
```

may override less serious interactions or allergies and continue to prescribe the medication. For example, if there is only one medication that will be effective in treating a life-threatening illness and the potential drug-to-drug interaction may result in a minor drop in blood pressure, the physician may determine that the need for the medication is worth the minor drop in blood pressure.

Challenges of E-Prescribing

Although e-prescribing affords many benefits to both patients and healthcare providers, there are also some challenges associated with the use of this technology. When EHRs were first implemented, the major challenge of fully implementing e-prescribing involved the dispensing of controlled substances. A **controlled substance** is a drug (primarily a narcotic) declared by US federal or state law to be illegal for sale or use by the general public but legal if dispensed per a healthcare provider's prescription. The basis for determining whether a drug is a controlled substance is the drug's potential for addiction, abuse, or harm.

Although US federal and state laws governing the distribution of controlled substances were in place prior to 1970, in that year the drug counterculture of the 1960s led the US government to enact stronger legislation regarding the manufacture and distribution of narcotics, stimulants, depressants, hallucinogens, anabolic steroids, and chemicals used in the illicit production of controlled substances. This legislation, known as the **Controlled Substances Act of 1970**, placed tight controls on the pharmaceutical and healthcare industries and outlined five schedules of controlled substances based on potential for harm. This legislation established additional procedures for healthcare providers writing prescriptions for controlled substances. These procedures required that prescribers use hard copy or printed prescriptions when ordering Schedule II controlled substances. Consequently, the use of e-prescriptions for these substances had to be approved by individual US state boards of pharmacy before this technology could be implemented. In August 2015, Vermont became the final state to permit e-prescribing for all medications, including all controlled substances.

Even though the legal barrier regarding controlled substances has been eliminated, using e-prescribing to order controlled substances is still a challenge because many EHR systems have not upgraded software to handle the e-prescribing of controlled substances. In addition, many providers are uncomfortable using e-prescribing for many of the frequently abused painkillers, such as oxycodone, hydrocodone, and morphine, fearing breaches in the security of the EHR may allow for fraudulent prescriptions.

Another challenge associated with e-prescribing is the lack of interoperability between healthcare facility EHR software and some pharmacy software. An e-prescription is not useful to a patient if he or she is unable to fill it at the pharmacy. If a pharmacy's software does not communicate with the healthcare facility's EHR, a traditional handwritten prescription must be used.

Tutorial 7.3

EHRNAVIGAT⊕R

Modifying a Patient's Prescription

Go to Navigator+ to launch Tutorial 7.3. As a physician, practice modifying a patient's prescription using the EHR Navigator.

Overriding a Drug Allergy Notification

Go to Navigator+ to launch Tutorial 7.4. As a physician assistant, practice adding an e-prescription and overriding a drug allergy notification using the EHR Navigator.

Consider This

Prescriptions that have been handwritten by physicians or other prescribers pose a number of potentially serious problems. The combination of handwriting style and the use of abbreviations can lead to difficulty in reading and filling the prescription accurately. This can result in mistaken drug names, dosages, and strengths. Another issue with handwritten prescriptions is that they can be easily altered by drug seekers. In light of these issues, how does the use of e-prescribing decrease the potential for medication errors and prescription forgeries?

CHECKP⊕INT 7.2

1. List three benefits of e-prescribing.

2. What legal barrier previously prevented e-prescribing from being fully implemented?

Clinical Results Reporting

Clinical reporting, also known as **clinical outputs**, contains data that can be extracted from a patient record and compiled in a meaningful way. For example, a physician might run a cumulative report of the laboratory results of a patient to easily determine if trends in laboratory values need to be addressed. The transcribed reports of an H&P as well as consultations and radiology reports are additional examples of clinical output. All clinicians involved in the patient's care can then use this data.

Data mining is the process of searching for and examining data to organize it into useful patterns and trends. Data mining and reporting of structured data can be accomplished quickly and easily using an EHR system because the fixed nature of structured data makes it easy to search for, query, and quantify. Data mining of unstructured data is a more challenging process that researchers and developers are working hard to simplify. A wealth of information is buried in the narrative provider notes of an EHR, waiting to be manipulated and studied.

Clinical results reporting is an EHR system function that allows healthcare providers to view laboratory and diagnostic test results immediately, provided there is an interface between the clinical results system and the EHR. This feature satisfies one of the National Patient Safety Goals (NPSGs) of The Joint Commission, an organization that surveys and accredits hospitals and other types of healthcare facilities. Hospitals accredited by The Joint Commission are required to comply with the NPSGs, which

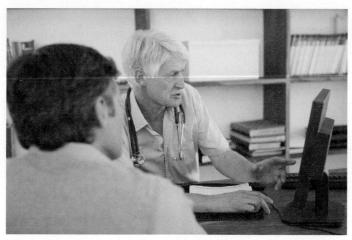

With clinical results reporting, clinicians are able to view and discuss lab results with patients immediately upon completion.

were established to help hospitals address specific areas of concern in regard to patient safety. The first set of NPSGs became effective on January 1, 2003, and the goals are annually updated by The Joint Commission based on the recommendations of the Patient Safety Advisory Group, a panel of widely recognized patient safety experts that includes nurses, physicians, pharmacists, risk managers, clinical engineers, and other professionals with hands-on experience in addressing patient safety issues. Reporting the critical results of tests and diagnostic procedures in a timely manner has been included in the NPSGs since 2005 and is likely to remain on the list of NPSGs for many years.

According to surveyors from The Joint Commission, "There is an increased awareness that poor communication is at the heart of medical errors and lawsuits, which is why The Joint Commission is emphasizing the role of communication in critical value reporting." This goal is meant to ensure that laboratories report important clinical results to healthcare personnel in a timely manner, thereby allowing them to expediently treat patients. Hospitals must have policies and procedures in place that specify the time frame during which healthcare providers must be advised of test results that are considered critical. Each healthcare organization is responsible for specifying the values and circumstances that define a critical test result. These specifications should be clearly defined in facility policy and medical staff bylaws. For example, the hematocrit laboratory value might be considered critical if it was below 18% or greater than 55% for an adult. A chest X-ray with a suspicious shadow may also be considered critical.

Automated Clinical Results Reporting

The clinical results reporting feature of EHR systems addresses a long-standing problem associated with phone and fax communications of test results, which is the inability for healthcare providers to receive these communications during times they are not in their offices (such as weekends, holidays, and nighttime hours). When EHR systems are able to interface with laboratory computers and other computers that output test results, healthcare providers can use personal computers or mobile devices to access test results and order medications, treatments, and further tests to address the reported results. This is an example of the **automatic method** of results entry. In addition, many EHR systems are able to generate email or text alerts to notify providers of critical test results or other important information.

Manual Method of Clinical Results Reporting

In an environment that does not have an EHR system interfaced with laboratory computers, the laboratory sends a printed report via fax to the prescriber's office, and then a staff member scans the report into the EHR. This is an example of the **manual method** of results entry. However, the preferred method for retrieving lab and test reports would be via automatic transmission or an interface between the laboratory systems and the EHR.

Eventually, most laboratory and other diagnostic company computers will be interfaced with all EHR systems, but this process will take many years to accomplish. In the meantime, telecommunications continues to be the best way to obtain test results for facilities whose laboratory computers cannot interface or transfer clinical results. Until total interface and interoperability is achieved, scanning of results is a manageable process and the best option available for some EHR users.

Tutorial 7.5

EHRNAVIGAT⊕R

Viewing Clinical Results

Go to Navigator+ to launch Tutorial 7.5. As a medical assistant, practice viewing a patient's lab results using the EHR Navigator.

Tutorial 7.6

EHRNAVIGAT⊕R

Signing a Scanned Diagnostic Report

Go to Navigator+ to launch Tutorial 7.6. As a physician, practice signing a scanned diagnostic report using the EHR Navigator.

Meaningful Use and Public Health Objectives

As you have learned throughout this text, there are core measures of meaningful use that must be achieved by healthcare organizations if they plan to receive incentive payments for EHR adoption. Stage 1 and 2 requirements of meaningful use have been implemented or are in the process of being implemented by healthcare organizations. EHR systems are able to demonstrate compliance with these requirements by collecting data and running reports that indicate core measure compliance. They also reveal noncompliance in core measures.

Stage 1 of meaningful use has three public health objectives that require the capability of the EHR system to submit electronic data to public health agencies for:

- Immunization registries

- Reportable laboratory results

- **Syndromic surveillance** (syndromic describes a group of symptoms that, when grouped together, are characteristic of a specific disorder or disease)

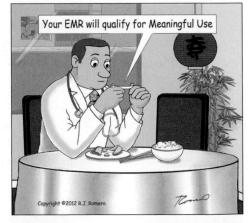

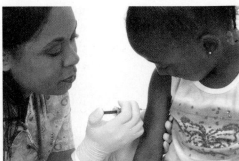

Immunization registries are part of Stage 1 of meaningful use.

EXPAND
YOUR LEARNING

To read about
engaged physicians
whose time commit-
ments to the EHR
implementation at
their practices have
resulted in positive
outcomes, visit
http://EHR2
.ParadigmEducation
.com/Physician
Commitment.

The US government included these meaningful use requirements for EHRs to improve collaboration between clinical and public health organizations at both the local and state levels. Consequently, these public health agencies (PHAs) may utilize the electronic data to improve the quality of health care, reduce healthcare disparities among various groups, and improve public health. An EHR system allows this data exchange to automatically occur with minimal interaction from healthcare personnel.

Immunization Registries

Healthcare clinics can report confidential, anonymous vaccination data about their patients to public health agencies. Immunization registries are important tools to help remind patients when vaccines are past due and consolidate immunization records for patients who may have multiple healthcare providers.

Tutorial 7.7   EHRNAVIGAT⊕R

Reporting an Immunization

Go to Navigator+ to launch Tutorial 7.7. As a medical assistant, practice reporting an immunization using the EHR Navigator.

EXPAND
YOUR LEARNING

For more information
on reportable condi-
tions, visit
http://EHR2
.ParadigmEducation
.com/Reportable
Conditions.

Reportable Laboratory Results

Reportable laboratory results for meaningful use is the electronic transfer of data from laboratories to PHAs. Reporting on conditions of concern to public health is a cornerstone of public health surveillance and includes the reporting of laboratory results that may indicate a notifiable condition. The Council of State and Territorial Epidemiologists determines the list of reportable conditions that are nationally notifiable on a voluntary basis to the Centers for Disease Control and Prevention (CDC) by state PHAs. Some examples of conditions that are reportable include anthrax, measles, rubella, polio, smallpox, and botulism.

Using the EHR system for laboratory results reporting has many benefits, including improved timeliness of reportable conditions, reduction of manual data entry errors, and more complete information provided to PHAs.

Syndromic Surveillance

Syndromic surveillance is the process of using near real-time health and health-related data to make information available on the health of a community. This information includes statistics on disease trends and community health behaviors. Syndromic surveillance is particularly useful to local, state, and federal PHAs for the awareness of public health trends, determining when emergency response is needed, and identifying an outbreak or potential outbreak of disease. Patient encounter data from healthcare settings are a critical input for syndromic surveillance, which is greatly enhanced with the transfer of patient data via EHRs. Clinical data are provided by hospitals and urgent care centers to PHAs for all patient encounters. The PHAs then use the Public Health Information Network, which is a national system for the electronic exchange of data operated by the CDC, to electronically exchange data and information across organizations and jurisdictions (e.g., clinical care to public health, public health to public health, and public health to other federal agencies).

Chapter Summary

Clinical documentation and reporting are at the core of the EHR system, making this system an interactive repository of timely, valuable, and possibly lifesaving data.

Data collection for the EHR occurs through a combination of manual and automated methods. Automated data collection is the preferred method of data capture, because it requires less personnel time, avoids repetitive requests of information from patients, and allows for more consistent data. Patient demographic data is usually entered manually at the patient's first encounter with the healthcare organization and is automated at subsequent visits. History and physical examination results, progress notes, assessments, consultations, and operative reports are examples of documents that may be manually or electronically added to the EHR. An area of concern related to EHR progress notes has been the increased use of cloned progress notes. Healthcare providers must ensure that their documentation is accurate at all times.

Diagnostic tests such as laboratory results are ideally transferred directly from the laboratory computer to the EHR. E-prescribing has greatly benefited patients and providers, with improved accuracy in medication administration and efficiencies related to communications and refills.

Without the capability for exchange of clinical data inputs and outputs, the EHR system would function merely as a static, electronic file folder. From filling e-prescriptions to the emergency review of laboratory results, the electronic exchange of clinical information has proven to be invaluable to patients and their caregivers.

Healthcare organizations must achieve core measures of meaningful use if they plan to receive incentive payments for EHR adoption. Stage 1 requires EHRs to have the ability to submit electronic data to public agencies for immunization registries, reportable laboratory results, and syndromic surveillance.

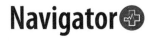

Navigator The following EHR Review, EHR Application, and EHR Evaluation activities are also available online in the Navigator+ learning management system. Your instructor may ask you to complete these activities online. Navigator+ also provides access to flash cards, study games, and practice quizzes to help strengthen your understanding of the chapter content.

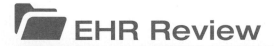

EHR Review

Acronyms/Initialisms

Study the following acronyms discussed in this chapter. Go to Navigator+ for flash cards of the acronyms and other chapter key terms.

CDC: Centers for Disease Control and Prevention

CPT®: Current Procedural Terminology

H&P: history and physical examination

HEENT: head, ears, eyes, nose, and throat

ICD: International Classification of Diseases

NPSG: National Patient Safety Goals

PHA: public health agency   **ROS:** review of systems
OIG: Office of Inspector General

Check Your Understanding

To check your understanding of this chapter's key concepts, answer the following questions.

1. *Uploading* is

    a. the transmission and filling of prescriptions.

    b. the process of transmitting a file from one computer to another.

    c. the auditing of computer files.

    d. the transmission of computer viruses.

2. Which document contains the results of the examination of a patient's body systems?

    a. operative report

    b. radiology report

    c. laboratory report

    d. history and physical examination (H&P)

3. Which of the following statements concerning e-prescribing are *true*?

    a. E-prescribing is the electronic generation and transmission of prescriptions.

    b. E-prescribing increases the efficiency of healthcare practices.

    c. E-prescribing assists prescribers by telling them which medication they should order for each diagnosis.

    d. Both *a* and *b* are true.

4. The abbreviation ROS means a

    a. review of systems on the history and physical examination.

    b. record of steroid use in e-prescribing.

    c. report of substance abuse.

    d. review of syndromic surveillance.

5. Which of the following is *not* one of the meaningful use Stage 1 public health objectives?

    a. immunization registries

    b. reportable laboratory results

    c. prescription fraud prevention

    d. syndromic surveillance

6. True/False: The e-prescribing feature of an EHR system is an optional meaningful use function.

7. True/False: A template is a preformatted file that provides prompts to obtain specific, consistent information.

8. True/False: If a physician's office does not interface with a laboratory's computer, there is no way to incorporate laboratory results into the EHR system.

9. True/False: A physician who copies and pastes documentation from one progress note to another is creating cloned notes.

10. True/False: Per US law, Schedule II controlled substances cannot be ordered via e-prescribing.

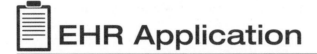

EHR Application

Go on the Record

To build on your understanding of the topics in this chapter, complete the following short-answer activities.

1. Explain why a healthcare provider might use cloned progress notes.

2. Describe the benefits of e-prescribing.

3. List three body systems examined during an H&P.

4. Describe the two elements of an H&P.

5. Explain how Northstar Medical Center can prove that its EHR system meets the core requirements of meaningful use.

Navigate the Field

To gain practice in handling challenging situations in the workplace, consider the following real-world scenarios and identify how you would respond to each.

1. You are the health information manager at a local hospital. A physician on the medical staff does not understand how to add H&P notes to a patient's EHR. He explains that he "always used to handwrite the H&P." You explain to the physician that he can no longer handwrite his H&P notes, and you give him two options of how he can add his H&P notes to the EHR. Describe these two options.

2. You are a laboratory manager at a local hospital. Your laboratory systems can interface with the hospital's EHR system to automatically provide test results. However, there are times when this process does not function properly and results have to be entered manually. As the laboratory manager, you want to develop a procedure for doing this. What steps might you include in this procedure? Write a one-page procedure for manually entering laboratory results into the hospital's EHR system when the laboratory computer cannot automatically transfer the laboratory results to the hospital's EHR system.

Think Critically

Continue to think critically about challenging concepts and complete the following activities.

1. As the quality manager at a local hospital, you are conducting an audit of physician progress notes to ensure that the progress notes accurately reflect the condition of the patient and are not simply cloned notes depicting inaccuracies.

   Patient Scenario #1: Progress note of 10/4/2030, 07:45: Infectious disease note: No fevers/chills. Tolerating antibiotics without difficulty. Lungs clear. Abdomen soft with positive bowel sounds. PICC without phlebitis. Vanc trough value of 10/2/2030 is 14.0.

   Which of the following progress notes is accurately written according to Patient Scenario #1 if the patient's status is completely the same as it was on 10/4/2030?

   _____ a. Progress note of 10/5/2030, 10:00: Infectious disease note: No changes from progress note of 10/4/2030, 07:45.

   _____ b. Progress note of 10/5/2030, 16:00: Infectious disease note: No fevers/chills. Tolerating antibiotics without difficulty. Lungs clear. Abdomen soft with positive bowel sounds. PICC without phlebitis. Vanc trough value of 10/2/2030 is 14.0.

   _____ c. Progress note of 10/5/2030, 14:00: Infectious disease note: Temp of 101.8°F today. Tolerating antibiotics without difficulty. Lungs clear. Abdomen soft with positive bowel sounds. PICC without phlebitis. Vanc trough value of 10/2/2030 is 14.0.

   Patient Scenario #2: Progress note of 04/12/2030, 08:10: Pulmonary note: Patient doing well on trach collar. Afebrile. Chest clear. No edema. Chronic respiratory failure. Change trach to #6 and start capping speech to evaluate for swallowing.

Which of the following progress notes is accurately written according to Patient Scenario #2 if the patient's status is completely the same as it was on 04/12/2030, except the patient now has a fever of 101.4°F?

_____ a. Progress note of 04/13/2030, 14:15: Pulmonary note: Patient doing well on trach collar. Fever of 101.4°F. Chest rales heard. No edema. Chronic respiratory failure. Change trach to #6 and start capping speech to evaluate for swallowing.

_____ b. Progress note of 04/13/2030, 14:10: Pulmonary note: Patient doing well on trach collar. Afebrile. Chest clear. No edema. Chronic respiratory failure. Change trach to #6 and start capping speech to evaluate for swallowing.

_____ c. Progress note of 04/13/2030, 11:10: Pulmonary note: Patient doing well on trach collar. Temp of 101.4°F. Chest clear. No edema. Chronic respiratory failure. Change trach to #6 and start capping speech to evaluate for swallowing.

2. Perform an Internet search to determine the laboratory results that must be reported to your state public health agency. Select another state and perform an Internet search to determine the laboratory results that must be reported to that state's public health agency. How do the required test results compare? What tests are in common? Which are different? Why do you think some required test results vary from state to state? Why are some tests similar?

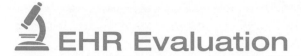
EHR Evaluation

Make Your Case

Consider the scenario and then complete the following project.

You are a nurse at a medical office committed to community outreach and education. Your office uses e-prescribing software and wants to conduct a meeting for patients and guests to explain this technology. Develop a presentation for the meeting that explains the functions and benefits of using e-prescribing.

Explore the Technology

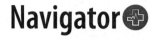

Complete the EHR Navigator practice assessments that align to each tutorial and the assessments that accompany Chapter 7 located on Navigator+.

Beyond the Record

- The International Classification of Diseases, Ninth Revision (ICD-9) classification system has 13,000 diagnosis codes, whereas the Tenth Revision (ICD-10) has almost 68,000 diagnosis codes.

The ICD-10 codes are updated to reflect the latest medical conditions. Because there are so many new codes, they may need to invent one for healthcare professionals spending a lot of time typing on a computer!

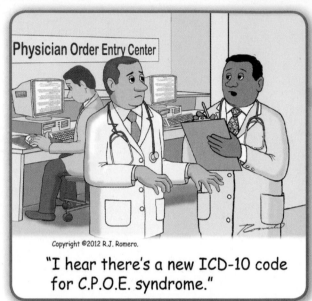

Copyright ©2012 R.J. Romero.

"I hear there's a new ICD-10 code for C.P.O.E. syndrome."

ICD Timeline

- **1837**—William Farr became the first medical statistician at the General Register Office of England and Wales. The office worked to secure better classifications of diseases and causes of death, and it pushed for international uniformity in these classifications.

- **1893**—French physician and statistician Jacques Bertillon presented the *Bertillon Classification of Causes of Death* at the International Statistical Institute of Chicago.

- **1900**—The first international conference convened to revise the *International List of Causes of Death*. Delegates from 29 countries reviewed the document and made revisions to the 179 causes of death.

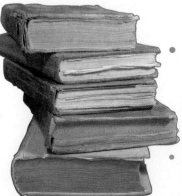

- **1948**—The World Health Organization endorsed the sixth revision of the classification and assumed responsibility for updating it every 10 years. The name was changed to *Manual of the International Statistical Classification of Diseases, Injuries, and Causes of Death*.

- **1955**—The seventh revision occurred in 1955 and resulted in the revised name International Classification of Diseases (ICD) that we continue to use today.

- **1965**—The eighth revision occurred in 1965.

This edition was more radical than the seventh but it did not change the structure of ICD.

- **1975**—The ninth revision (ICD-9) was published and contained many changes, including four-digit subcategories and five-digit subdivisions. The revision also included an optional alternative method of classifying diagnosing statements.

- **1979**—Clinical Modification codes (ICD-9-CM) are required for Medicare and Medicaid claims in the United States.

Chapter

8

Diagnostic and Procedural Coding

ICD-10 goes into much greater detail as to the types of injuries patients sustain, including some rather uncommon injuries, such as:

- Struck by a sea lion, initial encounter

- Pedestrian on foot injured in collision with roller skater, subsequent encounter

- Stabbed while crocheting

- Struck by a turtle, subsequent encounter

- Hurt at the opera

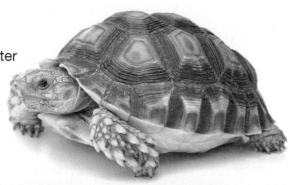

- **1990**—The tenth revision (ICD-10) was endorsed by the 43rd World Health Assembly.

- **2012**—The US Department of Health and Human Services proposed to delay the United States's adoption of ICD-10-CM and ICD-10-PCS from October 1, 2013, to October 1, 2014.

- **2014**—ICD-10-CM and ICD-10-PCS were delayed again to October 2015.

- **2015**—ICD-10-CM and ICD-10-PCS were finally implemented in the United States on October 1, 2015.

Field Notes

As a billing specialist, electronic health records (EHRs) have made it much easier to verify what we can bill for after a visit. Instead of having to hunt around for a paper chart in the shelves, I don't even have to leave my desk to find the documentation I need.

— Diana Schempp, Billing Specialist

The transition to EHRs in my clinic has been incredibly valuable for streamlining the patient experience of scheduling appointments, billing insurance, requesting records, and tracking patient visits. EHRs create a deeper sense of accountability of accuracy in documentation and also eliminate the constant search for runaway paper charts.

Kyle Meerkins, Volunteer Coordinator

8.1 Define *nomenclature* and identify its role in the electronic health record (EHR).

8.2 Define *classification systems* and identify specific classification systems used for coding for each healthcare delivery system.

8.3 Discuss the purposes of diagnostic and procedural coding.

8.4 Discuss the classification systems used to code diagnoses and procedures, including the *International Classification of Diseases*; Current Procedural Terminology; Healthcare Common Procedure Coding System; the *Diagnostic and Statistical Manual of Mental Disorders,* Fifth Edition; and Current Dental Terminology.

8.5 Discuss how EHRs affect coding processes.

8.6 Define and describe *computer-assisted coding*.

8.7 Define and discuss important coding concepts, such as *concurrent coding* and present on admission.

8.8 Discuss external and internal coding auditing.

8.9 Demonstrate coding processes utilizing EHR software.

Whether in an inpatient healthcare setting such as a hospital, nursing home, or long-term acute care hospital, or an outpatient setting such as an ambulatory surgical center or behavioral health clinic, there are individuals tasked with assigning and validating diagnostic and procedural codes to represent the patient's diseases or conditions and the treatment rendered. These individuals are known as **clinical coders**, medical coders, or coders, and they are responsible for assigning accurate codes based on health record documentation and coding guidelines. These codes are then used for reimbursement, research, decision-making, public health reporting, quality improvement, resource utilization, and healthcare policy and payment.

The practice of accurately coding diagnoses and procedures is a complicated process but can be facilitated by the use of electronic health records (EHRs). The adoption of an EHR system allows coders in every healthcare setting to easily access patient health data as well as billing and reimbursement systems. This improved access, along with the increased legibility of documentation, results in a more streamlined approach to coding and billing. However, EHRs will be of assistance in the reimbursement process only if clinical and support staff members are properly trained in complete and accurate documentation.

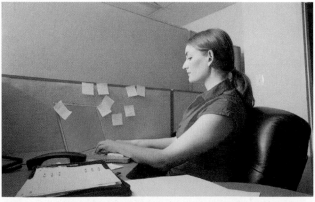

Clinical coders (or medical coders) are responsible for assigning and validating accurate codes based on health record documentation.

Nomenclature Systems

Nomenclatures and classification systems are two terms frequently—but incorrectly—used interchangeably. **Nomenclature** refers to a common system of naming things. When used in a discussion of EHRs, nomenclature refers to a system of common clinical and medical terms, with codes to represent diseases, procedures, symptoms, and medications. SNOMED-CT became a federally sanctioned nomenclature to be used with EHRs. Another common nomenclature system is MEDCIN. The term nomenclature is used interchangeably with terminology.

SNOMED-CT

EXPAND YOUR LEARNING

To learn more about SNOMED-CT and its applications with EHR systems, go to http://EHR2.ParadigmEducation.com/SNOMED to view an informational video.

SNOMED-CT is a standardized vocabulary of clinical terminology used by healthcare providers for clinical documentation and reporting, and it is considered the most comprehensive healthcare terminology in the world.

Federal and private developers of EHR systems can purchase a license to incorporate SNOMED-CT in their systems. SNOMED-CT was recommended and adopted as a federal Consolidated Health Informatics standard. However, even with the federal adoption of SNOMED-CT as a standard, EHR systems have not consistently implemented SNOMED-CT. For example, some facilities use the nomenclature system MEDCIN in their EHR systems.

MEDCIN

MEDCIN, which is a naming system primarily used in physicians' offices, was developed by Medicomp Systems Inc. and is derived from the US Centers for Medicare & Medicaid Services (CMS) guidelines for evaluation and management coding/charges. Because MEDCIN's vocabulary has been mapped to the evaluation and management Current Procedural Terminology (CPT®) codes that physicians use for billing their services, EHR systems using MEDCIN assist with the coding and billing processes. Physicians use nearly 300,000 clinical elements in MEDCIN at the point of patient care. In addition to a standard vocabulary, MEDCIN has a developed medical terminology interface that facilitates interoperability in regard to patient information exchange.

Classification Systems

A **classification system**, as used in health care, is a standardized coding method that organizes diagnoses and procedures into related groups to facilitate reimbursement, reporting, and clinical research. The two most widely used classification systems are the **International Classification of Diseases (ICD)** and **Current Procedural Terminology (CPT®)**. Hospitals, medical offices, long-term care facilities, ambulatory care centers, and many other healthcare institutions use ICD and CPT®. Other classification systems include the ***Diagnostic and Statistical Manual of Mental Disorders, Fifth Edition (DSM-5)***, used to classify psychiatric disorders; the **Healthcare Common Procedure Coding System (HCPCS)**, used to code ancillary services and procedures; and **Current Dental Terminology (CDT®)**, used to code dental procedures.

Under the Health Insurance Portability and Accountability Act of 1996 (HIPAA), the US government adopted specific code sets for diagnoses and procedures required of healthcare facilities for all billing transactions. These specific code sets include ICD for diagnosis coding in all settings and hospital inpatient procedure coding, CPT® for physician services procedures, CDT for dental claims, HCPCS for ancillary services and procedures, and National Drug Codes for drugs.

Purposes of Diagnostic and Procedural Coding

The use of standardized classification systems such as ICD and CPT® has a direct impact on health care, because the data is used for the following purposes:

- Reimbursement—enabling healthcare facilities and providers to bill for services and treatment rendered

- Research—helping researchers with studies and clinical trials

- Decision-making—supporting healthcare systems with operational and strategic planning

- Public health—assisting the Centers for Disease Control and Prevention (CDC) and other public health programs to monitor contagious diseases and other health risks

- Quality improvement—aiding healthcare providers with clinical, safety, financial, and operational quality improvement activities

- Resource utilization—supporting administrative and financial healthcare executives with tracking and monitoring use of resources

- Healthcare policy and payment—assisting government and private agencies with establishing and updating healthcare policies and payment systems

International Classification of Diseases Coding

The history of the ICD can be traced back to the eighteenth century, during which a classification system was developed in England and implemented for the statistical study of infant mortality rates. Although the classification system was rudimentary, it served its purpose at the time and accurately estimated an appalling trend: England's 36% child mortality rate before the age of six years. William Farr (1807–1883), one of the first medical statisticians, worked with the General Register Office in England and became interested in disease and mortality statistics. Farr used the classification system to categorize diseases by anatomic site and to monitor mortality rates.

Bertillon and the *International List of Causes of Death*

In 1891, the International Statistical Institute in Chicago commissioned Jacques Bertillon, chief of statistical services of the city of Paris, to create a classification system based on Farr's work. This new classification system, presented to the institute in 1893, became known as the *Bertillon Classification of Causes of Death* and was referenced as such until its first revision in 1900 when it was renamed the *International List of Causes of Death*. Twenty-six countries, including the United States, began to use and revise the *International List of Causes of Death*.

Emergence of the ICD

The *International List of Causes of Death* continued to evolve through several revisions until 1948, when the First World Health Assembly of the World Health Organization (WHO) endorsed the sixth revision of the classification system and renamed it the *Manual of the International Statistical Classification of Diseases, Injuries, and Causes of Death*. This sixth revision marked the beginning of a new era in international vital and health statistics. Governments began to establish national committees on vital and health statistics, correlate statistical activities within their countries, and coordinate statistical activities with other countries and the WHO.

The seventh revision occurred in 1955 and resulted in the revised name *International Classification of Diseases* (ICD), a title still used today. The eighth revision (ICD-8) was released in 1965, and the ninth revision (ICD-9) was published in 1975.

ICD-9

By 1977, the US National Center for Health Statistics convened a steering committee to provide expertise and advice in the development of a clinical modification of ICD-9 to be solely used by the United States. This clinical modification would make it more applicable to the diseases experienced by US patients and would include the level of detail requested by the country's researchers and statisticians. The US version was titled ICD-9, Clinical Modification (ICD-9-CM).

There have been annual updates to the 1977 version of ICD-9-CM to include new codes, delete codes, and modify existing codes. The Coordination and Maintenance Committee of the ICD-9-CM is responsible for maintaining the classification system and is composed of four cooperating parties: American Hospital Association (AHA), CMS, the American Health Information Management Association (AHIMA), and the National Center for Health Statistics. In addition to developing new and revised ICD-9-CM codes, the committee also provides coding guidance for ICD-9-CM and publishes clarifications of coding issues in *Coding Clinic*, published by the AHA. The clarifications of coding questions and issues that are published in *Coding Clinic* are considered official interpretations and guidance of coding issues and must be followed for accurate coding.

ICD-10

None of the revisions to ICD-9 and ICD-9-CM were extensive until the tenth revision (ICD-10) was adopted by the World Health Assembly in 1990. ICD-10 is vastly different from ICD-9. There were approximately 13,000 codes in ICD-9. Now there are approximately 68,000 codes in ICD-10 to allow for more specific coding and reporting of diagnoses and procedures. The format of the ICD-10 codes is also much different from that of the ICD-9 format. The codes in ICD-9 are primarily numeric (000.1–999.99), with combination alphanumeric codes being limited to three sections, namely the Morphology of Neoplasms (M codes), External Causes of Injury and Poisoning (E codes), and Factors Influencing Health Status and Contact with Health Services (V codes). All of the ICD-10 codes are alphanumeric (A00–T98, V01–Y98, and Z00–Z99). On October 1, 2015, the United States formally adopted a version of ICD-10 known as the International Classification of Diseases, 10th Revision, Clinical Modification (ICD-10-CM) to classify diseases and conditions in all healthcare settings. In conjunction with the adoption of ICD-10-CM, the United States also adopted a new system for classifying inpatient medical procedures and treatments. This new classification is called the International Classifications of Diseases, 10th Revision, Procedural Coding System (ICD-10-PCS). ICD-10 was originally scheduled for implementation in the United States in 2013. Both the AHA and the American Medical Association (AMA) requested a delay to allow healthcare providers and organizations time to fully prepare and test systems to ensure a smooth transition from ICD-9 to ICD-10. The implementation was then set for 2014 and again delayed to 2015. ICD-10-CM and ICD-10-PCS were finally implemented in 2015. Table 8.1 shows example ICD-9 codes and their corresponding ICD-10 codes.

Table 8.1 Example Codes

Diagnosis	ICD-9-CM Code	ICD-10-CM
Diabetes Mellitus, Type 2	250.00	E11.9
Fracture of neck of femur (fractured hip)	820.00	S72.019A

Procedure	ICD-9-CM	ICD-10-PCS
Percutaneous transluminal coronary angioplasty (PTCA)	Four codes are needed: 00.66, 36.07, 00.47, 00.41	One code includes all info: 0272342
Appendectomy	47.01	0DTJ4ZZ

ICD-11

ICD-11 is in development and will likely be implemented in the United States sometime around 2025. Experts have realized that waiting 38 years to update from ICD-9 to ICD-10 was not in the best interest of the healthcare industry or the population as a whole, and they are now committed to more frequent updates of the ICD classification system. Such updates are vital for keeping up with the progress of medicine and healthcare information technology, as well as for improving the foundation for international comparisons. Emerging diseases and scientific developments, combined with advances in service delivery, medical technologies, and health information systems, may require further revisions of this global classification system. One major need is to improve the relevance of the ICD system in primary care settings, such as clinics and physician offices, which are the sites where most people are treated. The process of developing the ICD-11 alpha draft began in 2009, and the beta draft was available soon after in 2011. The ICD-11 final draft was submitted to WHO in April 2015, with an expected worldwide implementation by October 2020. The United States will be an exception to the global adoption of ICD-11, because the country is not expected to implement ICD-11 until sometime after the year 2025. The reason for this delay is the projected time frame (five years or longer) to clinically modify (CM) WHO's version of ICD-11.

CPT Coding

CPT® is the classification system that describes medical, surgical, and diagnostic services, and it is used to report the procedures and services rendered to patients, including all surgical, radiologic, and anesthetic procedures, as well as other diagnostic screenings such as laboratory and pathology studies. The sites for these services include hospitals, nursing homes, ambulatory centers, medical offices, and other patient care facilities. CPT® codes are used to report procedures and services when billing both private and public insurance companies.

CPT® is published by the AMA and is updated every January. The AMA is also responsible for the creation and maintenance of CPT® codes. A CPT® editorial panel meets three times per year to discuss issues associated with new and emerging technologies as well as difficulties encountered with procedures and services and their relation to CPT® codes. The panel is composed of 17 members. Eleven are nominated by the AMA, and the remaining six individuals are nominated by entities such as private insurance companies or professional healthcare organizations.

Individuals who use CPT® codes must stay current and always use the most current manual to bill for services. There are more than 8,000 CPT® codes ranging from 00100 through 99607. In addition, two-digit modifiers may be added to certain CPT® codes to clarify or modify the description of the procedure.

Healthcare Common Procedure Coding System

CPT® codes are part of the Healthcare Common Procedure Coding System (HCPCS). HCPCS—pronounced "hick picks"—is divided into Levels I and II. Level I of HCPCS is composed of CPT® codes and is used to bill physician services and procedures. Level II of HCPCS is commonly referred to as National Codes and is primarily used to bill for products, supplies, and services not included in the CPT® codes, such as ambulance services, durable medical equipment, prosthetics, orthotics, and supplies. HCPCS codes are published annually by the CMS.

Current Dental Terminology Coding

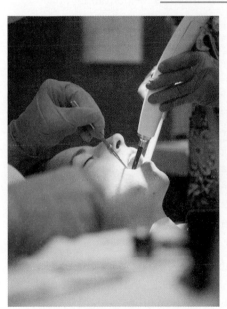

The code on dental procedures and nomenclatures that is used in the United States is Current Dental Terminology (CDT). CDT is maintained and published by the American Dental Association (ADA). CDT is a set of dental procedural codes used to report all dental services, with the exception of some oral surgery procedures. Dentists use ICD codes to report diagnoses and CDT to report the dental procedures and services. The ADA updates the CDT annually.

DSM-5 Coding

DSM-5 refers to the *Diagnostic and Statistical Manual of Mental Disorders*, Fifth Edition. DSM-5, published by the American Psychiatric Association (APA), is a manual that contains codes for every known behavioral health condition. The manual is designed to coincide with ICD, but the two coding systems are not identical. ICD diagnosis codes are used for billing purposes, but they are not detailed enough for researchers, clinicians, policy makers, health insurance companies, pharmaceutical companies, and psychiatric drug regulatory agencies.

Current Dental Terminology (CDT) is used to code dental services.

DSM codes are not included as an approved code in the HIPAA transaction and code set standards for electronic data interchange for billing purposes. Mental health providers rely on the DSM as a supportive diagnostic tool; to submit claims for reimbursement purposes, DSM codes are cross-walked to ICD codes. **Crosswalking** is the act of translating a code in one code set to a code in another code set.

WHO USES WHAT

ICD-9-CM/PCS and **ICD-10-CM/PCS** are used in the United States for diagnosis coding in all settings and hospital inpatient procedure coding.

CPT® is used in the United States to code outpatient procedures for facility coding, as well as all physician services rendered (regardless of the setting).

DSM-5 codes are used by the psychiatric community to more specifically code disorders such as major mental, learning, substance abuse, and personality disorders; intellectual disabilities; acute medical conditions; physical disorders; and psychosocial and environmental factors that contribute to the mental disorders for nonbilling purposes.

CDT is used to code dental procedures. The CDT codes are used with ICD codes for billing purposes.

Code Assignment

Traditionally, coders have used hard- or soft-cover coding manuals to assign ICD, CPT®, and DSM-5 diagnostic and procedure codes. Depending on the classification system, coders have used as many as three books at a time, such as when coding with ICD-9-CM. For those healthcare organizations with a low volume of health records to code, the use of coding manuals may be effective. However, with high volumes of health records to code, using several cumbersome manuals slows down the coding process.

Using Encoders versus Print Coding Manuals

To remedy the difficult process of coding from many different print manuals, clinical encoders/groupers were adopted by these high-volume facilities in the 1990s. A **clinical encoder** is a software program that helps coding professionals navigate coding pathways with the end result of assigning codes. It is important to note that many coding certification exams require the test taker to code from coding books. Therefore, classroom instruction often focuses on coding from manuals to ensure that students understand how the coding classification systems work and how to apply that knowledge when they take their certification exams. Coders must understand how to assign codes using encoder software and printed coding manuals.

Diagnosis-Related Groups

A **diagnosis-related group (DRG)** is a patient classification system that groups hospital inpatients of similar age, sex, diagnoses, and treatments. Each DRG is associated with a specific dollar amount that the hospital expects to be reimbursed for in relation to the treatment provided. The first DRG system, the Medicare **inpatient prospective payment system (IPPS)**, was implemented in 1983 to reimburse acute care hospitals for the treatment of Medicare patients. Since then, many other payers, such as Medicaid and commercial payers, have adopted the Medicare DRG system for the reimbursement of inpatient care of their insured members. The purpose of a DRG system is to relatively equalize payments to hospitals for providing the same care to patients with the same clinical characteristics. Prior to the implementation of the Medicare DRG system, acute care hospitals were reimbursed for whatever they charged Medicare or other payers. Take a look at a simplified example of pre-DRG and post-DRG payments for two patient scenarios in the following "Consider This" box.

Medicare and Medicaid patients may be grouped together using a diagnosis-related group classification system for coding purposes.

Consider This

Patient A
Final principal diagnosis:
acute respiratory failure
Principal procedure: mechanical ventilation, more than 96 hours

Patient B
Final principal diagnosis:
acute myocardial infarction
Principal procedure: coronary artery bypass

Hospital Name	Patient A Reimbursement Before Medicare DRG ($)	Patient A Reimbursement After Medicare DRG ($)	Patient B Reimbursement Before Medicare DRG ($)	Patient B Reimbursement After Medicare DRG ($)
City Hospital	63,588	47,184	24,160	33,238
Tender Care Hospital	52,140	47,184	44,321	33,238
Bayview Hospital	38,690	47,184	45,870	33,238
Grace Hospital	47,545	47,184	63,923	33,238

DRG = diagnostic-related group.

Analyze the table above. Why do reimbursement rates for Patients A and B vary among hospitals in the time before the Medicare DRG implementation? Why are the reimbursement rates the same for Patients A and B among the hospitals under the Medicare DRG system? Under the Medicare DRG system, why is the reimbursement for Patient A not the same as Patient B?

Consider This

Through the Medicare inpatient prospective payment system (IPPS), the US government spends more than $130 billion every year in payments to acute care hospitals for inpatient care. Because the IPPS depends on diagnostic and procedural coding to calculate the payments to acute care hospitals, what would happen if coding staff incorrectly coded charts 10% of the time?

Coding and the Electronic Health Record

The use of an EHR system has a positive impact on the coding of health records. It facilitates efficient concurrent and final coding processes, greater accuracy in code assignments, and improved access to health records.

The Coding Process

Healthcare facilities initiate the billing process for patient visits after each visit or admission. The healthcare facility prepares the claims to be sent to the insurance carrier, and upon submission, payments are made to the healthcare facility. A **medical coder**, a career option in the health information management field, plays a key role in the billing process by coding diagnoses and procedures in preparation for billing claims.

Medical coding is the process of assigning and validating standardized alphanumeric identifiers to the diagnoses and procedures documented in a health record. A **diagnosis** is a statement or conclusion that describes a patient's illness, disease, or health problem. A **medical procedure** is an activity performed on an individual to improve health, treat disease or injury, or identify a diagnosis. A **health record** is legal documentation in the form of a physical or electronic file in which doctors, nurses, and other healthcare professionals detail the diagnoses and procedures they provide to a particular patient. Health records also contain pertinent administrative and financial data about each patient.

When healthcare professionals document diagnoses and procedures in a health record, they do not always do so in a uniform way. For example, two physicians might describe the same condition in different terms, as shown in Figure 8.1. Assigning standardized alphanumeric codes to this medical data makes it easier to interpret immediately, share, compare, classify, and manipulate the data for reimbursement, research, and planning.

Coded data is used by healthcare providers to seek reimbursement from the government, private insurance companies, and other third-party payers. A **third-party payer** is an entity other than the patient that is financially responsible for payment of the medical bill. Patients who pay for the entire visit themselves are referred to as **self-pay patients**. Third-party payers are so named because there are typically three parties involved in the care of the patient:

- Party 1, the patient

- Party 2, the healthcare provider

- Party 3, the entity that pays the medical bill other than the patient

Coded data is also used in public health management to monitor the incidence and prevalence of diseases as well as death rates. To monitor health trends, nations track **morbidity**, which consists of illness statistics, and **mortality**, which consists of death statistics. Coded information enables the storage and retrieval of diagnostic information for clinical, epidemiological, and quality control purposes.

Figure 8.1 How Different Medical Notes Can Result in the Same Code

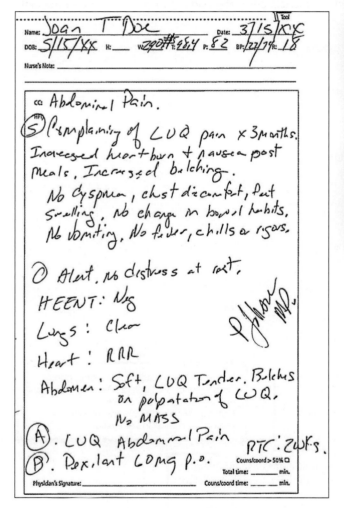

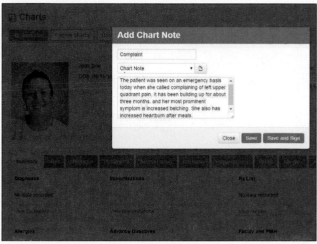

Reporting Codes from the Health Record

The health record and the documentation it contains is the starting point for reporting medical codes. An **operative report** is a form of clinical documentation that contains the details of a particular surgery or procedure performed on a patient. Figure 8.2 illustrates the different parts of an operative report for tarsorrhaphy, a procedure in which the eyelids are partially sewn together to narrow the opening.

The steps in reporting codes from an operative report are generally the following:

- Read the report and verify that the diagnosis and procedure listed at the top of the report are supported by the documentation of the procedure provided in the body of the report (sometimes called the operative technique).

- After verifying that everything matches, the coder uses several resources, such as codebooks and coding databases, to locate the correct codes for both the diagnosis and the procedure.

- If the documentation supports a different procedure or diagnosis than that listed by the physician, the coder should review the facility policies and procedures, which typically instruct the coder to query the provider for additional information.

- If working in a physician practice, enter the code(s) into the patient's financial account in the EHR.

- The coder enters the medical codes into the EHR to prepare the account for billing.

Figure 8.2 Example of an Ophthalmological Operative

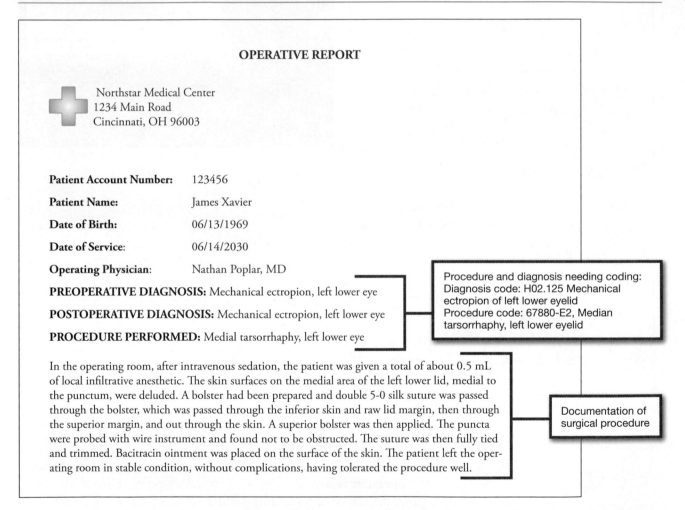

OPERATIVE REPORT

Northstar Medical Center
1234 Main Road
Cincinnati, OH 96003

Patient Account Number: 123456

Patient Name: James Xavier

Date of Birth: 06/13/1969

Date of Service: 06/14/2030

Operating Physician: Nathan Poplar, MD

PREOPERATIVE DIAGNOSIS: Mechanical ectropion, left lower eye

POSTOPERATIVE DIAGNOSIS: Mechanical ectropion, left lower eye

PROCEDURE PERFORMED: Medial tarsorrhaphy, left lower eye

> Procedure and diagnosis needing coding:
> Diagnosis code: H02.125 Mechanical ectropion of left lower eyelid
> Procedure code: 67880-E2, Median tarsorrhaphy, left lower eyelid

In the operating room, after intravenous sedation, the patient was given a total of about 0.5 mL of local infiltrative anesthetic. The skin surfaces on the medial area of the left lower lid, medial to the punctum, were deluded. A bolster had been prepared and double 5-0 silk suture was passed through the bolster, which was passed through the inferior skin and raw lid margin, then through the superior margin, and out through the skin. A superior bolster was then applied. The puncta were probed with wire instrument and found not to be obstructed. The suture was then fully tied and trimmed. Bacitracin ointment was placed on the surface of the skin. The patient left the operating room in stable condition, without complications, having tolerated the procedure well.

> Documentation of surgical procedure

Concurrent and Final Coding

Final bills are typically held in a suspended status for three days after patient discharge to allow for final charge entry, documentation, insurance verification, and final coding. Patient accounts not able to be final billed to the insurance company or responsible party because of a lack of final coding, insurance verification, or other data errors are considered **discharged not final billed (DNFB)**. These accounts are flagged as DNFB and are included on a data report produced by the EHR system. This report is monitored daily by health information managers, coders, and other staff members in healthcare organizations. For coders, this report highlights the oldest outstanding accounts and the accounts with the highest unbilled account balances. The EHR system further assists the coder by providing coding **work-list reports**. These reports present the patient accounts for coding in a priority order, beginning with the oldest accounts with the highest balances. For those coders who use physical paper records rather than an EHR system, a major contributor to a DNFB list is the delay in locating the paper record.

For coders, an EHR system can perform **concurrent coding**, which is the task of coding while a patient is still receiving treatment in a hospital. This concurrent coding process accelerates the final coding process that is completed upon discharge of the patient, by allowing coders to query healthcare providers for necessary documentation regarding diagnoses and procedures over the course of a particular patient's stay. Consequently, the coder has all the documentation needed upon patient discharge to allow for final coding.

The financial managers of healthcare organizations promote concurrent coding because the process speeds up final billing procedures, thereby reducing the number of unbilled accounts. Even though there are many contributing factors involved in the final billing process, health information management (HIM) departments and coding staff, in particular, are held accountable for the inability of an organization to produce final bills to payers due to a lack of final coding.

Accuracy in Code Assignments

As previously discussed in Chapters 1 and 2, EHRs eliminate the problems of illegible handwriting that exist in most paper health records. Illegible handwriting can result in inaccurate coding when coders miss or miscode diagnoses because they cannot read the healthcare provider's handwriting. The EHR also improves coding through more accurate documentation. Physicians may be prompted to enter more information based on the templates built in the EHR system. EHRs can therefore reduce the number of errors due to incomplete or vague diagnostic or procedural information.

Clinical encoder software windows are open and functional as the coder navigates through the EHR. As a result, the clinical coder can read and enter the patient's diagnoses and procedures rendered to a patient into the encoder resulting in the applicable codes. The coder may automatically generate physician queries and highlight or make notations to the EHR that do not change or affect the legality of the health record. A **physician query** is a request, typically from a coder or a case manager, to add documentation to the health record that clarifies a diagnosis or procedure performed. Physician queries may be issued to providers concurrently or retrospectively. AHIMA has published best practice guidance on the query process in its *Guidelines for Achieving a Compliant Query Practice*. In an EHR, all physician queries are automatically routed to the appropriate physician's message inbox and displayed when the physician logs in to the system.

The use of clinical encoders and physician queries assists coders in establishing the most accurate code assignments. Accurate code assignments, in turn, result in appropriate reimbursement for healthcare organizations. Although organizations must ensure that health record documentation is complete and accurate, its staff members cannot educate or encourage physicians to document simply for the purpose of claiming a higher-paying DRG and, therefore, increased reimbursement. This maneuver is referred to as **upcoding** and is illegal. Unintentional upcoding is considered **abuse**, whereas intentional upcoding is considered **fraud**. Those convicted of fraud or abuse may receive monetary fines or jail time.

Computer-Assisted Coding Programs

Some EHR systems incorporate **computer-assisted coding (CAC)** programs that automatically assign diagnosis and procedure codes based on electronic documentation, which can increase the productivity of a coder by up to 20%. However, the use of a CAC program does not mean that the coding process is completely automated. When CAC programs are used, the coder assumes the role of a reviewer or an auditor. The coder must validate the codes, ensure that coding guidelines have been followed, and validate whether or not the coded diagnoses were **present on admission (POA)**, meaning the patient had the diagnoses when he or she was admitted to the facility. All primary and secondary diagnoses require POA indicators to be reported on the Medicare claims of IPPS general acute care hospitals. POA indicator assignment is determined by the coder based on clinical documentation entered into the health record by the provider.

Coders must exercise care in assigning POA indicators. Medicare patients who experience diagnoses and conditions that are **hospital acquired**, meaning that they developed when the patient was an inpatient in the hospital, must not be reported as POA. The care and treatment of these hospital-acquired diagnoses and conditions (e.g., hospital-acquired pressure ulcer, urinary tract infection, pneumonia) are typically not reimbursed by Medicare.

Internal and External Auditing for Coding Compliance

To verify that a healthcare facility is coding accurately and following guidelines, they are often audited, either externally or internally.

External Coding Audits

External companies and organizations routinely conduct audits to verify coding accuracy. These external companies and organizations include insurance companies, auditing companies hired by insurance companies, and Medicare and Medicaid auditors. The purpose of the audits is to ensure that coders followed coding guidelines and regulations in the assignment of diagnosis and procedure codes.

Insurance Audits

Insurance audits are conducted by insurance companies or auditing companies hired to review coding assignments on behalf of insurance companies. They are routinely conducted for patient accounts that contain codes that are historically problematic for coders resulting in a high error rate. Insurance company audits also focus on patient accounts/bills that exceed a specific threshold. For example, CobaltCare might automatically conduct audits for any patient bill exceeding $100,000. Another insurance company may have a lower threshold of $80,000. Insurance companies also conduct more frequent coding audits on healthcare organizations that have historically had a higher coding error rate.

EXPAND YOUR LEARNING

To learn more about present on admission indicators and reduced Medicare reimbursement for hospital-acquired conditions, review the following websites:

http://EHR2
.ParadigmEducation
.com/MedicarePOA

http://EHR2
.ParadigmEducation
.com/MedicareHAC

Recovery Audit Contractor Program

The goal of a Recovery Audit Contractor (RAC) program is to identify improper payments made for healthcare services provided to Medicare beneficiaries. These improper payments include both overpayment and underpayment due to inaccurate coding. Any healthcare provider that bills Medicare Part A (inpatient services) or B (outpatient services) may be audited under the RAC program. These providers include hospitals, physician practices, nursing homes, home health agencies, durable medical equipment supplies, and any other provider or supplier that bills Medicare Part A or B charges. The Tax Relief and Health Care Act of 2006 required that a national RAC program be in place by January 1, 2010. The RAC program has resulted in millions of dollars being returned to the Medicare program. For example, in 2015 alone, more than $141 million was returned to the Medicare fund.

Internal Coding Audits

The best way for a healthcare provider to avoid having to repay insurance companies or Medicare for inaccurate coding and billing is to reduce the risk of coding errors. How can a healthcare provider accomplish this?

- Conduct internal coding audits—Instead of waiting for external organizations to identify coding errors, providers should routinely conduct their own audits to identify coding problem areas. EHR reporting capabilities can greatly enhance the auditing process, because reports can be quickly generated to the level of specificity desired by the auditor.

- Intensive coder training—As problematic coding scenarios are identified with internal audits, providers should conduct intensive, frequent coder training to reduce coding errors.

- Reaudit—Following coder training, the provider should reaudit the coding areas that were the subject of the coder training to ensure that coding accuracy has improved.

Improved Access to Health Records

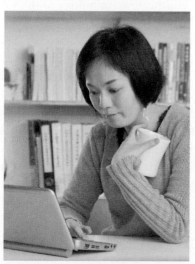

Remote coders are able to code from home using an EHR system.

For coders, an EHR system affords easy access to health records from any work site. Consequently, coding can be performed by **remote coders** who value the autonomy and flexibility of working from home. This work setup also benefits healthcare organizations by allowing hiring personnel to recruit top-notch coders from across the country.

Although implementation of an EHR system can be challenging for both healthcare organizations and personnel, the use of this type of technology can streamline coding as well as other record-keeping processes.

CHECKPOINT 8.2

1. List three ways in which the EHR benefits the coding process.

   a. _____

   b. _____

   c. _____

2. True or False: A successful healthcare organization uses upcoding to ensure that the best DRG is selected for billing. Discuss why you chose *true* or *false*.

   _____

   _____

Tutorial 8.1

EHRNAVIGATOR

Coding a Patient's Record

Go to Navigator+ to launch Tutorial 8.1. As an RHIT, practice coding a patient's record using the EHR Navigator.

Chapter Summary

Electronic health record (EHR) systems are revolutionizing the reimbursement, clinical coding, and billing processes. Some of the benefits of EHR implementation include easy access to clinical records by the coding and billing staff, more efficient methods of coding health records, a streamlined physician query process, improved documentation by providers, and improved fiscal management of healthcare organizations.

Nomenclature refers to a common system of common clinical and medical terms, with codes to represent diseases, procedures, symptoms, and medications. SNOMED-CT is a standardized vocabulary of clinical terminology used by healthcare providers for clinical documentation and reporting and is considered the most comprehensive healthcare terminology in the world. Another common nomenclature system is MEDCIN.

Classification systems are used for reimbursement, research, decision-making, public health, quality improvement, resource utilization, and healthcare policy and payment. The types of classification systems used depend on the types of services one is coding. Common coding classification systems include International Classification of Diseases (ICD), Current Procedural Terminology (CPT®), *Diagnostic and Statistical Manual of Mental Disorders*, Fifth Edition (DSM-5), and Current Dental Terminology (CDT).

ICD-10 was implemented in the United States in October 2015.

ICD-11 will likely be implemented in the United States around 2025.

CPT® is the classification system that describes medical, surgical, and diagnostic services and is used to report the procedures and services rendered to patients, including all surgical, radiologic, and anesthetic procedures, as well as other diagnostic screenings such as laboratory and pathology studies. CPT® is published by the AMA and is updated annually in January.

HCPCS, the Healthcare Common Procedure Coding System, is divided into Levels I and II. Level I is composed of CPT® codes and is used to bill physician services and procedures. Level II is primarily used to bill for products, supplies, and services not included in the CPT® codes such as ambulance services, durable medical equipment, prosthetics, orthotics, and supplies. HCPCS codes are published annually by CMS.

CDT is the Current Dental Terminology nomenclature that is used to report all dental services.

DSM-5 is published by the American Psychiatric Association and is used as a crosswalk to ICD-10 to bill for mental health services.

Crosswalking is the act of translating a code in one code set to a code in another code set.

To assist with the coding process, a coder may use a clinical encoder software program and classify patients by their diagnosis-related group (DRG). IPPS is the Medicare inpatient prospective payment system that reimburses acute care hospitals for the treatment of Medicare patients. Concurrent coding is the task of coding while a patient is still receiving treatment in a hospital. Patient accounts not able to be final billed to the insurance company or responsible party because of a lack of final coding, insurance verification, or other data errors are considered discharged not final billed (DNFB).

A physician query is a request to add documentation to the health record that clarifies a diagnosis or procedure performed.

Upcoding is the practice of using higher-paying but inaccurate DRGs in health records for the purpose of increasing reimbursement. Upcoding is illegal. Unintentional upcoding is considered abuse. Intentional upcoding is considered fraud.

Computer-assisted coding programs automatically assign diagnosis and procedure codes based on electronic documentation.

Present on admission (POA) are the diagnoses that are present upon admission to the hospital.

Hospital-acquired conditions are those that develop during a patient's hospital stay.

External coding audits are conducted by insurance companies, auditing companies hired by insurance companies, and Recovery Audit Contractors (RAC) for Medicare.

Checks and balances should be used in an EHR environment just as they should in a paper environment, because coders must still follow official coding guidelines, and physicians and healthcare providers must thoroughly and accurately document procedures and diagnoses.

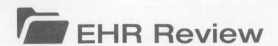

EHR Review

Navigator

The following EHR Review, EHR Application, and EHR Evaluation activities are also available online in the Navigator+ learning management system. Your instructor may ask you to complete these activities online. Navigator+ also provides access to flash cards, study games, and practice quizzes to help strengthen your understanding of the chapter content.

Acronyms/Initialisms

Study the following acronyms discussed in this chapter. Go to Navigator+ for flash cards of the acronyms and other chapter key terms.

ADA: American Dental Association

AHA: American Hospital Association

AHIMA: American Health Information Management Association

AMA: American Medical Association

CAC: computer-assisted coding

CDC: Centers for Disease Control and Prevention

CDT: Current Dental Terminology

CMS: Centers for Medicare & Medicaid Services

CPT®: Current Procedural Terminology

DNFB: discharged not final billed

DRG: diagnosis-related group

DSM-5: *Diagnostic and Statistical Manual of Mental Disorders*, Fifth Edition

HCPCS: Healthcare Common Procedure Coding System

HIM: health information management

ICD: International Classification of Diseases

IPPS: inpatient prospective payment system

POA: present on admission

RAC: Recovery Audit Contractor

SNOMED-CT: Systematized Nomenclature of Medicine—Clinical Terms

WHO: World Health Organization

Check Your Understanding

To check your understanding of this chapter's key concepts, answer the following questions.

1. The following are all examples of classification systems *except*

   a. MEDCIN

   b. *International Classification of Diseases* (ICD)

   c. Current Procedural Terminology (CPT®)

   d. *Diagnostic and Statistical Manual of Mental Disorders,* Fifth Edition (DSM-5)

2. Which of the following classification system is used to code outpatient procedures and inpatient and outpatient provider services?

   a. Current Dental Terminology

   b. ICD-10-CM

   c. DSM-5

   d. CPT®

3. How does the implementation of an electronic health record (EHR) system affect the process of coding health records?

   a. It allows for more efficient coding.

   b. It increases the accuracy of code assignments.

   c. It eliminates the physician query process.

   d. It allows for more efficient coding and increases the accuracy of code assignments.

4. When was ICD-10 implemented in the United States?

   a. October 1, 2012

   b. January 1, 2013

   c. January 1, 2014

   d. October 1, 2015

5. When is ICD-11 likely to be implemented in the United States?

   a. 2025

   b. 2020

   c. 2018

   d. Never

6. True/False: The term *nomenclature* refers to a standardized method of assigning codes to diagnoses and procedures.

7. True/False: Concurrent coding is an easy process to perform with paper records but is more difficult with an EHR system.

8. True/False: The RAC audits have not been successful in returning money to the Medicare fund.

9. True/False: Healthcare providers are best served by waiting for external auditors to show them where their coding problems exist.

10. True/False: The use of standardized classification systems has a direct impact on health care.

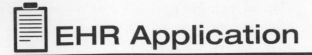 **EHR Application**

Go on the Record

To build on your understanding of the topics in this chapter, complete the following short-answer activities.

1. List and describe three purposes of diagnostic and procedural coding.

2. Discuss the differences between *nomenclature* and a *classification system*.

3. Define *clinical encoder* and discuss how this software program assists coding professionals.

4. List three ways in which the electronic health record (EHR) system improves work processes for a coder.

5. Define *physician query* and describe how the process is automated with the EHR system.

Navigate the Field

To gain practice in handling challenging situations in the workplace, consider the following real-world scenarios and identify how you would respond to each.

1. You are a coder for Northstar Medical Center. While coding diagnoses for a discharged patient's encounter, you notice that the attending physician has documented that the patient has type 1 diabetes mellitus, and a consulting physician has documented that the patient has type II diabetes mellitus. How would you handle this discrepancy?

2. As the lead coder for a large physician practice, you notice that a couple of the coders are not following the official coding guidelines. What steps should you take to ensure accurate coding?

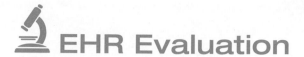

EHR Evaluation

Think Critically

Continue to think critically about challenging concepts and complete the following activities.

1. As the supervisor of coding at a large teaching hospital, you are concerned about the new interns and residents that rotate through the hospital every year. You have noticed that their documentation is not complete enough for coders to accurately code. What should you do to rectify this situation that is ongoing as the new interns and residents rotate through the organization?

2. Conduct an Internet search to identify two clinical encoders that can be interfaced with electronic health record systems. After examining the components of each system, write a proposal to the coding manager of Northstar Physicians that identifies the program you would select and discusses the reasoning behind your choice.

Make Your Case

Consider the scenario and then complete the following project.

As the coding manager for a hospital, you have been asked by the vice president of finance to prepare a short presentation for hospital administrators that addresses how the hospital's electronic health record (EHR) system has benefited the coding process of the hospital.

Explore the Technology

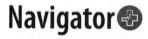

Complete the EHR Navigator practice assessments that align to each tutorial and the assessments that accompany Chapter 8 located on Navigator+.

Beyond the Record

- It is estimated that doctors in the United States leave approximately $125 billion on the table each year because of poor billing practices.

- The percentage of adults ages 18–64 with private insurance is 69.7%.

- The electronic health record (EHR) reduces the time and resources needed for manual charge entry, resulting in more accurate billing and reduction in lost charges.

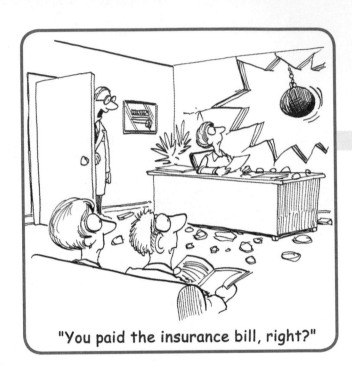

"You paid the insurance bill, right?"

Are You Ready?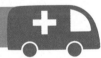

It can take as many as 250 people—from the nurse to the coder to the biller—to generate one medical bill from start to finish. Medical billers should possess good communication skills and be excellent problem solvers. Billing can sometimes be like a complicated puzzle— billers need to investigate and toubleshoot claims to ensure accurate billing. As you consider your future in health care, consider whether you would make a good biller.

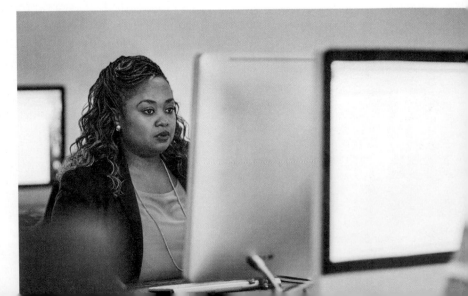

Managing Insurance, Billing, and Reimbursement

In the United States there are 12,871,500,000 medical claims transactions annually, which is about 410 transactions per year for every American.

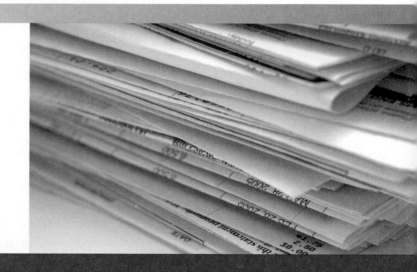

Insurance Time Line

- **1850**—Accident insurance first offered by Franklin Health Assurance Company of Massachusetts.
- **1911**—The first employer-sponsored group disability policy issued to replace lost wages.
- **1920s**—Hospitals offered services on a prepaid basis.

- **1930s**—Blue Cross organizations created. The Roosevelt Administration explored possibility of a national health organization.
- **1965**—Americans started receiving Medicare health coverage after President Lyndon B. Johnson signed legislation.

- **1973**—Congress passed the Health Maintenance Organization (HMO) Act, which provided grants to employers who set up HMOs.
- **1980**—Medicare Part C implemented.
- **1985**—Consolidated Omnibus Budget Reconciliation Act (COBRA) signed by President Ronald Reagan.

- **2003**—President George W. Bush signed into law the Medicare Prescription Drug Improvement and Modernization Act of 2003, adding an optional prescription drug benefit.
- **2010**—The Patient Protection and Affordable Care Act signed into law by President Barack Obama, expanding health insurance coverage for Americans.

9.1 Define *health insurance* and understand the concepts related to health coverage.

9.2 Discuss the evolution of health insurance.

9.3 Differentiate between indemnity, managed care, group, and individual insurance plans.

9.4 Define and discuss different types of government-sponsored health plans.

9.5 Discuss the importance and methods of verifying insurance.

9.6 Define *practice management* and explain how it relates to billing and electronic office billing systems.

9.7 Discuss how EHRs affect billing processes.

9.8 Demonstrate billing processes utilizing EHR software.

9.9 Demonstrate use of an electronic office billing system.

9.10 Demonstrate insurance claims processing.

9.11 Demonstrate use of practice management reports.

As with any business, to be successful, a healthcare organization must be financially stable. The financial stability of a healthcare organization results from the careful management of the health insurance, billing, and reimbursement process. In this chapter, we will explore the concepts of health insurance, billing, and reimbursement, and the role of the EHR in managing those transactions.

To understand health insurance, billing, and reimbursement, it is first important to understand **revenue cycle management**. The Healthcare Financial Management Association (HFMA) defines the revenue cycle as "all administrative and clinical functions that contribute to the capture, management, and collection of patient service revenue." The revenue cycle begins with the admission or registration of a patient and ends with collection and posting of payments. Figure 9.1 shows the revenue cycle management process. A healthcare organization that has a well-managed revenue cycle will experience a timelier, increased cash flow, which in turn translates into higher revenue.

Health Insurance

You are likely familiar with the concept of insurance because you most likely have car insurance, homeowner's insurance, or life insurance. With any type of insurance, an individual makes a specified number of consistent payments called a **premium** to a company in exchange for payment if something occurs, such as a car accident, death,

Figure 9.1 Revenue Cycle Management

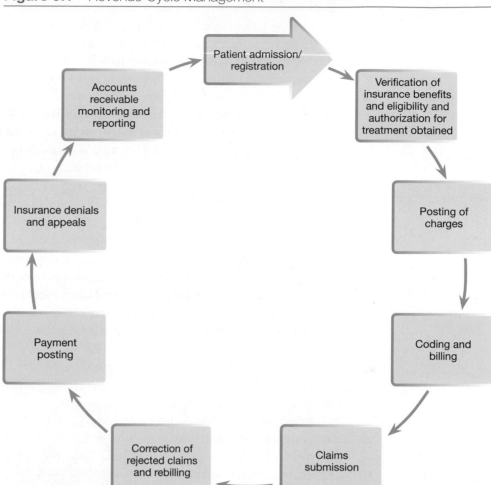

storm damage to a house, or healthcare treatment. Therefore, the definition of **health insurance** is a type of insurance that pays for healthcare services that are incurred by the insured person(s). In our discussion of health insurance, the third-party payer is the insurance company.

After patient admission or registration, the next step in revenue cycle management is to verify insurance benefits and eligibility. As you learned in Chapter 4, **admission/registration clerks** (sometimes also called *patient access specialists*) are generally responsible for entering insurance information into the EHR system at the time the patient is admitted to an inpatient hospital or scheduled for treatment at an outpatient facility or physician's office. Following insurance data entry, the admission/ registration clerk or **insurance verifier** must confirm with the insurance company the patient's insurance coverage. The purpose of this insurance verification process is twofold: (1) to ensure that the patient has active coverage, and (2) to determine important billing aspects of the insurance plan, such as the guarantor, guarantor information, covered dependents, copayments, deductibles, and any other limitations or payment rules. The verification process will be explored later in this chapter.

Understanding Health Coverage

Consider the following scenarios. Samuel Elliott is a retired army captain who recently saw his doctor for unexplained headaches. Angela Singh is an unemployed single parent with two children. She recently took her children to their pediatrician for their back-to-school checkups. Hazel Bellamy is an 83-year-old widow who is also a retired librarian. Hazel just made an appointment at the Coumadin clinic for a blood check. Matthew Foltz is a 25-year-old full-time manager at a small, family-owned company. He was recently injured at work and sought treatment at an urgent care facility. What do these people have in common? They have all recently received healthcare services. Whether they had an encounter with their primary care physician, a hospital, or an emergency room, they all received healthcare services and then all received a bill from the provider. How did they pay their bills? They all had some type of health coverage that paid all or a portion of their bills.

Health coverage is the legal entitlement to payment or reimbursement for healthcare costs, generally under a contract with a health insurance company, a group health plan offered in connection with employment, or a government program like Medicare, Medicaid, or the Children's Health Insurance Program (CHIP). When someone other than the patient pays for healthcare services, that entity is referred to as a **third-party payer**. In the group of scenarios discussed earlier, each individual has health coverage but different third-party payers. Samuel Elliott has health coverage through TRICARE, a federal program for retired military. Angela Singh has Medicaid, a state-administered health insurance program for low-income families and children. Hazel Bellamy has Medicare, a federal health insurance program for people who are age 65 or older. And Matthew Foltz is insured by a traditional health insurance company, in which his mother is the subscriber through her employer. Each of these types of health coverage will be discussed further in this chapter.

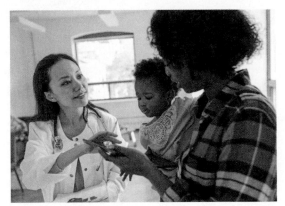

A checkup with a pediatrician can be covered by private insurance, Medicare, or the Children's Health Insurance Program (CHIP).

Evolution of Health Insurance

Over the course of the past century, there have been many significant advancements in the health insurance industry in the United States. The Affordable Care Act (ACA) is a recent, major legislative change in health insurance, but the discussion about a national health insurance system for Americans goes back much further.

History of National Health Insurance and Medicare

A discussion regarding how to deal with health insurance for Americans was part of President Theodore Roosevelt's platform when he ran for president in 1912, but the idea for a national health plan didn't gain steam until it was pushed by President Harry S. Truman. On November 19, 1945, seven months into his presidency, Truman sent a message to Congress, calling for creation of a national health insurance fund open to all Americans.

The plan Truman envisioned would provide health coverage to individuals, paying for typical expenses such as doctor visits, hospital visits, laboratory services, dental care, and nursing services. Although Truman fought to get a bill passed during his term, he was unsuccessful, and it was another 20 years before Medicare became a reality.

President John F. Kennedy made his own unsuccessful push for a national healthcare program for seniors after a national study showed that 56% of Americans over the age of 65 were not covered by health insurance, but it wasn't until 1965—after legislation was signed by President Lyndon B. Johnson—that eligible Americans started receiving Medicare health coverage.

In 1972, President Richard M. Nixon signed into the law the first major change to Medicare. The legislation expanded coverage to include individuals under the age of 65 with long-term disabilities and individuals with end-stage renal disease (ESRD).

In 1973, Congress passed the **Health Maintenance Organization (HMO) Act**, which provided grants to employers who set up HMOs.

When Congress passed the **Omnibus Reconciliation Act of 1980**, it expanded home health services. The bill also brought **Medigap**—or Medicare supplemental insurance—under federal oversight.

In 1982, **hospice services** for the terminally ill were added to a growing list of Medicare benefits. Also that year, other legislation gave those eligible for Medicare coverage more options on the private market when Medicare Part C, also known as Medicare Advantage, was implemented. Medicare Advantage gave more coverage options in the private insurance market and also added options such as prescription drug coverage for Medicare subscribers who wished to pay for additional coverage.

The Consolidated Omnibus Budget Reconciliation Act of 1985 (COBRA) is a health benefit act that Congress passed in 1986 requiring an employer to extend group health coverage to a terminated employee and his or her dependents at group rates for a specified time period.

In 1996, Congress required most employer-sponsored group health insurance plans to accept transfers from other group plans without imposing a preexisting condition clause as a part of the **Health Insurance Portability and Accountability Act (HIPAA)**.

In 2001, Congress expanded Medicare benefits to cover younger people with amyotrophic lateral sclerosis (ALS) upon diagnosis of the disease.

President George W. Bush signed into law the **Medicare Prescription Drug Improvement and Modernization Act of 2003**, adding an optional prescription drug benefit. Until this time, about 25% of those receiving Medicare coverage did not have a prescription drug plan.

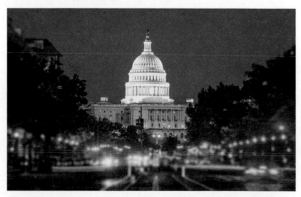

The discussion of health insurance has taken place in Washington for decades, from the creation of Medicare to the Affordable Care Act (ACA) to possible changes in the future.

In 2013, the federal government covered 26% of Americans' healthcare costs, individuals paid 28%, private businesses paid 21%, and local governments paid 17%. There have been some estimates that the federal government will pay 50% of health care in the United States by the year 2020.

Today, Medicare continues to provide health care for qualified individuals over the age of 65 and those with certain predetermined conditions. By the end of 2014, there were just under 50 million people receiving health coverage through a Medicare program. Benefits paid in 2013 amounted to $583 billion, which was about 14% of the federal budget.

Affordable Care Act

Federal legislation that has significantly affected health care and insurance industries is the **Affordable Care Act (ACA)**, also known as *Obamacare*. It was enacted in March 2010 with the goal of providing quality, affordable health care for all Americans. This comprehensive law was enacted in two parts: the **Patient Protection and Affordable Care Act** was signed into law on March 23, 2010, and was amended by the **Health Care and Education Reconciliation Act** on March 30, 2010. The name *Affordable Care Act* refers to the final, amended version of the law.

The ACA provides Americans with better health security by putting in place comprehensive health insurance reforms that:

- Expand coverage

- Hold insurance companies accountable

- Lower healthcare costs

- Guarantee more choice

- Enhance the quality of care for all Americans

To accomplish this, the ACA required immediate improvements in healthcare coverage for all Americans, preserved and expanded insurance coverage, and made insurance coverage available for all Americans. The specifics of the ACA have been controversial since the act was passed, primarily along political party lines. Democrats supported the ACA, and Republicans wanted it repealed and replaced with a different set of reforms. With the 2017 change in the US presidency and many US congressional seats, a replacement or significant changes to the ACA may occur.

Insurance Terminology

Insurance can be a difficult topic to navigate. It is important to be familiar with the different terms used when discussing insurance to give you a better understanding of health insurance concepts.

A **subscriber** is the person whose insurance coverage is used for acute or outpatient care. This is the person who usually pays for the health insurance (insurance premiums) and/or whose employment makes him or her eligible for enrollment in a health insurance plan. Again, using our group of insured individuals, Samuel Elliott and Hazel Bellamy are the subscribers for their health insurance. Angela Singh is the subscriber for herself and her two children, and Matthew's mother is the subscriber for his health insurance coverage.

EXPAND
YOUR LEARNING

Watch the video found at http://EHR2 .ParadigmEducation .com/ACA-Video to experience an overview of the ACA.

EXPAND
YOUR LEARNING

Have you ever thought about what goes into a medical bill? Many people find medical bills to be very complicated. The video "What Goes into a Medical Bill?" at http://EHR2 .ParadigmEducation .com/MedicalBill-Video helps to explain the components of a medical bill.

The insurance premium is the amount that the subscriber pays to the insurance company. The money is usually paid in regular installments, such as monthly, in exchange for insurance coverage.

Coinsurance is the insured person's share of the costs of a covered healthcare service, calculated as a percentage (for example, 20%) of the allowed amount for the service. The insured individual pays coinsurance plus any portion of the deductible he or she still owes. For example, if the plan's allowed amount for an office visit is $100 and the individual has met his or her deductible, the coinsurance payment of 20% would be $20. The plan pays the rest of the allowed amount.

A **copayment** is a fixed amount that an insured individual pays for a covered healthcare service, usually at the time the service is provided. For example, an individual may pay $15 for a visit to a physician. The amount can vary by the type of covered healthcare service, such as office visits, emergency room visits, or prescription medications.

The **out-of-pocket amount** includes expenses for medical care that are not reimbursed by the insurance company. Out-of-pocket costs include deductibles, coinsurance, and copayments for covered services plus all costs for services that are not covered.

The **allowed amount** is the maximum amount on which payment is based for covered healthcare services. The allowed amount is how much the insurance carrier has agreed to pay for the visit and is negotiated between the insurance carrier and provider. This amount may also be referred to as eligible expense, payment allowance, or negotiated rate. If the healthcare provider charges more than the allowed amount, the insured individual may have to pay the difference.

The **benefit year** is the year of insurance benefits coverage under an individual health insurance plan. January 1 to December 31 is a typical benefit year, although many plans may have benefit years that do not align with the calendar year, such as April 1 to March 31.

A cap on the benefits the insurance company will pay in a year is called the **annual limit**. These caps are sometimes placed on particular services such as prescriptions or hospitalizations. Annual limits may be placed on the dollar amount of covered services or on the number of visits that will be covered for a particular service. After an annual limit is reached, the insured individual must pay all associated healthcare costs for the rest of the year.

A cap on the total lifetime benefits an individual may receive from the insurance company is called a **lifetime limit**. An insurance company may impose a total lifetime dollar limit on benefits (such as a $1 million lifetime cap) or limits on specific benefits (such as a $200,000 lifetime cap on organ transplants or one gastric bypass per lifetime), or a combination of the two. After a lifetime limit is reached, the insurance plan may no longer pay for covered services. The ACA created policies that changed the ways some insurance companies handle lifetime limits.

The **guarantor** is the individual responsible for payment. An example might be a man who obtains health insurance coverage through his employer for himself as well as his spouse and children. In such an example, the man is the guarantor or subscriber, and the spouse and children are **covered dependents**.

A **deductible** is the amount an insured individual must pay out of pocket before the insurance will pay. This payment must be met before insurance coverage can be applied to healthcare services. For example, a family insurance plan may have a $25 copayment every time a parent takes his or her sick child to the pediatrician. That same family may have a deductible of $800 a year for healthcare services such as laboratory tests, X-rays, and hospitalizations before their insurance provider pays the remaining balance of any services rendered. Once the bill has been submitted to the insurance company, the deductible is calculated. The insurance company sends payment to the healthcare facility and sends the guarantor a copy of the explanation of benefits (EOB). The EOB describes the details of how the insurance company paid the healthcare bill. The healthcare facility subsequently bills the guarantor for the remaining balance of the bill that the insurance company did not pay.

Classification of Insurance Plans

Insurance plans are classified as either group health insurance plans or individual health insurance plans. An **individual health insurance plan** is an insurance plan that an individual purchases for himself or herself and/or his or her family. For example, John Smith's employer does not offer a group health insurance plan for its employees, so John purchases an individual health insurance plan to provide coverage for himself and his family. A **group health insurance plan** provides healthcare coverage to a specific group of people, typically based on an employer. For example, employees of ABC Chemical Manufacturing are the specific group of people that are eligible to sign up for the group health insurance plan offered by the company. There are three basic types of managed care plans: health maintenance organizations (HMOs), preferred provider organizations (PPOs), and point of service (POS). Coverage is determined by in-network or out-of-network use.

Health Maintenance Organization

A **health maintenance organization (HMO)** is a type of health insurance plan that usually limits coverage to include care only from doctors who work for or contract with the HMO. It generally will not cover out-of-network care except in an emergency. An HMO may require individuals to live or work in its service area to be eligible for coverage. A new approach to health care is called integrated care. **Integrated care** is the systematic coordination of health care. According to the World Health Organization, integrated care brings together inputs, delivery, management, and organization of services related to diagnosis, treatment, care, rehabilitation, and health promotion. HMOs often provide integrated care and focus on prevention and wellness.

Preferred Provider Organization

A **preferred provider organization (PPO)** is a type of health plan that contracts with medical providers, such as hospitals and doctors, to create a network of participating providers. Individuals pay less if they use providers that belong to the plan's network. They can use doctors, hospitals, and providers outside of the network for an additional cost.

Point of Service Plan

Point of service (POS) plans are considered to be a hybrid of HMOs and PPOs. The POS plans are considered to be the most flexible managed care insurance plans as they are less restrictive in the choice of providers and networks. For example, members do not have to choose an in-network physician, but they do need a referral from their primary care physician to go out of network. Another benefit of the POS plans is the national network of providers is available to members when they are traveling. POS plans are more flexible than HMOs and typically cost less than PPOs, making POS plans a good choice for many individuals looking for lower-cost insurance without sacrificing choice.

Health Savings Account

A **health savings account (HSA)** is a medical savings account available to taxpayers who are enrolled in a high-deductible health plan (HDHP). A **high-deductible health plan** has a higher annual deductible than a typical health plan and has a maximum limit on the out-of-pocket expenses that an insured individual or family would incur.

Consolidated Omnibus Budget Reconciliation Act

The **Consolidated Omnibus Budget Reconciliation Act (COBRA)** is a federal law that may allow individuals to temporarily keep health coverage after their employment ends, they lose coverage as a dependent of the covered employee, or another qualifying event occurs. If a person elects COBRA coverage, they pay 100% of the premiums, including the share the employer used to pay, plus a small administrative fee.

Insurance Classification of Healthcare Providers

Insurance coverage and costs are determined on the relationship of the insurance plan and the health providers. In this regard, health providers are separated into two categories: in network and out of network.

In Network

In network includes providers or healthcare facilities that are part of a health plan's group of providers with which it has negotiated a discount. Insured individuals usually pay less when using an in-network provider, because those networks provide services at a lower cost to the insurance companies they have contracts with.

Out of Network

Out of network usually refers to physicians, hospitals, or other healthcare providers who are considered nonparticipants in an insurance plan (usually an HMO or PPO). Depending on an individual's health insurance plan, expenses incurred from services provided by out-of-network health professionals may not be covered or may only be partially covered by an individual's insurance company.

Let's review some examples to make this concept clearer.

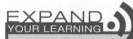

Healthcare services and treatment in the United States can be quite expensive as you may know from personal experience. Visit http://EHR2 .ParadigmEducation .com/BlueBook to identify the average costs of treatment.

- ABC City Hospital is located in a large metropolitan area in which there are nine hospitals within a 20-square-mile area. Cobalt Blue, a private payer, reduces costs of health care for the PPO plan it offers by only contracting with four of the nine hospitals in the area. ABC City Hospital is not one of the four hospitals that Cobalt Blue has contracted with, so ABC City Hospital is considered out of network. A patient with the Cobalt Blue PPO plan would most likely not want to receive healthcare services at ABC City Hospital, or the patient would likely be responsible for the entire hospital bill.

- Eloise Davis has healthcare insurance through an ApolloHealth HMO plan. Eloise should check the listing of physicians that have a contract with the ApolloHealth HMO plan before trying to schedule an office visit.

1. Name the type of health insurance plan that usually limits coverage to care from doctors who work for or contract with the insurance organization. _____

2. Name the type of health plan that contracts with medical providers, such as hospitals and doctors, to create a network of participating providers. _____

3. Name the federal law that may allow individuals to temporarily keep health coverage after employment ends. _____

Government-Sponsored Healthcare Programs

The US government sponsors five major healthcare programs: Medicare, Medicaid, TRICARE, CHAMPVA, and workers' compensation. There are specific eligibility requirements for each of these programs.

Medicare

Medicare is a federal health insurance program for people who are age 65 or older and certain younger people with disabilities. It also covers people with end-stage renal disease (permanent kidney failure requiring dialysis or a transplant, sometimes called ESRD). Medicare has four parts: Part A, Part B, Part C, and Part D.

Part A Hospital Insurance **Medicare Part A** (hospital insurance) helps cover inpatient care in hospitals, including critical access hospitals and skilled nursing facilities (not custodial or long-term care). It also helps cover hospice care and some home health care. Most people don't pay a premium for Part A because they or their spouses have already paid for it through their payroll taxes while working. Beneficiaries must meet certain conditions to receive these benefits.

Part B Medical Insurance **Medicare Part B** (medical insurance) helps cover doctors' services and outpatient care. It also covers some other medical services that Part A doesn't cover, such as physical and occupational therapists and some home health care. Part B helps pay for covered services and supplies when they are medically necessary. Most people pay a monthly premium for Part B.

Medicare Part C **Medicare Part C** is also known as *Medicare Advantage Plans*, or *MA Plans*. These plans are offered through private companies approved by the Centers for Medicare and Medicaid Services (CMS). People who select a Medicare

EXPAND YOUR LEARNING

The Medicare Learning Network (MLN) is a free source of education, information, and resources for the healthcare professional community. Navigate to this link to discover the many video and audio educational resources available regarding Medicare. http://EHR2 .ParadigmEducation .com/ MedicareLearning

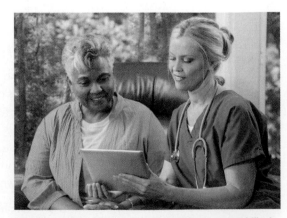

Medicare Part A helps cover inpatient care, skilled nursing facility care, and some home health care for people age 65 or older.

Advantage Plan will have Medicare Part A and Part B through their Advantage Plan and not CMS.

Medicare Part D **Medicare Part D** is a program that helps pay for prescription drugs for Medicare beneficiaries who have a plan that includes Medicare prescription drug coverage. There are two ways to get Medicare prescription drug coverage: through a Medicare Prescription Drug Plan or a Medicare Advantage Plan that includes drug coverage. Both these plans are offered by insurance companies and other private companies approved by Medicare.

Medicaid

Medicaid is a state-administered health insurance program for low-income families and children, pregnant women, the elderly, people with disabilities, and in some states, other qualified adults. The federal government provides a portion of the funding for Medicaid and sets guidelines for the program. States also have choices in how they design their programs, so Medicaid benefits vary state by state and may have a different name in your state.

EXPAND YOUR LEARNING

TRICARE has 9.6 million beneficiaries. The weekly health care sought by these beneficiaries results in 20,000 hospital admissions, 1.9 million outpatient visits, 122,000 dental visits, 2.6 million prescriptions, and 2,372 births. It's incredible that these are just weekly numbers! Watch the video "What is TRICARE?" at http://EHR2.ParadigmEducation.com/Tricare-Video to learn more about TRICARE.

CHAMPVA and TRICARE

Due to the similarity between CHAMPVA (Civilian Health and Medical Program of the Department of Veterans Affairs) and the Department of Defense (DoD) TRICARE program (sometimes referred to by its old name, CHAMPUS), the two are often mistaken for each other. **CHAMPVA** is a comprehensive healthcare benefits program in which the Department of Veterans Affairs (VA) shares the cost of covered healthcare services and supplies with eligible beneficiaries. **TRICARE** is a DoD regionally managed healthcare program for active duty and retired members of the uniformed services, their families, and survivors.

Workers' Compensation

Workers' compensation is an insurance plan that employers are required to have to cover employees who get sick or injured on the job. Workers' compensation is managed by state governments, and rules and guidelines vary from state to state.

States will typically reimburse injured employees covered by workers' compensation with four types of payment, which include income replacement benefits, healthcare treatment, mileage reimbursement, and burial and death benefits.

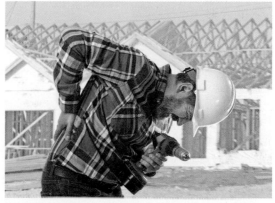

For those who are injured while on the job, workers' compensation can provide income replacement benefits.

Income Replacement Benefits With income replacement benefits, states categorize the lost income of injured employees in one of four ways. These include **temporary total disability (TTD) benefits**, **temporary partial disability (TPD) benefits**, **permanent total disability (PTD) benefits**, and **permanent partial disability (PPD) benefits**. TTD benefits are paid when an employee has been injured at work and cannot perform his or her work duties. TPD benefits are paid when an employee works in a reduced capacity but cannot work to the same extent as he or she could before his or her injury or illness. PTD benefits are paid when the worker's injury permanently prevents the worker from returning to his or her former occupation. PPD benefits are paid when medical maximum improvement has been achieved and a worker may be able to work in some capacity, but the injury has caused damage for an indefinite period and he or she cannot return to his or her old occupation. As mentioned previously, benefits vary from state to state. For example, an injured worker in Ohio qualifying for TTD benefits would be paid for 12 weeks at 72% of the preinjury average weekly wage, and after the first 12 weeks, the worker would receive 66% of the weekly wage. If this same injured worker qualified for the same workers' compensation benefits in California, the worker would receive approximately 66% of the preinjury average weekly wages for the entire covered period.

Healthcare Treatment With the workers' compensation payment for **healthcare treatment**, the medical provider who treats the work-related injury or illness will be paid directly by the patient's employer's insurer.

Mileage Reimbursement Employees injured at work who must travel to their medical appointments will receive **mileage reimbursement** from their employers for the mileage cost and for some of the wages they lose while in transit to and from and during their appointments.

Burial and Death Dependents of an employee who dies from a work-related illness or injury are entitled to **burial and death benefits**. Death benefits are used to replace a portion of the employee's lost income due to the work-related illness or injury. A surviving spouse, minor children, and other dependents of the deceased employee may receive eligible death benefits. Death benefits are typically 75% of the employee's average weekly wages. Burial benefits may be paid to the person who paid for the deceased employee's burial expenses.

CHECKP✚INT 9.2

1. Name the five major healthcare programs that are government sponsored.

_____

_____

_____

_____

_____

2. Name the federal health insurance program for people who are age 65 or older and certain younger people with disabilities.

_____

3. List the four types of payment covered by workers' compensation.

_____

_____

_____

_____

Verification of Insurance Coverage and Benefits

Major insurance plans have web pages for online eligibility requests to determine coverage and benefits for their subscribers (called eligibility databases). In addition, providers may choose to partner with vendors that provide online responses to queries about all major insurance plans. Medicare and Medicaid also have online eligibility databases for providers to query their patients' eligibility, benefits, and in the case of Medicare, the number of coverage days in categories such as inpatient and skilled nursing facility. The Medicare eligibility database application is called the **HIPAA Eligibility Transaction System (HETS)**. The application provides access to Medicare beneficiary eligibility data in a real-time environment. Figure 9.2 is an example of a portion of a typical response from a search in the HETS. The actual response would continue for several additional pages.

Figure 9.2 HETS Eligibility Response

```
□0000004511□
ISA*00* *00* *ZZ*CMS *ZZ*SUBMITTERID *150127*0758*^*00501*111111111*0*P*|~
GS*HB*CMS*SUBMITTERID*20150127*07580000*1*X*005010X279A1~
ST*271*0001*005010X279A1~
BHT*0022*11*TRANSA*20150127*07582355~
HL*1**20*1~
NM1*PR*2*CMS*****PI*CMS~
PER*IC**UR*http://www.cms.gov/HETSHelp/*UR*http://www.cms.gov/center/provider.asp~
HL*2*1*21*1~
NM1*1P*2*IRNAME*****XX*1234567893~
HL*3*2*22*0~
TRN*2*TRACKNUM*ABCDEFGHIJ~
NM1*IL*1*LNAME*FNAME*M***MI*123456789A~
N3*ADDRESSLINE1*ADDRESSLINE2~
N4*CITY*ST*ZIPCODE~
DMG*D8*19400401*F~
DTP*307*RD8*20150101-20150327~
EB*6**30~
DTP*307*RD8*20150101-20150108~
EB*I**41^54~
EB*1**88~
EB*1**30^10^42^45^48^49^69^76^83^A5^A7^AG^BT^BU^BV*MA~
DTP*291*D8*20050401~
EB*C**30*MA**26*1260~
DTP*291*RD8*20150101-20151231~
EB*C**30*MA**29*1260~
DTP*291*RD8*20150101-20151231~
EB*C**30*MA**29*0~
DTP*291*RD8*20150116-20150120~
```

Due to the difficulty of deciphering the HETS response, many providers choose to subscribe to a third-party vendor for Medicare inquiries. These vendors provide the data in a format that is easier to read.

Coverage and benefits for patients who have veterans' benefits can be verified with the US Department of Veterans Affairs (VA) at 1-800-827-1000 or by visiting www.va.gov.

Coverage and benefits for TRICARE subscribers can be verified at 1-866-773-0404 or by visiting www.tricare.osd.mil.

Medicaid eligibility is verified with each state medical assistance (Medicaid) office.

In Chapter 4, you learned how to read an insurance card as presented by a patient and how to enter this information into the EHR. Figure 9.3 shows an example of a Medicare subscriber's insurance card.

EHR systems have a listing of the insurance plans that the provider accepts and from which they will receive reimbursement. Figure 9.4 illustrates the drop-down screen of accepted insurance providers in the EHR Navigator.

Figure 9.3 Medicare Card

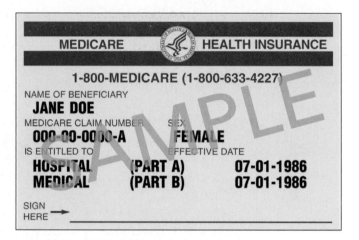

Figure 9.4 Insurance Companies in EHR Navigator

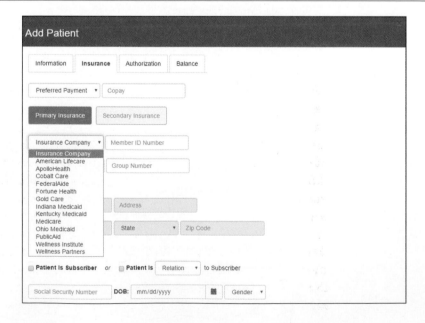

A provider of healthcare services must be eligible to receive reimbursement from an insurance payer, as not all healthcare providers are able to receive reimbursement from all insurance payers.

The Billing Process

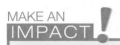
Practice management is the day-to-day operations of a medical practice. An important function in a medical practice is the coding and billing for medical services rendered to patients.

The billing aspect of a medical practice is intricate and includes claims processing, claims management, revenue management, and reporting. Successful practice management in today's medical practice most often uses an electronic office billing system. Electronic office billing systems are used to process insurance claims. Billing staff members also need to follow up on the claims that have been billed and learn how to manage the revenue cycle. Electronic office billing systems include many practice management reports that are useful to the practice managers and owners, which will be discussed in this chapter in greater detail.

As you learned in Chapter 4, accurate data gathering must begin before or upon the delivery of healthcare services. This typically begins at the time the patient is scheduled for a visit or treatment. Patient data—including demographics, insurance, and payment information—must be updated to ensure accurate billing and reimbursement. The method of payment (such as self-payment or insurance) must be verified and entered into the electronic health record (EHR) system.

Following the provision of healthcare treatment or services, a healthcare provider should receive payment for these services.

It is imperative that all staff of a healthcare provider, such as a physician office or hospital, understand the importance of the coordination of timely and accurate patient data entry, billing, and reimbursement. Receipt of monies due for services rendered is required to keep a healthcare organization financially stable and viable.

Electronic Billing

An EHR system may have a billing software component built in, or the EHR system may interface with a separate billing software program. EHR Navigator has billing software built directly into the EHR system so no computer interface is necessary. This is the preferred method because potential communication problems between the EHR system and the billing software are eliminated.

The **electronic superbill** is an itemized form that allows charges to be captured from a patient visit. The provider selects the appropriate reason for the visit and treatment rendered. A superbill typically consists of provider information, patient demographic and insurance information, and details regarding the visit, such as the diagnosis and procedure codes.

The process of entering medical codes into the billing system is called **charge entry**. Staff members can enter charges they are responsible for, or that the provider missed during the electronic superbill entry, via the Add Charges button.

Once charge entry is complete, electronic claims are produced for insurance reimbursement for patients who have insurance coverage, and bills are produced for patients who do not have insurance coverage.

It is important that a provider's billing staff understand basic insurance terms and how to effectively navigate an electronic billing system.

Figure 9.5 shows an example of an encounter form that may be used in an orthopedic office. The master encounter form includes the set fee schedule for the physician office. These fees are typically slightly higher than the highest payer fee schedule.

Figure 9.5 Encounter Form

Patient Identification			Insurance Identification
Date:			COMPANY NAME:
Name:			Insurance #:
Student ID #:			
DOB:		Gender:	Provider name/NPI:
Confidential visit today? ❑ Yes ❑ No		SHQ needed today? ❑ Yes ❑ No	Provider signature:

OFFICE VISIT / **ON-SITE LAB TESTS**

ESTAB	NEW		X	CPT	DESCRIPTION
99211		Minimal eval.			No labs given
99212	99201	Problem focused		80061	Lipid panel
99213	99202	Expanded problem focused		81000	Urinalysis – dip stick
99214	99203	Detailed		81001	Urinalysis, auto. – microscopy
	99204	Comprehensive, mod. complexity, 45 min.		81002	Urinalysis, non-auto. – no microscopy
99215	99205	Comprehensive, high complexity		81003	Urinalysis, auto – no microscopy
99354	99354	**Add-on code to 99215 or 99205** Prolonged service; with patient contact; beyond 30-74 min.		81015	Urine – microscopic only

EPSDT WELL CHILD EXAM / PREVENTIVE MEDICINE

ESTAB	NEW	Consider use of Modifier 25 (write in +25 after code)		81025	Urine pregnancy test-by visual color
99391	99381	Infant		82270	Guiac, occult blood
99392	99382	1-4 years		82465	Cholesterol, total
99393	99383	5-11 years		82947	Glucose; quantitative; blood
99394	99384	12-17 years		82948	Glucose fingerstick
99395	99385	18+ years		82962	Glucose monitoring device
				84703	hCG preg. test (urine) – qualitative

NUTRITION

				85013	Hematocrit
97802		Medical nutritional therapy, initial assessment and intervention, individual, each 15 min		85018	Hemoglobin
97803		Medical nutritional therapy, re-assessment and intervention, individual, each 15 min.		86308	Mono-spot screen
				86677	H. pylori antibody

PSYCHIATRIC THERAPEUTIC PROCEDURES

			87210	Wet mount (e.g., saline) for infectious agents
90832	Psychotherapy, 30 minutes with patient and/or family member		87430	Streptococcus, group A (culture nonbillable)
90833	Psychotherapy, 30 minutes with patient and/or family member when performed with an evaluation and management service - add-on code		87491	Urine CT/GC – amplified probe nonbillable
90834	Psychotherapy, 45 minutes with patient and/or family member		87880	Streptococcus, group A (rapid strep test)
90836	Psychotherapy, 45 minutes with patient and/or family member when performed with an evaluation and management service - add-on code		Q0091	PAP smear, obtaining/preparation **Man. care only**
90837	Psychotherapy, 60 minutes with patient and/or family member		Q0111	Web prep, obtaining/preparation
90838	Psychotherapy, 60 minutes with patient and/or family member when performed with an evaluation and management service - add-on code		92567	Tympanometry – impedance testing

PROCEDURES

				10060	I&D simple

MEDICATIONS, SUPPLIES, AND DURABLE MEDICAL EQUIPMENT

				10120	I&D of foreign body, subcutaneous (simple)
J0170	Adrenaline, epinephrine up to 1 ml	J7603	Albuterol, unit dose form, 1 mg	11730	Nail avulsion
J0560	Penicillin G, up to 600,000 units	A4614	Peak flow meter, hand-held	11740	Evacuation of subungual hematoma
J0570	Penicillin G, up to 1,200,000 units	A4266	Diaphragm device	11750	Excision of nail and nail maxtix, partial or complete, for permanent removal
J0580	Penicillin G, up to 2,400,000 units	A4261	Cervical cap for contraceptive use		
J0696	Ceftriaxone 250 mg. IM per vial	A4267	Condom, male	12001	Suturing – specify body part:
J1055	Depo Provera 150 mg. IM	A4268	Condom, female	12031	Layer closure of wounds of scalp, axillae, trunk, and/ or extremities (excluding hands and feet) 2.5 cm
J1056	Medroxyprogesterone	A4269	Spermicidal agent		
J2550	Promethazine HCl, injection up to 50 mg	J8499 **U1**	Plan B or similar emergency contraception	16000	Initial tx – first-degree burn (local), doc. % coverage and depth
J7300	Intrauterine copper contraceptive	J7307	Etenogestrel contraceptive implant system		
J7302	Levonorgesterel-releasing intrauterine (Mirena)	S4989	IUD other than above (Progestacert)	17110	Wart removal
J7303	Hormone-containing vaginal ring (Nuvaring)	S4993	Contraceptive pills for birth control	26641	Closed tx of carpometacarpal (thumb) dislocation
J7304	Hormone-containing patch (OrthoEvra)	Q0144	Azithromycin oral powder 1 gm **Man. care only**	28190	Removal of foreign body, foot, subcutaneous
J7602	Albuterol, concentrated form, 1 mg			29130	Application of finger splint (static)

IMMUNIZATIONS / **IMMUNIZATION ADMINISTRATION**

				30300	Removal of foreign body, intranasal
90471	One immunization **Managed care only**	90472	Each additional vaccine **Managed care only**	36415	Venipuncture

VACCINATIONS

				54050	Destruction of lesion(s), penis
90633	Hep A	90702	DT	56501	Destruction of lesion(s), vulva
90645	HIB(HbOC) [HibTITER]	90707	Measles, Mumps, Rubella	57170	Diaphragm fitting
90646	HIB(PRP-D) [ProHIBIT]	90712	Poliovirus	58300	IUD insertion
90647	HIB(PRP-OMP) [PedvaxHIB]	90713	IPV (polio)	58301	IUD removal
90648	HIB(PRP-T) ActHIB or Omni HIB]	90715	Tdap	69200	Removal foreign body from external auditory canal
90649 **HB**	HPV females 9-10 and 19-26	90716	Varicella SQ	69210	Removal impacted cerumen (one or both ears)
90649	HPV females 11-18	90718	Tetanus and Diphtheria (Td)	87220	KOH for skin/hair/nails
90657	Influenza (split virus 6-35 mo.)	90732	Pneumococcal polyvalent, SQ or IM	94640	Nebulizer treatment
90658	Influenza (split virus 3 yrs+)	907033	Meningococcal (polysaccharide, SQ)	94010	Spirometry
90669	Pneumococcal conjugate, IM <5 yrs	90734	Meningococcal conjugate vaccine, sero-groups A, C, Y, and W-135 (tetravalent)		
90700	DTaP				
90701	DT	90744	Hep B 3 dose IM		
90660	Influenza virus vaccine, live, for intranasal use	90748	Heb B/Hib Combination IM		TELEHEALTH SERVICE

FOLLOW-UP / **REFERRAL**

			Q3014	Telehealth originating site facility fee
Return to EMC (follow-up date):	To:			
To provider:				

DIAGNOSIS (ICD-9)

Code # and name	

EMC Medical Center

CMS-1500 and UB-04 Forms

Traditionally, insurance companies were billed for services provided in a physician's office using a paper billing form called the CMS-1500. The **CMS-1500** is a universal claim form accepted by Medicare, Medicaid, and most insurance payers. Figure 9.6 shows an example of the CMS-1500 claim form.

Figure 9.6   CMS-1500 (02-12) Universal Billing Form for Physician Services

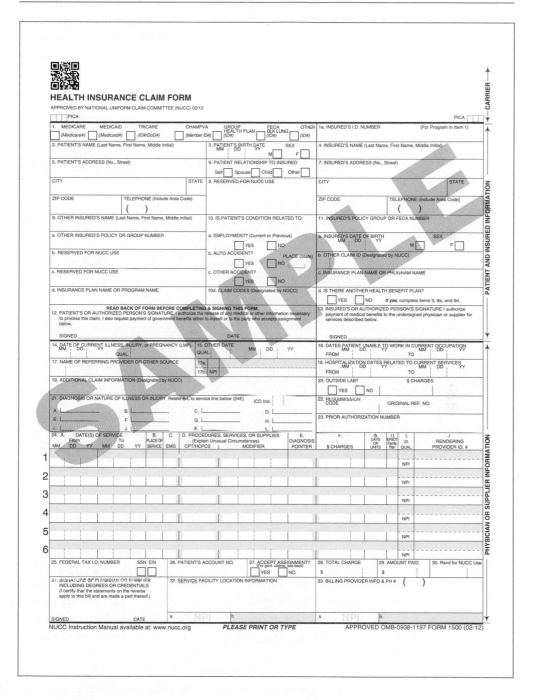

HIPAA regulations require that most claims now be processed electronically using the **HIPAA X12 837 Healthcare Claim**, typically called the 837 Claim or the HIPAA Claim. The 837 Claim file is generated by the software and then transmitted to appropriate insurance payers. Depending on the volume of patients treated by the practice, claims may be filed weekly or even daily. Frequent claims processing should occur to keep cash flow steady.

In an inpatient facility, the UB-04 (also known as the CMS-1450) is the paper form used to bill Medicare. It is also used for billing of institutional/hospital charges to most Medicaid state agencies. The UB-04 contains pertinent information regarding the patient's insurance coverage, medical provider, services provider, and diagnosis. It also contains information that allows for the billing of outpatient services. Figure 9.7 illustrates a UB-04 form.

Tutorial 9.1   EHRNAVIGAT⊕R

Populating a CMS-1500 Form
Go to Navigator+ to launch Tutorial 9.1. Practice populating a CMS-1500 form.

Tutorial 9.2   EHRNAVIGAT⊕R

Populating a UB-04 Form
Go to Navigator+ to launch Tutorial 9.2. Practice populating a UB-04 form.

CHECKP⊕INT 9.3

1. Define practice management.

   _____

   _____

2. Traditionally, insurance companies were billed for physician services using this paper billing form. _____

3. Describe the 837 Claim file:

   _____

   _____

   _____

Benefits of Using an EHR for Billing Operations

Most EHR systems have a billing software component that may or may not be used by the healthcare organization. The decision to use the EHR's billing component depends on the sophistication of the organization's current billing software. Smaller healthcare organizations and physician practices are more likely to utilize the billing software component that comes with the EHR system that they implement. Hospitals and large physician practices are likely to already have a well-functioning billing system and may choose to interface it with the EHR system instead. An **interface** provides communication flow between two or more computer systems. If a healthcare organization chooses to interface the EHR system with the current billing/financial system, the patient record is easily accessible, which is an advantage to the

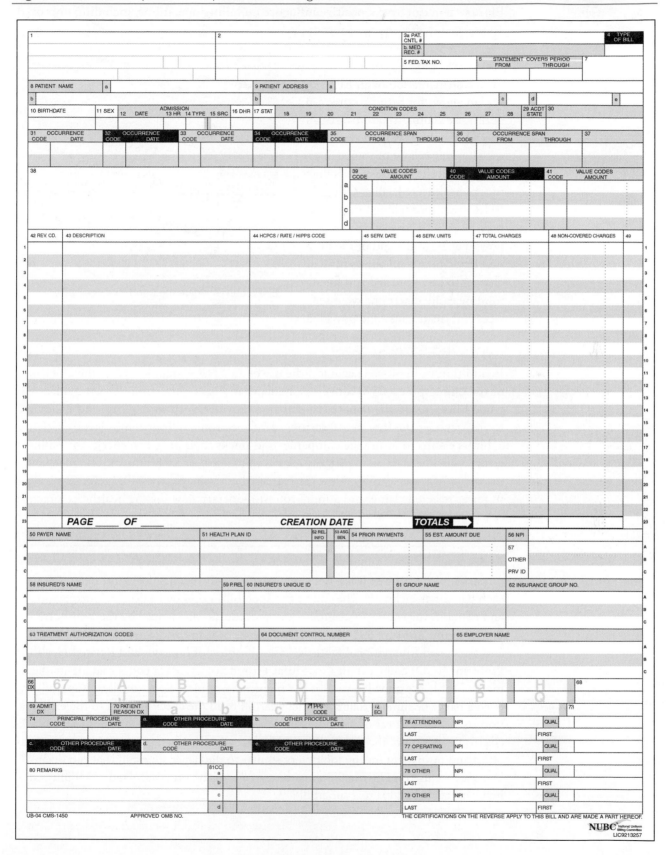

billing staff. Regardless of which approach a healthcare organization chooses, an EHR system can have a positive influence on billing operations, including improved accuracy and efficiency of procedures.

Improved Accuracy

The implementation of an EHR system allows for better accuracy in healthcare claims. The software can check for billing errors as well as speed up the billing process. Faster billing typically improves cash flow for the healthcare facility. Using the EHR system for billing purposes may also eliminate having to chase down papers at the end of the business day. The system allows for daily charges to be reconciled and for staff to more easily determine what services and treatments were provided.

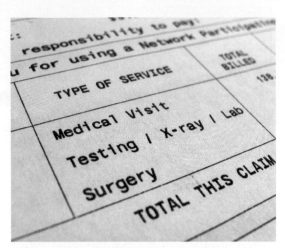

EHRs can eliminate the need for paper bills, improving efficiency of the billing process.

Improved Efficiency

In addition to improved accuracy, the use of an EHR system increases the efficiency of the billing process. No longer are patients and insurance companies provided with paper bills sent via the mail. EHR software provides electronic billing and insurance forms, accesses the Internet to securely send electronic bills or reminders to patients, submits claims to insurance companies and tracks their progress, checks for billing errors, provides data analysis tools related to medical office billing and finance, and more. All of these features allow for increased efficiency of the billing cycle, resulting in fewer rejected claims and a more robust monetary flow for the healthcare practice.

Superbills

As discussed earlier, a superbill (also known as an *encounter form*) is a staple of every physician office because it is a document that records the diagnosis and treatment for each patient at each visit. The content of superbills varies by healthcare organization and contains the common diagnoses and procedures experienced by the healthcare organization. The superbill contains checkboxes next to the diagnoses, procedures, and associated International Statistical Classification of Diseases and Related Health Problems (ICD) and Current Procedural Terminology (CPT®) codes that are marked by the healthcare provider, such as the physician or nurse. Traditionally, a superbill has been a paper document that the patient carries from the check-in desk to the examination room and to areas of testing such as the laboratory and radiology department. The electronic version of the superbill found in many EHR systems for use in the physician office and outpatient setting looks very similar to the paper superbill that physicians and staff are used to. Figure 9.8 illustrates an electronic superbill. Figure 9.9 illustrates how charges are added to a superbill.

Figure 9.8 Completed Electronic Superbill in the EHR Navigator

View Billing Information

Patient Name: Yang,Sophia
Account Number:
Service Date: 04/15/2016

Office | Labs/Supplies/Immunizations

Office Visit - New

QTY	Charges Procedure Code	Charges Procedure Description	Modifiers		
	99201	Office Visit - New, Problem Focused	24	25	57
	99202	Office Visit - New, Expanded	24	25	57
	99203	Office Visit - New, Detailed	24	25	57
	99204	Office Visit - New, Comprehensive	24	25	57
	99205	Office Visit - New, Complex	24	25	57

Office Visit - Established

QTY	Charges Procedure Code	Charges Procedure Description	Modifiers		
	99211	Office Visit - Established, Minimal	24	25	57
	99212	Office Visit - Established, Problem Focused	24	25	57
	99213	Office Visit - Established, Expanded	24	25	57
1	99214	Office Visit - Established, Detailed	24	25	57
	99215	Office Visit - Established, Comprehensive	24	25	57

Figure 9.9 Adding Charges to a Superbill in the EHR Navigator

Edit Billing Information

Patient Name: Yang,Sophia
Account Number:
Service Date: 04/15/2016

Office | Labs/Supplies/Immunizations

Office Visit - New

QTY	Charges Procedure Code	Charges Procedure Description	Modifiers		
	99201	Office Visit - New, Problem Focused	24	25	57
1	99202	Office Visit - New, Expanded	24	25	57
	99203	Office Visit - New, Detailed	24	25	57
	99204	Office Visit - New, Comprehensive	24	25	57
	99205	Office Visit - New, Complex	24	25	57

Office Visit - Established

QTY	Charges Procedure Code	Charges Procedure Description	Modifiers		
	99211	Office Visit - Established, Minimal	24	25	57
	99212	Office Visit - Established, Problem Focused	24	25	57
	99213	Office Visit - Established, Expanded	24	25	57
1	99214	Office Visit - Established, Detailed	24	25	57

When used correctly, the superbill is a useful tool in coding compliance activities. With the selection of the ICD and CPT® codes placed in the hands of the individual providing the healthcare service or treatment, coding should be accurate and consistent. When superbills are used, there must still be a review of the healthcare provider's documentation to ensure that the documentation supports the diagnoses and procedures selected on the superbill. A coder performs this review, and there must be frequent communication between the coder and the provider to ensure that the provider's superbill documentation and health record documentation are in sync.

Tutorial 9.3

EHRNAVIGATOR

Adding a Superbill

Go to Navigator+ to launch Tutorial 9.3. As a biller, practice adding a superbill in the EHR Navigator.

Transmitting Claims

The claims should be reviewed for accuracy and marked as "Ready for Final Billing" before transmission. This review of claims before billing is a proactive approach that saves staff from spending time correcting errors, thus speeding up payment processing. Figure 9.10 demonstrates where claims are marked "Ready for Final Billing" in the EHR Navigator.

Figure 9.10   Ready for Final Billing in EHR Navigator

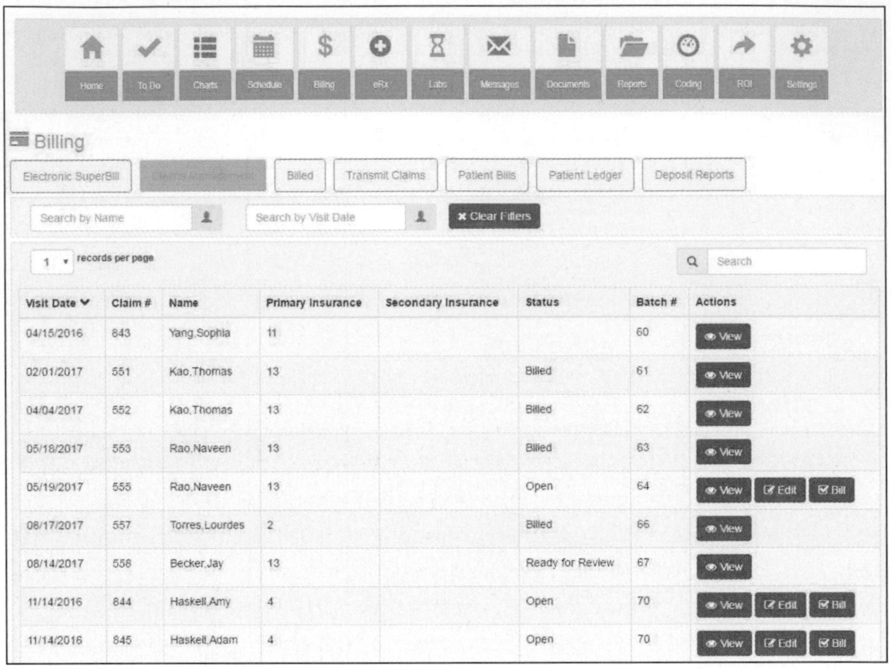

Claim Scrubbing

Before transmission to the insurance companies, patient bills are checked for errors via a process called **claim scrubbing**. Claim scrubbing is the process of checking claims for errors before transmitting them to insurance companies. The number of times a claim is scrubbed before transmission to the insurance company or other payer depends on the policies of the healthcare organization and the level of sophistication of its billing or EHR system. After performing the claim scrubbing process according to its policies and procedures, the healthcare provider then corrects any errors identified by its in-house claim scrubbing report and either transmits the claims directly to the appropriate payer or transmits the claims to a clearinghouse. A medical claims **clearinghouse** is a company that accepts electronic claims from healthcare providers, scrubs the claims, transmits the clean claims to the appropriate payer, and returns the claims that have errors to the healthcare provider. **Clean claims** are those without errors. Why don't healthcare providers just scrub and transmit the claims themselves instead of having to pay a clearinghouse to do this for them? Most healthcare providers do not have claim scrubbing and transmission software sophisticated enough to perform the thousands of error checks, including billing rules, official coding guidelines, and specific insurance carrier rules required to ensure clean claims. In addition, with the hundreds of insurance companies and payers, all with their own billing and claims requirements, it is a monumental job to keep up with all the billing regulations and requirements. Smaller healthcare organizations, including most physician practices, do not have the resources, including software and staff to perform the same functions as a clearinghouse; therefore, the clearinghouses play a significant role in facilitating fast, accurate billing and reimbursement.

The healthcare providers that perform claim scrubbing in house utilize their EHR and billing systems to perform a set of edits on the claims that are ready to be final billed. In the EHR Navigator, you can run reports that show which claims contain errors and then correct those errors for final billing.

Tutorial 9.4   EHRNAVIGAT⊕R

Running a Claim Scrubbing Report and Editing the Claims

Go to Navigator+ to launch Tutorial 9.4. As a biller, practice running a claim scrubbing report. Then identify the errors on the report and correct them in the EHR Navigator.

Final Billing

Following transmission of the clean claim, also known as the *final bill*, to the payer, the EHR system automatically updates to reflect the name of the payer, date, and amount billed. The billing supervisor of the physician practice receives a report automatically delivered to an email address that lists the accounts that were final billed.

When the review of claims is complete and the claims have been marked for final billing, the claims are electronically transmitted to payers or the clearinghouse, and patient bills are printed and mailed or emailed. Since the bills have already been reviewed and marked for final billing, they are in a holding file awaiting the electronic transfer. To accomplish this, the medical biller needs to select the "Transmit Claims" button in the EHR Navigator. The claims that are transferred electronically are either sent to the appropriate insurance payer or the clearinghouse. Amounts that are the patients' responsibility are either printed for postal mailing or generated and sent via email, depending on the patients' preferences. In the EHR Navigator, this is accomplished by selecting the "Patient Bills" button.

Reimbursement Methodology

Reimbursement is the act of compensating a person for services rendered. In the healthcare industry, medical providers treat patients before receiving payment. Fees may not be collected before the patient receives treatment because the necessary treatment is not yet known. There are many different reimbursement methods within health care. The following section reviews the most common methods.

Fee-for-Service Reimbursement

Fee-for-service is a reimbursement method that requests payment for each service or procedure. Each service or procedure has a set fee or charge. Providers are reimbursed only the allowed amount as listed on the third-party payer fee schedule.

Fee Schedules

A **fee schedule** is a price list of services and procedures. Each payer has its own customized fee schedule. However, many healthcare providers base their fees on the **CMS Medicare Physician Fee Schedule (MPFS)**. Medicare uses the **resource-based relative value scale (RBRVS)** to create the MPFS. The RBRVS sets fees for CPT® and HCPCS codes. To calculate the value of a service or procedure, the RBRVS uses three factors:

1. **Relative value units (RVU)** calculated for three components:

   - Work RVU—the amount of work needed to render the treatment

   - Practice expense RVU—the expense to the practice to facilitate the treatment

   - Malpractice RVU—the risk of malpractice associated with the treatment

2. **Geographic practice cost indices (GPCI)** are adjustments applied to the RVU values to account for variations in the costs of practicing medicine in specific geographic regions.

3. **Conversion factor (CF)** is a fiscal year monetary amount that is adjusted annually and is derived from a formula set by the US Congress to convert the GPCI into a dollar amount that reflects several elements:

   - The category of services (medical, surgical, or nonsurgical)

   - The percentage of changes to the Medicare Economic Index

   - Physician expenditures

   - Access to health care

   - Quality of health care

Examples of the calculations are provided in Tables 9.1 and 9.2.

Table 9.1   Example of a National (Standard) RVU Calculation

CPT®/HCPCS Code	RVU Component			Total RVU
	Work	Practice Expense	Malpractice	
49540	$10.74	$6.18	$2.51	$19.43

Table 9.2   Calculation of RVUs for Los Angeles, California, and Red Banks, Mississippi, Using GPCI

City	CPT®/HCPCS Code	RVU Component GPCI Value			Total RVU Value
		Work	Expense	Malpractice	
Los Angeles, CA	49540	$11.24	$7.17	$2.28	$20.69
Red Banks, MS	49540	$10.74	$5.34	$1.53	$17.61

The national RVU provides the base value for CPT® and HCPCS codes. Table 9.1 shows the use of the RVU formula for code 49540, *Repair lumbar hernia*. The three RVU components—work, practice expense, and malpractice—are given set values. The values are added together to determine the national (standard) RVU for the procedure: $10.74 + $6.18 + $2.51 = $19.43.

However, a procedure performed in a major metropolitan area such as Los Angeles, California, will have higher work, practice expenses, and malpractice costs than the same procedure in a smaller city, such as Red Banks, Mississippi. The RVU is geographically adjusted by the GPCI (informally referred to as the *gypsy*). Table 9.2 compares the RVUs for the two cities for code 49540, calculated as:

$$\text{Los Angeles} = \$11.24 + \$7.17 + \$2.28 = \$20.69$$
$$\text{Red Banks} = \$10.74 + \$5.34 + \$1.53 = \$17.61$$

To convert the GPCI into a dollar amount, the total RVU is multiplied by a monetary CF. CFs differ based on the category of services (medical, surgical, or nonsurgical).

Using a CF of 35.7547 and the values in Table 9.2, the fees for code 49540 in Los Angeles and Red Banks are calculated by multiplying their respective GPCI-adjusted, total RVUs by the CF:

$$\text{Los Angeles} = \$20.69 \times 35.7547 = \$739.76$$
$$\text{Red Banks} = \$17.61 \times 35.7547 = \$629.64$$

Rounding the results to the nearest penny shows that the procedure has a Medicare monetary value of $739.76 in Los Angeles and $629.64 in Red Banks.

The MPFS lists RVUs on the CMS website. The MPFS is updated on April 15 of each year. The formulas used to establish RVUs and GPCIs are published in the *Federal Register*, the US government's daily publication of final and administrative regulations for federal agencies. Coders reference the *Federal Register* to stay current on changes that affect healthcare regulations and Medicare.

Health insurance companies base their fees on the MPFS. Physician offices may also use the MPFS to establish a fixed fee schedule for the office, which lists all services and procedures offered at that practice. However, the fees set by the practice do not determine reimbursement amounts from third-party payers. Hospitals compile all procedures, services, supplies, and drugs that are billed to insurance payers into a computer database called a **hospital chargemaster**. Most hospital chargemasters include several thousand line items that are reviewed and updated annually by a medical coder who has the title of chargemaster. Physician offices incorporate their most common procedure and diagnosis codes into the superbill.

Posting payments, insurance appeals, and collections is the last step in the billing or revenue cycle. At this point in the revenue cycle, the focus is on making sure the healthcare organization receives the correct amount of reimbursement for the treatment and services rendered. When insurance companies do not pay correctly, healthcare organizations go through an appeals process to request additional payment from the insurance companies. When individuals owe the healthcare organization monies and do not pay in a timely manner, the healthcare organizations initiate a formal collections process.

Let's look at CPT® code 20610, *Arthrocentesis, aspiration and/or injection, major joint or bursa (e.g., shoulder, hip, knee, subacromial bursa); without ultrasound guidance*. Code 20610 may be reported for the removal of fluid from a major joint or bursa. It may also be reported for the injection of drugs into a major joint or bursa. Physician offices typically accept patients with Medicare, Medicaid, and commercial insurance. The physician, who is contracted with the payers, has access to the fee schedules for each payer. The following is a list of the payers' fees for code 20610 as well as the office fee:

Payers' Fee Schedule for Code 20610:

Medicare	$61.14
Medicaid	$58.12
Commercial payer	$78.28

Physician Office Fee Schedule:

Code 20610	$85.00

The fee schedule shows that each payer has a different allowable fee for code 20610. The commercial payer fee represents a single amount despite the range of fees set by the many different commercial payers that all have their own fee schedules. Rather than looking up the exact fee for each payer, billing is expedited if the physician's office has one set fee for code 20610, typically set a few dollars above the highest listed fee on the commercial payers' fee schedules. If the fee is set lower than what is listed on the fee schedule, and the reimbursement is approved, the payer will pay only the amount requested. In our example, the physician office sets a fee of $85.00 for code 20610.

Practice Management Reports

Frequent and routine monitoring of billing and collections reports is necessary to ensure the practice is receiving the correct monies owed. One such report is the **billing/payment status report**. This report lists the status of every patient account, allowing the billing staff to identify claims that need to be billed or rebilled and insurance payers that need to be contacted regarding lack of payment. Figure 9.11 illustrates the billing/payment status report in the EHR Navigator. Payments from payers may come in the form of electronic funds transfer or a check. The billing supervisor receives a **remittance advice (RA)** report that lists the patient's information and amount paid by Medicare or other payer to the physician practice.

Tutorial 9.5

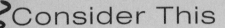

Posting a Payment from a Remittance Advice

Go to Navigator+ to launch Tutorial 9.5. As a billing supervisor, practice posting a payment from a remittance advice using the EHR Navigator.

Figure 9.11 Billing/Payment Status Report

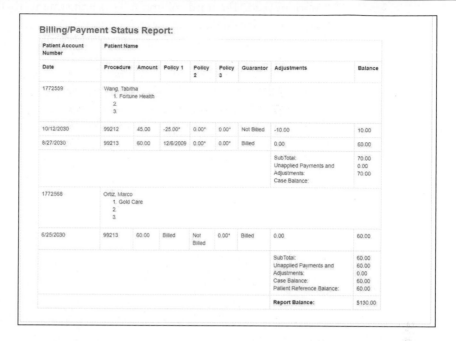

Production Reports

The EHR system is able to generate valuable financial and statistical **production reports** to assist the practice manager with budgeting and revenue management. These reports assist the practice manager in daily, weekly, monthly, and yearly financial reconciliations of billed charges, receipts, and adjustments. Reports should be generated and reviewed routinely by the practice manager for opportunities to improve the management of practice revenues and expenses, as well as billing, accounts receivable, and collections processes. Let's take a look at some of these reports.

Production by Provider Report

The **production by provider report** shows how many patients are treated within a specified period of time by each provider in a practice, along with the revenue generated. These are important statistics to track over time and may be used for a variety of reasons, including the following:

- Calculating provider salaries if based on number of patients treated

- Calculating the number of appointment slots needed for each provider

- Scheduling staff

- Ordering supplies

Figure 9.12 is a sample production by provider report, illustrating the incoming revenue for each provider. This report reflects both month-to-date totals and year-to-date totals. In the first column, you see the ID number of the provider; the second column is the name of the provider; then there are three columns for month-to-date totals and three columns for year-to-date totals. The first of these three columns in each section reflects the amount of charges generated. The second column reflects the amount paid. The third column reflects adjustments that were made to the patient's account. There are many reasons for adjustments, such as refunds or overpayments, differences between the amount billed and the allowed amount per the insurance contract, and nonpayment by a patient.

Figure 9.12 Production by Provider Report

Production by Provider:
Date: 11/01/2030 - 11/30/2030

Doctor ID	Doctor ⌄	Month To Date			Year to Date		
		Charges	Payments	Adjustments	Charges	Payments	Adjustments
1	Corners, Bonnie	$150	$15	$0	$150	$15	$0
2	Merck, Colotta	$42	$10	$0	$42	$10	$0
10	Connor, Marcia	$175	$100	$0	$175	$100	$0
15	Roman, Silvia	$42	$20	$0	$1746	$595	$0
16	Dapkins, Thomas	$150	$20	$0	$1672	$320	$0
17	Hill, Geoff	$42	$50	$0	$1142	$340	$0
22	Petterson, Opal	$42	$50	$0	$409	$240	$0
24	Goldman, Ryan	$150	$50	$0	$300	$65	$0
27	Goodson, Michelle	$375	$15	$0	$525	$25	$0
28	Montague, Roberta	$150	$50	$0	$150	$50	$0
29	Kyee, Nicolas	$42	$30	$0	$1938	$897	$47
30	Feltner, Alana	$150	$0	$0	$2362	$795	$0
31	Turrell, Avis	$150	$50	$0	$1454	$505	$0
32	Gertz, Lester	$150	$0	$0	$2716	$510	$0
33	Vandenbosch, Ricardo	$80	$10	$0	$80	$10	$0
34	Holzer, Gregory	$150	$50	$0	$2971	$770	$0
35	Dowling, Linda	$150	$70	$0	$4552	$1135	$25

Calculating Provider Salaries If a provider's salary at Northstar Physicians is based partially or totally on how much revenue is produced by the provider, you would use the Payments column to calculate the provider's salary since that is the actual revenue that was received. In the previous example, if we look at the year-to-date totals, Dr. Gertz would earn the highest salary. Dr. Alana Feltner would earn the lowest salary, since she generated the least amount of revenue for the practice.

Calculating Appointment Slots and Scheduling Staff Using this same report, an office manager is able to see at a glance which providers need the most appointment slots available for scheduling and the most scheduled medical assistants and staff available to assist them.

Ordering Supplies Because the use of supplies would also be expected to fluctuate with the amount of patient activity, an office manager is able to use this report to gauge supply use and ordering.

Production by Procedure Report

The **production by procedure report** reflects the number of procedures performed during a specific time period along with the associated revenue. Figure 9.13 is an example of one page of a production by procedure report. This report lists the Current Procedural Terminology (CPT®) code that was billed along with the description of the CPT® code, the associated charge for the procedure, the number of procedures performed during the time period specified, the total amount billed, the expected payment amount to be received, the actual payment amount that was received, and the actual adjustment in the patients' accounts that needed to be made. Another useful data sort would be by *actual payment amount*. A **data sort** is arranging data in a particular sequence, from high to low or low to high.

Figure 9.14 illustrates the production by procedure report sorted in ascending numerical order by CPT® code. However, another useful data sort of this report would be by number of procedures performed, in descending order, so the practice manager would be able to report the most common procedures performed by the practice. In Figure 9.14, you can see the most common procedure performed/billed by the practice is 99212, *Office Visit–Established Patient 10 minutes.*

Figure 9.13   Production by Procedure Report

Production by Procedure Report-Summary:
Report includes Data From: 11/01/2030 Through: 11/30/2030

CPT Procedure Code ˅	Procedure Description	Charge	Number of Procedures Performed	Total Billed Amount	Expected Payment Amount	Actual Payment Amount	Actual Adjustment
80048	Metabolic panel, basic	$80	20	$1600	$848	$752	$22
81000	UA	$90	17	$1530	$895	$635	$0
85025	CBC, w auto differential	$42	33	$1386	$-11	$1397	$12
87088	Urine culture	$380	15	$5700	$4985	$715	$0
99201	Office Visit - New, Problem Focused	$150	10	$1500	$995	$505	$0
99204	Office Visit - New, Comprehensive	$375	11	$4125	$3745	$380	$0
99212	Office Visit - Established, Problem Focused	$150	74	$11100	$8190	$2910	$75
99213	Office Visit - Established, Expanded	$175	13	$2275	$1715	$560	$0
Totals:			193	$21664	$21362	$7854	$109

Figure 9.14   Production by Procedure Report Sorted by Procedure

Production by Procedure Report-Summary:
Report includes Data From:
06/01/2030 Through: 06/30/2030

CPT Procedure Code	Procedure Description ˅	Charge	Number of Procedures Performed	Total Billed Amount	Expected Payment Amount	Actual Payment Amount	Actual Adjustment
88141	Cervical Pap Smear	$31.38	49	$1,537.62	$922.57	$872.40	$665.22
99212	Office Visit-Established Patient 10 minutes	$110.00	309	$33,990.00	$20,394.00	$19,420.00	$14,570.00
99213	Office Visit-Established Patient 15 minutes	$160.00	283	$45,280.00	$27,168.00	$25,723.00	$19,557.00
99214	Office Visit-Established Patient 25 minutes	$260.00	55	$14,300.00	$8,580.00	$8,450.00	$5,850.00
99215	Office Visit-Established Patient 40 minutes	$305.00	108	$32,940.00	$19,764.00	$19,140.00	$13,800.00
99211	Office Visit-Established Patient 5 minutes	$54.00	200	$10,800.00	$6,480.00	$6,320.00	$4,480.00
99201	Office Visit-New Patient 10 minutes	$92.00	0	$0.00	$0.00	$0.00	$0.00
99202	Office Visit-New Patient 20 minutes	$180.00	46	$8,280.00	$4,968.00	$5,110.00	$3,170.00
99203	Office Visit-New Patient 30 minutes	$250.00	38	$9,500.00	$5,700.00	$5,610.00	$3,890.00
99204	Office Visit-New Patient 45 minutes	$355.00	18	$6,390.00	$3,834.00	$3,800.00	$2,590.00
99205	Office Visit-New Patient 60 minutes	$441.00	12	$5,292.00	$3,175.20	$3,250.00	$2,042.00
87070	Throat Culture	$173.00	58	$10,034.00	$6,020.40	$5,110.00	$4,924.00

Figure 9.15 is an example of the production of procedure report sorted by actual payment amount. This report shows that the most revenue for the month of June was generated by CPT® procedure code 99213, *Office Visit—Established Patient 15 minutes.*

Figure 9.15 Production by Procedure Report Sorted by Actual Amount

Production by Procedure Report-Summary:
Report includes Data From:
06/01/2030 Through: 06/30/2030

CPT Procedure Code	Procedure Description	Charge	Number of Procedures Performed	Total Billed Amount	Expected Payment Amount	Actual Payment Amount ⌄	Actual Adjustment
99201	Office Visit-New Patient 10 minutes	$92.00	0	$0.00	$0.00	$0.00	$0.00
99215	Office Visit-Established Patient 40 minutes	$305.00	108	$32,940.00	$19,764.00	$19,140.00	$13,800.00
99212	Office Visit-Established Patient 10 minutes	$110.00	309	$33,990.00	$20,394.00	$19,420.00	$14,570.00
99213	Office Visit-Established Patient 15 minutes	$160.00	283	$45,280.00	$27,168.00	$25,723.00	$19,557.00
99205	Office Visit-New Patient 60 minutes	$441.00	12	$5,292.00	$3,175.20	$3,250.00	$2,042.00
99204	Office Visit-New Patient 45 minutes	$355.00	18	$6,390.00	$3,834.00	$3,800.00	$2,590.00
99202	Office Visit-New Patient 20 minutes	$180.00	46	$8,280.00	$4,968.00	$5,110.00	$3,170.00
87070	Throat Culture	$173.00	58	$10,034.00	$6,020.40	$5,110.00	$4,924.00
99203	Office Visit-New Patient 30 minutes	$250.00	38	$9,500.00	$5,700.00	$5,610.00	$3,890.00
99211	Office Visit-Established Patient 5 minutes	$54.00	200	$10,800.00	$6,480.00	$6,320.00	$4,480.00
99214	Office Visit-Established Patient 25 minutes	$260.00	55	$14,300.00	$8,580.00	$8,450.00	$5,850.00
88141	Cervical Pap Smear	$31.38	49	$1,537.62	$922.57	$872.40	$665.22

Production by Insurance Report

Another useful production report is a **production by insurance report**. This report reflects the amount of revenue generated by each insurance carrier. As you can see by the sample report found in Figure 9.16, ApolloHealth has generated the most revenue for Northstar Physicians year to date, with Cobalt Care generating the least amount.

Figure 9.16 Production by Insurance Report

Production by Insurance:
Date: 11/01/2030 - 11/30/2030

Company ID ⌄	Company	Month To Date			Year to Date		
		Charges	Payments	Adjustments	Charges	Payments	Adjustments
1	American Lifecare	$NaN	$360	$12	$1404	$NaN	$12
2	Cobalt Care	$3090	$1125	$25	$4250	$1310	$25
3	PublicAid	$579	$370	$0	$979	$400	$0
4	ApolloHealth	$1496	$305	$0	$1871	$375	$0
5	FederalAide	$545	$250	$0	$795	$250	$0
6	Medicare	$1352	$640	$0	$2032	$680	$0
7	Wellness Partners	$NaN	$360	$0	$1928	$480	$0
8	Fortune Health	$1769	$555	$0	$2539	$620	$0
9	Gold Care	$1372	$325	$0	$1727	$355	$0
10		$470	$275	$25	$920	$300	$25
11	Ohio Medicaid	$501	$195	$0	$876	$225	$0
12	Indiana Medicaid	$2153	$780	$0	$3053	$900	$0
13	Kentucky Medicaid	$4173	$870	$47	$4643	$1072	$47
14	Wellness Institute	$2056	$385	$0	$2511	$455	$0
Totals		$NaN	$6795	$109	$29528	$NaN	$109

Tutorial 9.6

Running Production Reports

Go to Navigator+ to launch Tutorial 9.6. Practice running various production reports in the EHR Navigator.

CHECKP✛INT 9.4

1. Why is a billing/status report generated?

_____

2. Name and describe a report that may assist the practice in revenue cycle management.

_____

3. Describe why a production by provider report is used. _____

_____

Day Sheets

Besides production reports, which may be generated for different time periods and focus, there are several other reports that are useful in practice management. One such report is a day sheet. A **day sheet** is a report of practice activity for a 24-hour period that is used to reconcile patient accounts on a daily basis to ensure that no fraud, abuse, or theft is occurring. To accomplish this daily reconciliation or balancing, the most common type of day sheet used is the **patient day sheet**. The format of a patient day sheet may vary but usually contains the patient name, patient account number, description of activity (such as charge, payment, adjustment), provider, transaction code (such as the CPT® code for a charge, type of payment, or reason for adjustment), amount, and end-of-report totals. Figure 9.17 illustrates the way different criteria can be selected to show various day sheets in the EHR Navigator.

Two other day sheet reports that may prove useful with a practice's daily activity reconciliation are the payment day sheet and the procedure day sheet. The **payment day sheet** is similar to the patient day sheet, except that it lists only the payments made during the 24-hour period. Likewise, the **procedure day sheet** is similar to the patient day sheet but just lists the procedures charged during the 24-hour period.

Tutorial 9.7

Running Day Sheets

Go to Navigator+ and launch Tutorial 9.7. Practice running various day sheets in the EHR Navigator.

Figure 9.17 Patient Day Sheet Report

Patient Day Sheet -- Report Date: 12/02/2030

Patient Account Number ⌄	Name	Activity	Transaction Date	Diagnosis	TX Code	Amount
1772573	Jennifer Barl	Adjustment	12/02/2030	N39	99214	-31
1772544	Tyler Mulligan	Adjustment	12/02/2030	R21	99213	-25
1772500	Vance Donaldson	Adjustment	12/02/2030	I10	99213	-16
1772503	Lily Nguyen	Adjustment	12/02/2030	B35 .1,99213		-45
1772563	Henry Tran	Adjustment	12/02/2030	J01	99212	-15
1772513	Todd Jackson	Adjustment	12/02/2030	J44.9	99214	-5
1772573	Jennifer Barl	Adjustment	12/02/2030	R32	90714	-8
1772569	Kenji Wantabe	Adjustment	12/02/2030	E10.9	99213	-22
1772541	Stephanie Miller	Adjustment	12/02/2030	Q05.8	97010	-18
1772519	Simona Brushfield	Adjustment	12/02/2030	Z23	99213	-25
1772540	Bette Goldman	Adjustment	12/02/2030	I10	90782	-20
1772532	Sophia Yang	Charge	12/02/2030	Z00.00	97010	-25
1772551	Rhonda Taylor	Charge	12/02/2030	E66.9	99214	-15
1772531	Mason Fernandez	Charge	12/02/2030	A53.9	97010	-20
1772561	Benjamin Fowler	Charge	12/02/2030	I70.501	90781	-20
1772506	Miguel Esparza	Charge	12/02/2030	A54.21	90714	-30
1772543	Franklin Romero	Charge	12/02/2030	K57.32	90714	-15
1772568	Marco Ortiz	Charge	12/02/2030	K57.32	99213	-26
1772519	Simona Brushfield	Charge	12/02/2030	I10	90782	-25

Deposit Reports

Two types of deposit reports may be generated daily, weekly, monthly, and yearly for the deposits made from insurance payers and from patient payments. The reports reflect the totals for payments made in cash, checks, credit cards, and electronic direct deposit. The **deposit report** may be filtered by several categories as noted below. A filter limits the records that are included in the report. For example, if the deposit report is filtered by the Payer Type of Patient, then only the payments made by patients would be included in the report, whereas payments from insurance companies would not be included.

Filters on this report include the following:

- *Payment Date:* From and To

- *Payer type:* Insurance or Patient

- *Payer:* All Insurance Payers or Patients or Specific Insurance Payer or Patient

- *Provider:* A specific provider or all providers

A typical deposit report is illustrated in Figure 9.18.

Figure 9.18 Deposit Report

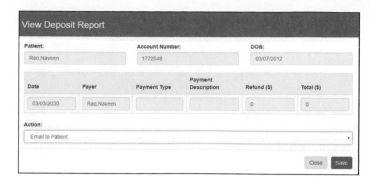

Patient Ledger

The **patient ledger** is a report that reflects the patient's financial status in summary and/or in detail. Charges, ledger notes, billings, payments, and adjustments are all shown in both the summarized and detailed status. The status of each charge is listed, as well as insurance payments that have been made and the amount for which the patient or guarantor is responsible. Figure 9.19 shows a patient ledger.

Figure 9.19 Patient Ledger

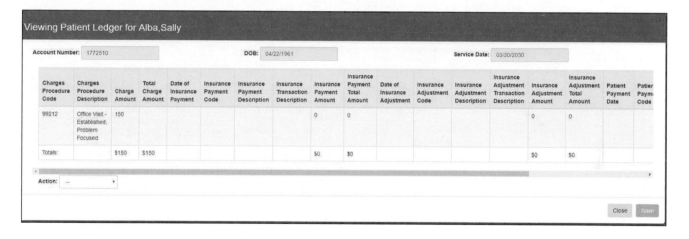

Patient Aging Report

A **patient aging report** is an accounts receivable report that shows how long patients have owed money to the practice. A provider's staff may use this report to follow up with patients regarding payment of past due balances. This report is separated by the length of time outstanding, such as 15 days, 21 days, 30 days, 45 days, 60 days, over 90 days, or over 120 days. A typical patient aging report is shown in Figure 9.20.

Figure 9.20 Patient Aging Report

Patient Aging Report:

Medical Record # ⌄	Patient Account #	Last Name	First Name	Current 0-30 days	31-60 days	61-90 days	91-120 days	121+ days	Total Balance Due
585108	1772559	Wang	Tabitha	$0.00	$15.00	$0.00	$0.00	$0.00	$15.00
585109	1772560	Chan	Brian	$0.00	$0.00	$20.00	$0.00	$0.00	$20.00
585110	1772561	Fowler	Benjamin	$0.00	$0.00	$0.00	$0.00	$0.00	$0.00
585111	1772562	Santos	Sebastian	$0.00	$55.00	$0.00	$0.00	$0.00	$55.00
585112	1772563	Tran	Henry	$0.00	$0.00	$0.00	$80.00	$0.00	$80.00
585113	1772564	Blackwater	Jake	$0.00	$0.00	$66.00	$0.00	$0.00	$66.00
585114	1772565	Yang	Mia	$0.00	$0.00	$0.00	$0.00	$55.00	$55.00
585115	1772566	Tambe	Sandeep	$0.00	$10.00	$0.00	$0.00	$0.00	$10.00
585116	1772567	Singh	Manhesh	$25.00	$0.00	$30.00	$0.00	$0.00	$55.00
585117	1772568	Ortiz	Marco	$0.00	$120.00	$0.00	$25.00	$0.00	$145.00
585118	1772569	Watanabe	Kenji	$0.00	$0.00	$0.00	$0.00	$0.00	$0.00
585119	1772570	Saito	Minako	$0.00	$0.00	$48.00	$50.00	$0.00	$98.00
585121	1772571	Walker	Marjorie	$10.00	$0.00	$0.00	$0.00	$0.00	$10.00
585121	1772572	Oberg	Ingrid	$0.00	$0.00	$40.00	$0.00	$0.00	$40.00
585122	1772573	Bari	Jennifer	$0.00	$0.00	$0.00	$240.00	$0.00	$240.00
585123	1772574	Smith	Emmanuel	$0.00	$30.00	$0.00	$0.00	$0.00	$30.00
585124	1772575	Castanza	Joyce	$25.00	$0.00	$0.00	$0.00	$0.00	$25.00
585125	1772576	Smith	Nathaniel	$0.00	$75.00	$0.00	$0.00	$0.00	$75.00
585126	1772577	Smith	Emmanuel	$0.00	$15.00	$0.00	$0.00	$0.00	$15.00
Totals				$60.00	$320.00	$204.00	$395.00	$55.00	$1,034.00

Chapter Summary

Healthcare service providers must have accurate insurance information to be able to accurately bill for their services. Health insurance is a type of insurance that pays for healthcare services that are incurred by the insured person(s). The discussion of national health insurance has been going on for many decades and includes the creation on Medicare and the Affordable Care Act (ACA). There are many third-party payers with which medical billers will work. These include government-sponsored plans (including Medicare, Medicaid, TRICARE, CHAMPVA, and workers' compensation), private payers, and self-funded health plans. Patient insurance eligibility and coverage is verified to ensure accurate insurance information for billing. There are many detailed steps the billing staff must perform in the practice to ensure the accurate and timely payment for healthcare treatment and services. Most healthcare providers are required to electronically transmit claims to insurance payers. The practice billing system that is part of the EHR or that interfaces with the practice's EHR assists in billing and claims processing as well as revenue cycle management. The electronic superbill is used by providers to document the treatment and procedures that are to be billed. Standard practice management reports must be generated and monitored routinely.

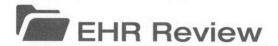 EHR Review

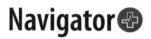
Acronyms/Initialisms

Study the following acronyms discussed in this chapter. Go to Navigator+ for flash cards of the acronyms and other chapter key terms.

ACA: Affordable Care Act

ALS: amyotrophic lateral sclerosis

CF: conversion factor

CHAMPVA: Civilian Health and Medical Program of the Department of Veterans Affairs

CHIP: Children's Health Insurance Program

COBRA: Consolidated Omnibus Budget Reconciliation Act

DoD: Department of Defense

EOB: Explanation of Benefits

ESRD: end-stage renal disease

GPCI: Geographic Practice Cost Indices

HETS: HIPAA Eligibility Transaction System

HFMA: Healthcare Financial Management Association

HIPAA: Health Insurance Portability and Accountability Act

HMO: Health Maintenance Organization (Act)

HSA: health savings account

MA: Medicare Advantage

MPFS: Medicare Physician Fee Schedule

POS: Point of Service

PPD: permanent partial disability

PPO: Preferred Provider Organization

PTD: permanent total disability

RA: remittance advice

RBRVS: Resource-Based Relative Value Scale

RVU: Relative Value Unit

TPD: temporary partial disability

TTD: temporary total disability

VA: Veterans Affairs

Check Your Understanding

To check your understanding of this chapter's key concepts, answer the following questions.

1. The following are all considered government-sponsored healthcare programs *except*

    a. TRICARE.

    b. Medicare.

    c. UnitedHealth.

    d. CHAMPVA.

2. Medicare Part A helps cover all of the following *except*

    a. inpatient care in hospitals.

    b. physician office visits.

    c. critical access hospital care.

    d. skilled nursing facility care.

3. Which of the following is NOT a goal of the Affordable Care Act?

    a. expand coverage

    b. limit choice

    c. lower healthcare costs

    d. enhance quality of care

4. In 2013, the federal government accounted for paying which percentage of the healthcare costs of Americans?

    a. 26%

    b. 40%

    c. 50%

    d. 20%

5. Which of the following describes TRICARE?

   a. a healthcare program for active-duty and retired uniformed services members and their families

   b. an insurance plan that employers are required to have to cover employees who get sick or injured on the job

   c. a state-administered health insurance program for low-income families and children

   d. a program that helps pay for prescription drugs for people with Medicare

6. True/False: The definition of health coverage is "a type of insurance that pays for healthcare services that are incurred by the person(s) that are insured."

7. True/False: A managed care plan is a type of insurance offered by a carrier who has negotiated and contracted with healthcare providers to provide healthcare services for their subscribers.

8. True/False: Medicare Part A helps cover doctors' services and outpatient care.

9. True/False: An HMO is a type of health insurance plan that usually limits coverage to care from doctors who work for or contract with the HMO.

10. True/False: COBRA is a federal law that may allow individuals to temporarily keep health coverage after their employment ends.

11. True/False: The electronic superbill is how charges are captured for a patient visit.

12. True/False: Insurance claims should be filed monthly.

13. True/False: Office managers may choose to bill insurance companies either via paper or electronically.

14. True/False: The Add Charges screen does not provide an opportunity to enter charges that were missed.

15. True/False: A patient aging report is a listing of all the patients' ages and dates of birth.

16. True/False: There are two types of deposit reports: insurance payers and patient payments.

17. Three production reports that are useful in managing a practice include production by

   a. patient, procedure, and provider.

   b. provider, procedure, and insurance.

   c. guarantor, insurance, and medicare.

   d. patient aging, insurance, provider.

18. Which of the following reports is used to reconcile a practice's daily activity?

   a. patient ledger

   b. insurance manual

   c. patient day sheet

   d. patient aging report

19. All of the following data elements are found on the patient ledger *except* a

   a. diagnosis code.

   b. date of service.

   c. procedure code.

   d. patient marital status.

20. It is necessary to reconcile accounts on a daily basis for all of the following reasons *except*

   a. fraud.

   b. abuse.

   c. theft.

   d. privacy.

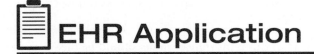

EHR Application

Go on the Record

To build on your understanding of the topics in this chapter, complete the following short-answer activities.

1. Explain the difference between in-network and out-of-network providers.

2. List the five comprehensive health insurance reforms of the ACA.

3. Discuss the difference between coinsurance and copayment.

4. Give an example of a government-sponsored health program and a private payer.

5. What are the major differences between Medicare and Medicaid?

6. Explain how charges are captured for a patient visit.

7. Before the transmission of claims, what procedure should be completed?

8. Discuss two reasons why production reports are used.

9. Explain the difference between the patient day sheet and payment day sheet.

10. Describe the patient aging reports.

Navigate the Field

To gain practice in handling challenging situations in the workplace, consider the following real-world scenarios and identify how you would respond to each.

1. You are the medical biller for a large physician practice and experience frequent difficulties deciphering eligibility responses from Medicare's HETS. What might you suggest to the supervisor of your billing department that would help you, and the other billing staff, obtain Medicare insurance verifications that are easier to read?

2. You are the office manager of a physician practice, and you would like your staff to become more familiar with Medicare. Search the Medicare Learning Network and identify a training program that you would like your staff to review. Here is the website for your reference: http://EHR2 .ParadigmEducation.com/MLNch9Activity.

3. You are the office manager for a large physician practice, and for the past week, the daily deposits have not matched the day sheets. Why should you be concerned?

4. You are a medical assistant in a small rural physician practice, and you have noticed that the physician you work with has, in your opinion, been marking the electronic superbill incorrectly. For example, the physician has spending 10 minutes with the patient yet marks 99205 new PT Level 5. How would you address this with the physician?

EHR Evaluation

Think Critically

Continue to think critically about challenging concepts and complete the following activities.

1. Apply the knowledge that you have gained about healthcare insurance, and research current articles about the future of health insurance in the United States. Summarize your findings in a two-page paper.

2. Compare and contrast the workers' compensation coverage and benefits in your home state with two other states of your choice. The following website will likely assist with your review: http://EHR2.ParadigmEducation.com/ WorkersComp.

3. You are a medical assistant working for a physician practice that currently outsources its medical billing. Because of the high cost of outsourcing, the physicians have decided to bring the medical billing process in house. Since you are interested in the position, you have been asked to write the job description. Based on the knowledge acquired in this chapter, write a detailed job description for a medical biller.

4. Go to the Medicare Learning Network (MLN) Suite of Products and Resources for Billers at http://EHR2.ParadigmEducation.com/MLNBillers and explore the Medicare Learning Network. Identify three resources that you would find useful if you were a medical biller. Prepare a one-page summary of your findings.

Make Your Case

Consider the scenario and then complete the following projects.

1. As the office manager, you have been asked to prepare a presentation for your office on HIPAA regulations as related to electronic billing.

2. Describe the main components of the Affordable Care Act. You may find the following website helpful in your research: http://EHR2.ParadigmEducation.com/ACAComponents.

Explore the Technology

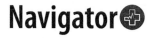

Complete the EHR Navigator practice assessments that align to each tutorial and the assessments that accompany Chapter 9 located on Navigator+.

> " Machines don't make the essential and important connections among data, and they don't create information. Humans do. "
>
> —Jim Stikeleather, Dell

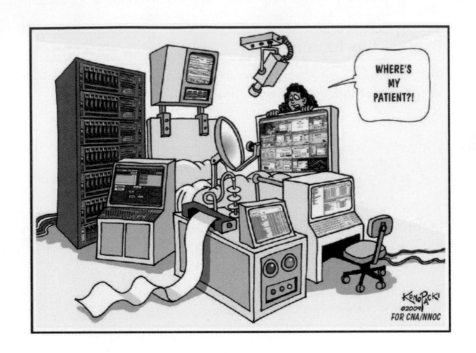

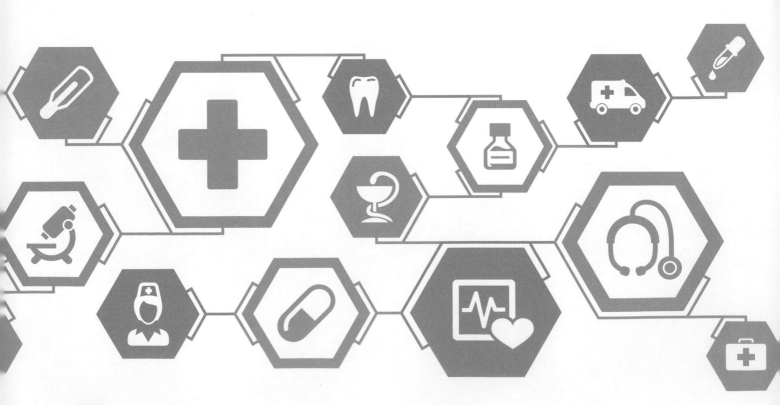

Chapter 10

Data Management and Analytics

How Big Data Is Transforming Health Care

1 Big data creates value for patients by making information personal and accurate.

2 Big data improves quality of life to help treat and manage patients' current conditions.

3 Big data reduces medical errors with evidence-based and personalized care.

4 Big data provides cost effectiveness to healthcare facilities by helping to eliminate fraud and abuse.

5 Big data improves innovation by analyzing data from past trials and current health trends.

Learning Objectives

10.1 Identify data elements in the electronic health record.

10.2 Identify primary and secondary data sources.

10.3 Discuss the concepts and standards of data integrity.

10.4 Define and explain the term *data mapping*.

10.5 Define and identify data dictionary elements.

10.6 Explain how data collection and tools are used in maintaining health data.

10.7 Identify data sets, databases, and indices used in health care.

10.8 Define and explain the term *data warehouse*.

10.9 Explain data governance.

10.10 Identify the eight principles of data quality management.

10.11 Examine the role that data plays in decision-making.

10.12 Discuss big data in health care.

10.13 Define and differentiate informatics and health informatics.

Data is invaluable in every industry, because data turns into information, and information is priceless if managed and analyzed appropriately. The healthcare industry is experiencing an enormous accumulation of data and information because the electronic health record (EHR) captures this. Whether you are a medical assistant entering a patient's vital signs, a physician entering assessments and diagnoses, a nurse scanning medication barcodes and documenting the results of medication administration, a lab technician entering information about a blood draw, or a coder entering diagnosis and procedure codes, you are helping to build a repository of a patient's health information within the EHR.

The data and information from the EHR play a critical role in health care because they can be analyzed to create personalized care and improve the quality and delivery of health care. Furthermore, data and information are used by healthcare organizations, state and federal agencies, public health organizations, and research organizations to make decisions regarding expansions in service, public policy, medical protocols, and more importantly, influencing the quality of the healthcare industry and the services provided.

Recall that in Chapter 2, you learned that data plays a vital role in the health record. This chapter will provide a more in-depth examination of data, its importance in the EHR, its role in healthcare organizations, the roles of the healthcare providers in the creation of data, and how this data is used.

Data Elements

Data is defined as descriptive or numeric attributes of one or more variables. Often the term *data* is referred to as a data element in the EHR. A data element can be one single detail. In the EHR, examples of data elements include date of birth, race, ethnicity, gender, and laboratory test results. In Chapter 2, you learned that data is collected and analyzed to become information. To expand on this idea, data elements are combined into meaningful information about a specific group of patients. Data is stored in the EHR, personal health record, databases, and registries, which will be explored later in this chapter.

Internal and External Data

There are two types of data used in health care to improve the quality of care as well as to facilitate decision-making. They are internal data and external data. **Internal data** is data that is accessed from within the healthcare organization. An example of internal data may be patient financial information. **External data** is data that comes from outside the organization. Sources of external data include Centers for Medicare and Medicaid Services (CMS) and Hospital Compare. **Hospital Compare** is part of the CMS's Hospital Quality Initiative. The goal of Hospital Compare is to provide data to examine how well a hospital delivers quality care and how healthcare organizations can improve. An example of data from Hospital Compare is the readmission rate after a hip and knee replacement by state. The data may be used to compare two healthcare organizations.

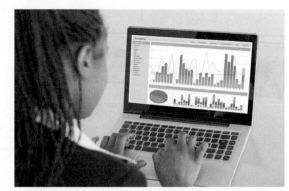

Internal data is accessed within the healthcare organization.

Data Sources

There are two kinds of data sources, primary and secondary. These sources are important to recognize when using and reporting data. Primary data is the original collection or original data found in the health record. Secondary data sources are data that is collected by someone else or data that already exists. It is important to use a combination of the two data sources, primary and secondary, to help researchers predict outcomes based on available data.

Primary

Primary sources of health information are data and information from the patient's EHR. For example, data entered into the EHR in the course of treating the patient would be considered a primary source of data. Types of primary data sources found in the EHR include administrative data, clinical notes, diagnosis and procedure codes, and laboratory procedures. Primary data may be used to document a patient visit and to bill insurance.

Secondary

Secondary data sources are indexes and registries. The data is taken from the patient's health record and reported to cancer registries or vital statistics such as birth records. Secondary data can be used for research, marketing, and public health monitoring, such as the number of cases of Zika virus disease or influenza.

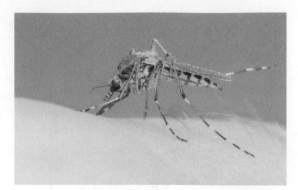

Secondary data can help monitor public health issues, such as the spread of the Zika virus.

CHECKPOINT 10.1

1. Name four data elements.

   a. _____-_____

   b. _____-_____

   c. _____-_____

   d. _____-_____

2. What is the difference between primary and secondary data sources?

   _____

   _____

   _____

Data Integrity

Data integrity refers to the accuracy, completeness, and reliability of data in the EHR. The EHR includes data from multiples sources, including primary and secondary sources as discussed earlier in the chapter. When data is generated by multiple sources, it increases the likelihood that errors will be present in the EHR. Data integrity can be compromised when the content of the data element is entered incorrectly or when the EHR system protections do not work properly. For example, a nurse does not enter a patient's medication allergy correctly in the EHR, which results in an alert either not working correctly or being ignored. The result of incorrect data is that the patient may be harmed. To prevent incorrect data, policies and procedures for data standards should be implemented.

MAKE AN IMPACT!

You may have heard about a career as a healthcare data analyst. What does a healthcare data analyst really do? Watch the video about a day in the life of a healthcare data analyst.
http://EHR2
.ParadigmEducation
.com/DataLife

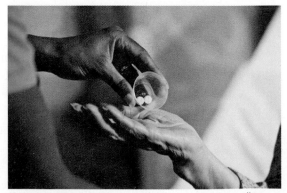

If data is entered into the EHR incorrectly, medication errors can occur.

Standards

Data standards are agreed-upon definitions and formats of data. Interoperability is a key component to data standards. Chapter 1 explains interoperability in relation to the EHR. Chapter 1 also addresses common data standards such as Health Level Seven International (HL7). Data standards are important for bringing data into a common format to allow for sharing, which aids in patient care. Data standards help to create the exchange, transfer, and transmission of data between different systems.

Policies and Procedures

Policies are principles or guidelines that are agreed upon by the organization. **Procedures** are methods used to put policies in action within the healthcare organization. Together, policies and procedures provide an explanation to employees of the healthcare organization about how to handle data operations. Policies and procedures provide a framework to identify the data standards for a healthcare organization. Policies and procedures also detail the use of data, such as the policies and procedures of using data in relation to privacy and confidentiality.

Data Dictionary

A **data dictionary** is a document that describes the content, format, and structure of data elements within a database. A data dictionary is important to data standards because it provides a way to prevent inconsistencies, define elements and their meanings, and also provide consistency and enforce data standards. Common data elements that may be found in a data dictionary include the data field name, definition, data type, format, data field size, and data values. Figure 10.1 illustrates an example of a data dictionary table.

Figure 10.1 Data Dictionary Table

Table List of Candidate Values

Variable Name	Value	Description
SurgID	varchar	surgery identifier
SurgTime	date	date of surgery
PtID	varchar	patient identifier
SurgType	varchar	{CABG, HERNIA, HIP, KNEE}
SSI	integer	{0 for absent, 1 for present}
SSI_type	varchar	{superficial, deep, organ}
WBC	number	highest wbc postop day 3-30
PercNeu	number	highest % neutrophils post op day 3-30
ESR	number	highest ESR postop day 3-30
CRP	number	highest CRP (in mg/dL) postop day 3-30
Fever	number	highest temp (in Fahrenheit) postop day 3-30
Cx_Sent	integer	whether a culture was sent postop day 3-30
Cx_Pos	integer	whether postop cx was positive
Path_Org	varchar	s. aureus, P. aeruginosa, enterobacteriaceae, etc.
Cx_Site_Match	integer	for example culture site hip for hip operation
Re_Admit	integer	readmission on postop day ____; null if no readmission
PostOp_Abx	integer	postop day 3-30 but no preop day 1 to 7

Data Mapping

Data mapping is a special type of data dictionary. Data mapping is a method that is used to connect data from one system to data of another system. Data is analyzed in the original or source system to match data in the other or target system. Mapping the data is key to accurate data connection. Data mapping can be matched through the data dictionary or data sets. There can be challenges with data mapping when the source and target data do not match. An example of when this issue may arise is when the source system uses ICD-9 codes and the target system requires ICD-10 codes.

Data Collection

As discussed in Chapter 7, **data collection** is important to capture and maintain the accuracy and completeness of data. Data collection consists of both manual and automated data collection. The collection of information can then be shared to provide quality care to the patient. Manual data collection is data collected by a staff member or entered by the patient. Manual data collection can take place through a paper or digital form completed by an employee or the patient. Automated data collection is the reuse of data that was initially captured for other purposes.

CHECKP✚INT 10.2

1. Explain why policies and procedures are important to data standards.

_____

_____

_____

2. Why is a data dictionary important to data standards?

_____

_____

_____

3. Explain data mapping.

_____

_____

_____

Data Sets

A **data set** is a structured collection of related data elements. These data elements have standard definitions to provide consistent data for all users. Data sets used in health care are frequently created to relate to a specific area of health care, such as inpatient care, outpatient care, long-term care, and home health care. Healthcare data sets are also frequently used for clinical areas, such as cardiology, gastroenterology, and pediatrics. Several data sets that are commonly used in health care are defined next.

Uniform Hospital Discharge Data Set

Initially discussed in Chapter 4, the **Uniform Hospital Discharge Data Set (UHDDS)** began with 14 data elements and applied only to acute care hospitals. Since then, 6 additional data elements have been added for a total of 20 data elements. These data elements are required by the US Department of Health and Human Services (HHS) to be abstracted for Medicare and Medicaid inpatients only. However, most hospitals abstract the UHDDS for all inpatients, as this information is vital for organizational planning. Use of the UHDDS made the implementation of the prospective payment system possible for acute care hospitals. The UHDDS has been revised over the years to accommodate changes in data required by users and agencies.

In 2006, long-term care hospitals (LTCHs; or long-term acute care hospitals [LTACs]) were required to use the UHDDS to facilitate implementation of the LTCH prospective payment system (PPS). The UHDDS has been revised over the years to accommodate changes in data required by users and agencies. The below reflects alternative care settings.

Uniform Ambulatory Care Data Set

As presented in Chapter 4, the US National Committee on Vital and Health Statistics recommended a data set for ambulatory care records. These 16 data elements represented the uniform minimum basic data set for ambulatory records. The uniform minimum basic data set for ambulatory records was revised and titled the **Uniform Ambulatory Care Data Set (UACDS)**. Like the UHDDS, the UACDS contains data elements that identify the patient, provider, place, and reason for the encounter as well as the services provided and patient disposition.

Minimum Data Set

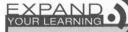

Visit this Medicare site showing data that allows consumers to compare nursing homes:

http://CHIR2 .ParadigmEducation .com/NursingHome.

The **Minimum Data Set (MDS)** is a core set of screening, clinical, and functional status elements required to be completed for all residents of nursing homes certified by Medicare or Medicaid. Table 10.1 lists some of these core data elements from the MDS. The MDS is part of the Resident Assessment Instrument (RAI). The primary purpose of the RAI tool is to identify resident care problems that are addressed in an individualized care plan; however, use of the RAI has expanded. Data collected from MDS assessments is used for the Skilled Nursing Facility Prospective Payment System (SNF PPS) Medicare reimbursement system and many state Medicaid reimbursement systems. Data is also used for monitoring the quality of care provided to nursing home residents. A sampling of the Minimum Data Set Version 3.0 Resident Assessment and Care Screening is illustrated in Figure 10.2.

Table 10.1 Minimum Data Set Core Elements

Core Elements
Facility provider numbers
Type of provider
Type of assessment
Unit certification or licensure designation
Preadmission screening and resident review
Identification information
Hearing, speech, and vision
Cognitive patterns
Mood
Behavior
Preferences for customary routine and activities
Functional status
Functional abilities and goals
Bladder and bowel
Active diagnoses
Health conditions
Swallowing/nutritional status
Oral dental
Skin conditions
Medications
Special treatments, procedures, and programs
Restraints
Participation in assessment and goal setting
Care area assessment summary
Correction request
Assessment administration

Outcomes and Assessment Information Set and OASIS-2

The **Outcome and Assessment Information Set (OASIS)** is a group of data elements that represent core items of a comprehensive assessment for an adult home care patient. OASIS is the basis for measuring patient outcomes to analyze and improve the quality of care for home care patients. Just like the previous data sets discussed in this section, OASIS is also a requirement of the Medicare and Medicaid certified home health agencies (HHAs). The use of OASIS data began in 1999, and since October 2000, OASIS has been used to reimburse HHAs for the care rendered to Medicare beneficiaries and participating states for Medicaid clients.

OASIS was updated in January 2017 and is now titled OASIS-2. The reason for the update is to meet requirements of the Improving Medicare Post-Acute Care Transformation (IMPACT) Act of 2014. OASIS-2 increases standardization with assessment item sets for other post-acute care (PAC) settings.

Figure 10.2 Minimum Data Set Version 3.0 Resident Assessment and Care Screening

Resident _____ Identifier _____ Date _____

MINIMUM DATA SET (MDS) - Version 3.0
RESIDENT ASSESSMENT AND CARE SCREENING
Nursing Home Comprehensive (NC) Item Set

Section A	Identification Information

A0050. Type of Record

Enter Code ☐
1. **Add new record** → Continue to A0100, Facility Provider Numbers
2. **Modify existing record** → Continue to A0100, Facility Provider Numbers
3. **Inactivate existing record** → Skip to X0150, Type of Provider

A0100. Facility Provider Numbers

A. **National Provider Identifier (NPI):**
☐☐☐☐☐☐☐☐☐☐

B. **CMS Certification Number (CCN):**
☐☐☐☐☐☐☐☐☐☐

C. **State Provider Number:**
☐☐☐☐☐☐☐☐☐☐☐☐

A0200. Type of Provider

Enter Code ☐
Type of provider
1. **Nursing home (SNF/NF)**
2. **Swing Bed**

A0310. Type of Assessment

Enter Code ☐☐
A. **Federal OBRA Reason for Assessment**
01. **Admission** assessment (required by day 14)
02. **Quarterly** review assessment
03. **Annual** assessment
04. **Significant change in status** assessment
05. **Significant correction** to **prior comprehensive** assessment
06. **Significant correction** to **prior quarterly** assessment
99. **None of the above**

Enter Code ☐☐
B. **PPS Assessment**
PPS Scheduled Assessments for a Medicare Part A Stay
01. **5-day** scheduled assessment
02. **14-day** scheduled assessment
03. **30-day** scheduled assessment
04. **60-day** scheduled assessment
05. **90-day** scheduled assessment
PPS Unscheduled Assessments for a Medicare Part A Stay
07. **Unscheduled assessment used for PPS** (OMRA, significant or clinical change, or significant correction assessment)
Not PPS Assessment
99. **None of the above**

Enter Code ☐
C. **PPS Other Medicare Required Assessment - OMRA**
0. **No**
1. **Start of therapy** assessment
2. **End of therapy** assessment
3. **Both Start and End of therapy** assessment
4. **Change of therapy** assessment

Enter Code ☐
D. **Is this a Swing Bed clinical change assessment?** Complete only if A0200 = 2
0. **No**
1. **Yes**

Enter Code ☐
E. **Is this assessment the first assessment** (OBRA, Scheduled PPS, or Discharge) **since the most recent admission/entry or reentry?**
0. **No**
1. **Yes**

MDS 3.0 Nursing Home Comprehensive (NC) Corrected Version 1.14.0 DRAFT   Page 1 of 45

OASIS data regarding the assessment of the condition of the patient as well as treatment and services rendered are collected at the following time points:

- Start of care
- Resumption of care following inpatient facility stay
- Recertification within the last 5 days of each 60-day recertification period
- Other follow-up during the home health episode of care
- Transfer to inpatient facility

- Discharge from home care

- Death at home

In 2017, CMS, with the goal of reducing the data collection burden for OASIS, identified 35 OASIS items to eliminate from the data set. If the data items were not:

- used to calculate a measure finalized for the Home Health Quality Reporting Program (HH QRP),

- used in the Home Health Prospective Payment System (PPS),

- used in the survey process for Medicare certification,

- used to calculate a measure in the Home Health Value-Based Purchasing (HH VPB) demonstration,

- used as a critical risk adjustment factor, or

- incorporated into OASIS to fulfill a data category as part of the Conditions of Participation,

they will be eliminated as of January 1, 2019. Eliminating these 35 OASIS items reduces the collection of 247 fewer data elements at certain time points in the OASIS process. A few examples of the data elements to be eliminated includes the following:

- Vision

- Ability to hear

- Understanding of verbal content

- Pressure ulcer assessment

- Formal pain assessment

Data Elements for Emergency Department Systems

In 1997, the National Center for Injury Prevention and Control developed **Data Elements for Emergency Department Systems (DEEDS)**, which are uniform specifications for data entered into emergency department (ED) patient records. There are 156 data elements in this data set, and the number of data elements used to complete a patient's record will vary according to the complexity of the patient's problem and the extent of care rendered during the ED visit. DEEDS focuses on the detailed clinical condition of the patient along with a very thorough reporting of the treatments rendered, including all medications, which significantly increases the number of data elements as compared to the UHDDS and UACDS.

Essential Medical Data Set

The Essential Medical Data Set (EMDS) complements DEEDS, because it provides the data elements for the history of the emergency room patient, whereas DEEDS provides the data elements for the specific emergency department encounter by the patient.

Databases

A **database** is a collection of data that is organized in rows, columns, and tables. The data is indexed. **Indexes** in a database are used to find data without searching every row. The data is combined to form information that can be analyzed, managed, and updated. The EHR is a database that collects the healthcare organization and patient data. Healthcare organizations use data from databases to improve delivery and quality of care. Many types of databases are used by healthcare organizations. A few of the most frequently used databases are HealthData.gov, the Healthcare Cost and Utilization Project, Medicare Provider Analysis and Review, and National Practitioner Data Bank.

HealthData.gov

HealthData.gov (shown in Figure 10.3) provides access to health data with the hope of improving healthcare quality. Healthcare data is collected from various sources, such as CMS, the Centers for Disease Control and Prevention (CDC), US Food and Drug Administration (FDA), and the National Institutes of Health (NIH). The database is used by innovators who are developing new applications and services that can improve the quality and delivery of health care. The goal of HealthData.gov is to permit private sector innovators to access data collected by HHS.

Figure 10.3 HealthData.gov Site

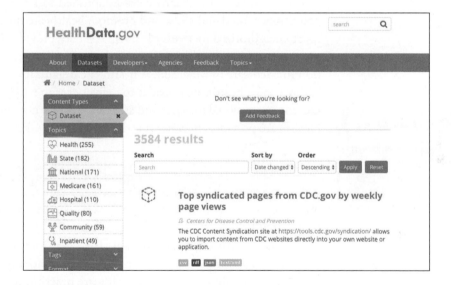

The Healthcare Cost and Utilization Project

The **Healthcare Cost and Utilization Project (HCUP)** is a collection of databases that is sponsored by the Agency for Healthcare Research and Quality (AHRQ). The collection of databases contains data from state organizations, hospitals, private data organizations, and the federal government to create a national resource of encounter level healthcare data. The database contains all payer encounter level information dating back to 1988. HCUP contains a variety of databases, including the National Inpatient Sample (NIS), the Kids' Inpatient Database (KID), the Nationwide Emergency Department Sample (NEDS), the Nationwide Readmissions Database (NRD), the

State Inpatient Databases (SID), the State Ambulatory Surgery and Services Databases (SASD), and the State Emergency Department Databases (SEDD). HCUP data is primarily used by researchers and policymakers; however, this data is publicly available. The collection of data is an information resource of patient-level healthcare data that is used to identify, track, and analyze trends in healthcare use, including access, quality, and outcomes.

Medicare Provider Analysis and Review

Medicare Provider Analysis and Review, known as MEDPAR, is a database that contains inpatient hospital and skilled nursing facility records for all Medicare beneficiaries. MEDPAR contains procedures, diagnoses, and diagnosis-related groups (DRGs); length of stay; beneficiary and Medicare payment amounts; and summarized revenue center charge amounts. The data is organized by state and then by DRG. The data fields include total charges, covered charges, Medicare reimbursement, total days, number of discharges, and average total days. This data set contains data on older patients, since they are most likely Medicare patients.

National Practitioner Data Bank

The **National Practitioner Data Bank (NPDB)** is a database that contains information on medical malpractice payments and actions against healthcare practitioners, providers, and suppliers. The database was established in 1986 by the US Congress to deter practitioner fraud and abuse and promote healthcare quality. A user of this database must be authorized to access the data. The data provides information on healthcare providers, including malpractice awards, loss of license, and exclusion from participation in Medicare or Medicaid. A healthcare organization accesses the NPDB prior to authorizing a healthcare provider to deliver care to patients. Other users of this database include professional societies and state and federal licensing and certification agencies. Healthcare providers may use this database to view their own information.

Data Warehouse

A **data warehouse** is a database that accesses data from multiple databases that are integrated to be used for analytic purposes. The data warehouse is viewed as the trusted source that brings together all the data from the EHR and other data generators and gathers them within the organization. The data from the warehouse can provide information on a single patient or a related group of patients. The goal of analyzing data from a data warehouse is to help healthcare practitioners and organizations provide better care.

Data Indices

International Classification of Diseases (ICD) was discussed in Chapter 8. Recall that ICD is an index that is used to classify and code all diagnoses, symptoms, and procedures in combination with a patient's inpatient or hospital care.

Current Procedural Terminology (CPT®) was discussed in Chapter 8. Remember that CPT® is an index of medical, surgical, and diagnostic procedure codes used by healthcare providers in delivery of outpatient care.

EXPAND
YOUR LEARNING

To analyze population health, healthcare organizations look at data from hospitals, payers, primary care providers, specialists, pharmacies, public health organizations, and patients. Read the article "Which Healthcare Data is Important for Population Health Management?" to better understand the various data sources that are used in managing population health.
http://EHR2.ParadigmEducation.com/Analytics

Data Registries

An EHR is used to collect various clinical and demographic data about each patient for every healthcare encounter. A registry is more specific, as it is used to collect data about certain diseases or conditions. In the future, once interoperability between systems is in place, an EHR may populate the registry. Currently, technology is being developed to integrate registries into the EHR. Meanwhile, registries provide valuable information regarding the health status of patients.

The National Vital Statistics System is an example of data sharing in public health by collecting data from the National Center for Health Statistics (NCHS) and vital registration systems. State laws require birth certificates to be submitted for all births. Federal law requires the national collection and publication of births. A birth registry contains information about the newborn, mother and father, and health information. The registry contains information on live births, infant deaths, and fetal deaths.

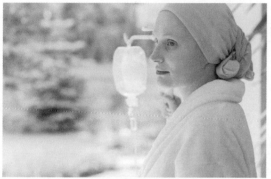

All patients with cancer in the United States are added to a cancer registry.

Cancer Registries

A **cancer registry** is a collection of data focusing on cancer and tumor diseases. The data is collected by cancer registrars who collect information such as patient history, diagnosis, treatment, and status. The registry contains this information for every patient that has been diagnosed with cancer by a healthcare provider in the United States. Healthcare organizations are required to report new cancer cases to their state cancer registries. The data may be submitted electronically or by paper. The registry helps to report cancer incidences as well as evaluate experience and quality of treatment.

Clinical Trials

ClinicalTrials.gov is a registry that provides access to information on publicly and privately funded clinical studies. Clinical trials evaluate new laboratory findings that may advance diagnosis, treatment, or prevention in humans. A clinical trial is a study that uses human volunteers. These studies assign interventions based on a plan and then evaluate the health effect and outcome. The registry is maintained by the National Library of Medicine at the NIH. Clinical trials can be based on new treatments, different drugs, or changes in diet.

Trauma Registries

A **trauma registry** includes the collection, storage, and reporting of patient trauma data. Trauma data that is collected for the registry is based on serious bodily injury. An example of trauma that may be reported would be a person who is seriously injured in a car accident and if the patient was wearing a seat belt. The registry collects data about an injured patient who meets a specific criteria. The data consists of demographic, injury, and trauma outcome data. The registry helps to analyze injuries, establish prevention programs, evaluate major trauma outcomes, and provide research and education.

Information Governance

One of the major challenges in the management of healthcare information is creating an effective framework for the access and use of healthcare data. This framework is known as **information governance** and includes the policies, procedures, and processes for data and information creation, storage, access, use, analysis, archival, and deletion.

Information governance is a relatively new concept in health care. It took the implementation of EHR systems for many healthcare executives to recognize the vast amount of data and information available to their organizations and the need for governance of this data and information. Healthcare executives typically turn to their information technology (IT) departments and/or health information management (HIM) departments for assistance with information governance.

An effective information governance system should include the following components:

- Data governance committee
- Strategic plans for using and expanding data
- Management of data quality
- Appropriate access to data
- Resources for users to correctly interpret the data

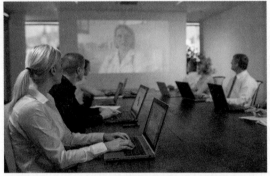

All departments in a healthcare facility should be represented on a data governance committee.

Data Governance Committee

One of the first steps in establishing a data governance program is to create a data governance committee made up of a broad representation of the organization's stakeholders. A broad representation promotes the establishment of processes, policies, and procedures that apply to the organization, avoiding those that are narrow in scope. For example, if only IT and HIM staff serve on the data governance committee, many clinical needs could be ignored, whereas including representatives from clinical departments enhances the committee's membership.

Strategic Plans for Using and Expanding Data

The data governance program should be a fluid program that is constantly growing and changing to meet the needs of the organization. An essential component of a data governance program is to establish a strategic plan. A **strategic plan** is an organization's process of defining its direction by including goals or objectives and a sequence of steps to achieve each goal and objective. Establishment of strategic plans, both short term and long term, helps to keep the data governance program on track and relevant to the needs of the organization.

Management of Data Quality

In the discussion of the importance of data quality earlier in this chapter, you learned how important it is to an organization to have accurate data. A successful data governance program should have specific auditing programs in place to ensure data accuracy.

A key data auditing program that will be discussed in Chapter 11 is a clinical documentation improvement (CDI) program. In addition to the auditing and correcting of clinical data, data quality auditing should also be conducted for financial and demographic data.

Appropriate Access to Data

As we have discussed in previous chapters, there is a need for data security as well as a process of minimum use in which each user of the organization's data has access to only the minimum amount of data necessary for completion of his or her job role. Considering the heightened focus on the security of health data in the daily news, there is a tendency to keep a tight control on all data. However, a well-functioning data governance program should encourage the use of data while keeping security protocols in mind. To facilitate appropriate access to data, an organization should consider merging committees dealing with IT privacy, security, and data governance.

Resources for Users to Correctly Interpret Data

Data users must have the necessary resources to correctly interpret data. Otherwise, poor decisions could result. For example, the concept of the data dictionary, which was discussed earlier in this chapter, is a perfect example of a necessary resource. Consider this example. The CEO of a hospital asks the director of radiology to provide the actual cost of a chest X-ray performed at the hospital over the past year. The director of radiology queries the database, requesting the number of chest X-rays performed on the admissions for the past year as one of the numbers needed in his calculation. By requesting data based on admissions, the director of radiology is missing the number of chest X-rays performed during the year on outpatients. The presence of a data dictionary would assist the director in accurately interpreting this data.

AHIMA Information Governance Principles for Healthcare

According to the American Health Information Management Association (AHIMA), the foundation of data and information governance is accomplished with the implementation of eight key principles. These eight key principles form the AHIMA Information Governance Principles for Healthcare (IGPHC) and are described here.

1. "Accountability: Designation or identification of a senior member of leadership responsible for the development and oversight of the IG Program.

2. Transparency: Documentation of processes and activities related to IG are visible and readily available for review by stakeholders.

3. Integrity: Systems evidence trustworthiness in the authentication, timeliness, accuracy, and completion of information.

4. Protection: Program protects private and confidential information from loss, breach, and corruption.

5. Compliance: Program ensures compliance with local, state, and federal regulations, accrediting agencies' standards and healthcare organizations' policies and procedures and ethical practices.

6. Availability: Structure and accessibility of data allows for timely and efficient retrieval by authorized personnel.

7. Retention: Lifespan of information is defined and regulated by a schedule in compliance with legal requirements and ethical considerations.

8. Disposition: Process ensures the legal and ethical disposition of information including, but not limited to, record destruction and transfer."

Source: Davoudi, Sion; Dooling, Julie A.; Glondys, Barbara; Jones, Theresa D.; Kadlec, Lesley; Overgaard, Shauna M.; Ruben, Kerry; Wendicke, Annemarie. "Data Quality Management Model (2015 Update)" Journal of AHIMA 86, no. 10 (October 2015): expanded web version.

CHECKPOINT 10.3

1. Explain the difference between a data set, database, registry, and index.

_____

_____

2. List the eight principles of the AHIMA Information Governance Principles for Healthcare.

_____

_____

Data and Decisions

There has been a great deal of information presented in this chapter about the importance of data in health care. Healthcare data is important for making decisions about patient care. Healthcare data provides information about patients, which can in turn identify treatments to improve and create patient-centered quality care. Analyzing a patient's data may also help to identify warning signs of serious illness to provide treatment at an early stage, which can also be less expensive. Other ways data influences decisions include helping to predict epidemics, cure diseases, and avoid preventable deaths.

Big Data

The term *big data* is often discussed in health care today. What is big data? **Big data** is large data sets that are analyzed to reveal trends and patterns. Healthcare decisions are being made based on data. Big data is being used to learn as much as possible about the patient to pick up on warning signs as early as possible. This approach can lead to earlier treatment and decreased costs.

Healthcare organizations are large and complex. The healthcare industry has been slow to adopt use of data to improve the quality and delivery of health care. The question is, what could healthcare organizations do to use data to improve the quality and delivery of health care?

Medication errors have been a big problem in the delivery of health care. Because humans can make errors, patients may end up with incorrect medications, which could lead to adverse effects. Using data can help reduce errors by analyzing the patient's health record and medication list. Analyzing the data could help flag any medications that appear to be out of place. Another way healthcare organizations could use data to improve delivery of care is by identifying high-risk patients. Currently, many patients still repeatedly use the ED. Using the ED for care increases the cost of health care and often does not lead to better outcomes. One way data could be used to improve outcomes for patients is by predicting high-risk patients, reducing ED visits, and offering patient-centric care.

Analyzing healthcare data could be used to reduce wait times. Data can be used to analyze and track the wait times and overall visit times of patients. Analysts can look at procedures and healthcare providers to analyze efficiencies and identify holdups. The data from the EHR can alert staff if a patient has been waiting too long. Data can be used to identify and prevent security breaches. Data can be used to analyze websites, tracking pages and application interfaces to catch attacks and analyze uncharacteristic access patterns as well as complete security forensics. Finally, data from wearable technology, if shared with healthcare providers, can improve patient engagement and outcomes. The data can be analyzed to help patients remain independent and reduce office visits. The EHR has become easier for healthcare professionals to access and analyze data. There is still room for improvement with analyzing the available data. What other ways do you think healthcare organizations can use data to improve the quality and delivery of health care?

EXPAND YOUR LEARNING

Watch a five-part series of short videos on big data in health care, starting with part 1 at

http://EHR2.Paradigm Education.com/ BigData.

Informatics

Informatics is a growing and evolving multidisciplinary field that focuses on technology and information. **Informatics** is defined as the science of processing data for storage and retrieval. There are many subspecialties of informatics, including health care, pharmacy, public health, nursing, and biomedical research. The goal of informatics is to examine the data to serve as information to increase knowledge between individuals and groups.

Healthcare Informatics

Healthcare informatics is the study of managing health information. Healthcare informatics includes health systems such as the electronic health record (EHR), data standards such as HL7, terminologies including Systematized Nomenclature of Medicine-Clinical Terms (SNOMED-CT), and health data collected through personal digital devices. Healthcare informatics is used to evaluate the patient's data to improve the quality and delivery of health care.

Tutorial 10.1

Running a Vaccine Effectiveness Report

Go to Navigator+ to launch Tutorial 10.1. As an office manager, practice running and printing a vaccine effectiveness report using the EHR Navigator.

Tutorial 10.2

Running a Lab Values Report

Go to Navigator+ to launch Tutorial 10.2. As an office manager, practice running and printing a lab values report using the EHR Navigator.

Tutorial 10.3

Running a Diagnostic Test Report

Go to Navigator+ to launch Tutorial 10.3. As an office manager, practice running and printing a diagnostic test report using the EHR Navigator.

Tutorial 10.4

Running a Postoperative Readmission Report

Go to Navigator+ to launch Tutorial 10.4. As an admission clerk, practice running and printing a postoperative readmission report using the EHR Navigator.

Tutorial 10.5

Running an Emergency Department Report

Go to Navigator+ to launch Tutorial 10.5. As an admission clerk, practice running and printing an emergency department report using the EHR Navigator.

Chapter Summary

Data is invaluable in the healthcare industry. As healthcare providers enter patient data into the EHR, they are participating in the accumulation of vast amounts of data and information about patients, their health statuses, and treatments rendered.

Data is defined as descriptive or numeric attributes of one or more variables, and the term *data* is frequently referred to as a data element in the EHR. The two types of data that are used in health care to improve quality and care and to facilitate decision-making are known as *internal* and *external data*. There are two kinds of data sources, primary and secondary. The accuracy, completeness, and reliability of this data in the EHR, also known as *data integrity*, is vital for organizations to achieve their goals of providing high-quality care and making good decisions for their patients. It is important for healthcare organizations to establish policies and procedures for their employees to follow regarding data usage and operations. A data dictionary is one such policy, as the data dictionary describes the contents, format, and structure of elements within a database. A data set is a structured collection of related data elements that have standard definitions. Healthcare data sets include UHDDS, UACDC, MDS, OASIS, DEEDS, and EMDS. Healthcare databases, a collection of data that is organized in rows, columns, and tables, include HealthData.gov, the Healthcare Cost and Utilization Project (HCUP), Medicare Provider Analysis and Review (MEDPAR), and National Practitioner Data Bank (NPDB). Data registries are databases focused on a collection of information about a specific condition or disease. Examples include cancer registries, birth registries, and trauma registries. A data warehouse is a database that accesses data from multiple databases to be used for analytic purposes. The goal of analyzing the data is to help healthcare providers and organizations provide better care.

One of the major challenges in the management of healthcare information is information governance, which is an effective framework for the access and use of healthcare data. An effective information governance system should include a data governance committee, strategic plans for using and expanding data, management of data quality, appropriate access to data, and resources for users to correctly interpret the data.

The term *big data* is often used in health care today, and it refers to the large data sets that are used to reveal trends and patterns, such as predicting epidemics, curing diseases, and avoiding preventable deaths.

Informatics is the science of processing data for storage and retrieval and is a growing and evolving multidisciplinary field that focuses on technology and information.

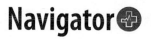

Navigator The following EHR Review, EHR Application, and EHR Evaluation activities are also available online in the Navigator+ learning management system. Your instructor may ask you to complete these activities online. Navigator+ also provides access to flash cards, study games, and practice quizzes to help strengthen your understanding of the chapter content.

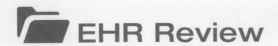

EHR Review

Acronyms/Initialisms

Study the following acronyms discussed in this chapter. Go to Navigator+ for flash cards of the acronyms and other chapter key terms.

AHRQ: Agency for Healthcare Research and Quality

CDC: Centers for Disease Control and Prevention

CDI: clinical documentation improvement

CMS: Centers for Medicare and Medicaid Services

DEEDS: Data Elements for Emergency Department Systems

EMDS: Essential Medical Data Set

FDA: US Food and Drug Administration

HCUP: Healthcare Cost and Utilization Project

HH QRP: Home Health Quality Reporting Program

HH VBP: Home Health Value-Based Purchasing

IGPHC: Information Governance Principles for Healthcare (AHIMA)

IMPACT: Medicare Post-Acute Care Transformation Act

KID: Kids' Inpatient Database

LTAC: long-term acute care hospital

LTCH: long-term care hospital

MDS: Minimum Data Set

MEDPAR: Medicare Provider Analysis and Review

NCHS: National Center for Health Statistics

NEDS: Nationwide Emergency Department Sample

NIH: National Institutes of Health

NIS: National Inpatient Sample

NPDB: National Practitioner Data Bank

NRD: Nationwide Readmissions Databases

OASIS: Outcomes and Assessment Information Set

PPS: Prospective Payment System

RAI: Resident Assessment Instrument

SEDD: State Emergency Department Databases

UACDS: Uniform Ambulatory Care Data Set

UHDDS: Uniform Hospital Discharge Data Set

Check Your Understanding

To check your understanding of this chapter's key concepts, answer the following questions.

1. Which of the following is an example of data integrity being compromised?

    a. a medication allergy entered incorrectly in a patient's EHR

    b. a medical coder selecting the wrong principal diagnosis for billing

    c. a health information management department staff member releasing a patient's record with a patient authorization

    d. a physician entering an order for a lab test

2. The MDS is a core set of screening, clinical, and functional status elements that is required to be completed for which of the following?

    a. All residents of nursing homes certified by Medicare and Medicaid

    b. All home health patients using Medicare or Medicaid as their payment source

    c. All Medicare and Medicaid patients, both inpatient and outpatient

    d. All inpatients and outpatients covered by Medicare or Medicaid

3. All of the statements about the Outcome and Assessment Information Set (OASIS) are true *except*

    a. OASIS is a requirement of Medicare and Medicaid.

    b. the OASIS is a group of data elements that represent core items of a comprehensive assessment.

    c. the OASIS is used to reimburse home health agencies.

    d. the OASIS was updated in January 2017 to meet HIPAA requirements.

4. The Healthcare Cost and Utilization Project is a collection of databases that is sponsored by the

    a. AHRQ.

    b. SID.

    c. HIMSS.

    d. CMS.

5. MEDPAR contains all the following data *except*

    a. diagnoses.

    b. procedures.

    c. social history.

    d. revenue center charge amounts.

6. NPDB is a database that contains information on which of the following?

   a. Medicare beneficiaries

   b. patients' vital statistics such as births and deaths

   c. cancer and tumor diseases

   d. medical malpractice payments against healthcare providers

7. A database that accesses data from multiple databases that are integrated to be used for analytic purposes is the definition of

   a. data warehouse.

   b. external data sources.

   c. information governance.

   d. healthcare cost and utilization project.

8. An organization's process of defining its direction by including goals or objectives and a sequence of steps to achieve each goal and objective is known as

   a. management of data quality.

   b. data governance committee.

   c. strategic plan.

   d. big data.

9. An effective information governance system should include all *except*

   a. appropriate access to data.

   b. management of data quality.

   c. data governance committee.

   d. data warehousing.

10. Documentation of processes and activities related to information governance need to be visible and readily available for review by stakeholders. This is one of the eight key principles of the AHIMA Information Governance Principles for Healthcare and is called

    a. protection.

    b. transparency.

    c. availability.

    d. retention.

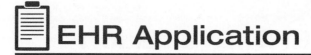

EHR Application

Go on the Record

To build on your understanding of the topics in this chapter, complete the following short-answer exercises.

1. Explain the difference between the two types of primary and secondary data. Include examples of each data type.

2. Explain why standards, policies, and procedures are important elements of data integrity.

3. Describe three different data sets.

4. List and describe three registries.

5. Explain the components that should be included in an information governance system.

Navigate the Field

To gain practice in handling challenging situations in the workplace, consider the following real-world scenarios and identify how you would respond to each.

1. You are the chair of the Information Governance Committee at Northstar Medical Center. You have been asked to educate physicians on the importance of health information governance. Prepare an outline that lists the components of health information governance you will include in your training to the physicians.

2. You are the IT administrator. You have been instructed to create a data dictionary for Wellness Hospital. You are to identify the Field Name, Data Type, and Description. Create a table and include the following fields: Patient first name, Patient last name, Date of birth, Patient ID, Diagnosis, Admission date, Discharge date, Encounter type, Procedure ID, Clinical date, Procedure code, Antibiotic name, Antibiotic dose, Antibiotic frequency, Vital sign temperature, Lab ID, Lab test name, and Lab test result.

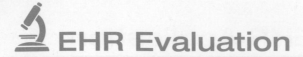

EHR Evaluation

Think Critically

Continue to think critically about challenging concepts and complete the following activities.

1. You are a data analyst with Northstar Medical Center. You have been asked to review the National 2014 Emergency Department statistics to make some comparisons. Go to http://EHR2.ParadigmEducation.com/HCUPNET. Under HCUP Products, select HCUPnet. Then select Get Quick Statistics Tables. Select Emergency Department. Select National. Select 2014 for the year. Select No for the question regarding data on specific diagnosis or condition. Then select Create Analysis. How are the statistics broken down? What type of statistics are included in the table? Is the information helpful? Submit the tables and explanation in a Word document.

2. Investigate an entry-level career focusing on healthcare data.

   a. Select an entry-level position that you might be interested in pursuing.

   b. Describe the position along with promotional and transitional career.

   c. Describe how data plays an important role in this career.

Make Your Case

Consider the scenario and then complete the following project.

You are presenting to Northstar Medical Center about a clinical trial you helped create. Create a presentation of your clinical trial. Go to http://EHR2.ParadigmEducation .com/ClinicalTrials. Select a condition/disease of your choice. Select United States for the country. Click Search All Studies. Review the possible clinical trials. Select a clinical trial that has a status of recruiting. Prepare a presentation that includes the following elements: title of clinical trial, purpose, study type, study design, summary of clinical trial, primary and secondary outcome measures, estimated enrollment, anticipated study start and completion date, eligibility, criteria, and location. Include any other information that is important to share about the clinical trial.

Explore the Technology

To expand your mastery of EHRs, explore the technology by completing the following online activities.

1. Perform an Internet search and identify and explain three different ways data is collected with the EHR.

2. Locate the top 10 cancers in 2014 by going to http://EHR2 .ParadigmEducation.com/NPCR. Click on United States Cancer Statistics. Click on Top Ten Cancers. Submit the graphs to your instructor by ethnicity. Is there anything that surprises you? Are there any interesting trends? Then search again to determine the states with the highest occurrences of cancer. Why do you think certain states have a high occurrence of cancer? Are there any trends you can identify from the data?

3. Conduct an Internet search to identify how data collected through personal digital devices is improving health outcomes.

4. Research how health informatics is being used to improve the quality and delivery of health care.

Explore the Technology

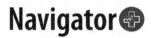

Complete the EHR Navigator practice assessments that align to each tutorial and the assessments that accompany Chapter 10 located on Navigator+.

Are You Ready?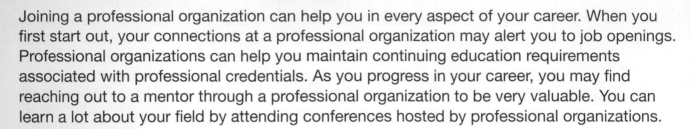

Joining a professional organization can help you in every aspect of your career. When you first start out, your connections at a professional organization may alert you to job openings. Professional organizations can help you maintain continuing education requirements associated with professional credentials. As you progress in your career, you may find reaching out to a mentor through a professional organization to be very valuable. You can learn a lot about your field by attending conferences hosted by professional organizations.

What professional organizations serve the health information technology/health information management industry?

What organizations exist for allied health professionals?

Be sure to review the credentialing opportunities and careers found on the American Health Information Management Association website, www.AHIMA.org.

Beyond the Record

- Some common clinical decision support systems (CDSSs) include:
  - ESAGIL
  - CADUCEUS
  - DiagnosisPro
  - DXplain
  - MYCIN
  - RODIA

- A 2005 review of 100 studies showed that CDSSs improved practitioner performance in 65% of the studies.
- CDSSs improved patient outcomes in 13% of the studies.

Field Notes

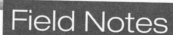

EHR has drastically improved communication and continuity for our pulmonary patients. This integrative technology has allowed clinicians to thoroughly review ventilator weaning tolerance from previous facilities and implement achievable goals in improving patient outcomes.

— *Tom Frye, RRT*
Manager, Respiratory Therapy

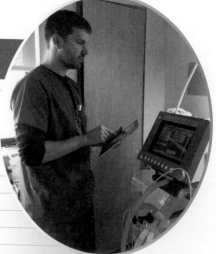

Chapter 11

Clinical Decision Support Systems and Quality Improvement

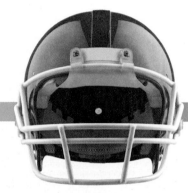

EHRs in the News

The National Football League (NFL) has implemented an interoperable electronic health record (EHR) system for its 32 teams. This NFL-wide EHR system allows records for all NFL players to be accessed, no matter where they are playing or for which team they are playing. This system includes features unique to the NFL, such as video footage of injuries occurring and a sideline concussion assessment tool. This EHR allows players to be treated immediately, with a comprehensive health record that includes a player's history, medications, and video footage of the injury(s).

11.1 Define *clinical decision support system (CDSS)*.

11.2 Define the two types of CDSSs.

11.3 Discuss the knowledge-based CDSS.

11.4 Discuss the advantages and disadvantages of using a CDSS.

11.5 List the most common uses of clinical decision support in health care.

11.6 Explain the requirements of the Centers for Medicare and Medicaid Services (CMS) for the clinical decision support rule as part of meaningful use core measures.

11.7 Demonstrate clinical decision support activities in electronic health record (EHR) software, and discuss the role of EHRs in clinical decision support.

11.8 Discuss the role of the EHR in quality improvement.

11.9 Explain the importance of National Quality Measures of the Joint Commission.

11.10 Define and discuss eCQI.

As you have learned throughout this text, electronic health records (EHRs) improve the quality of patient care in many different ways. One of the most significant ways is through the incorporation of clinical decision support systems. A **clinical decision support system (CDSS)** assists healthcare providers with decision-making tasks such as determining diagnoses, choosing the best medications for a patient, and selecting proper diagnostic tests. The CDSS filters EHR data available for a specific patient, producing information based on current healthcare knowledge and interactions among physicians and other healthcare providers to assist them in making decisions that will result in the highest quality of care. This chapter will discuss CDSSs in detail and explore the federal mandates that require healthcare providers to use EHR systems with CDSSs.

In addition to CDSSs, the role of EHRs in healthcare quality improvement activities will be discussed. Healthcare providers and organizations constantly strive to improve processes, policies, and

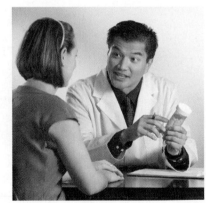
A CDSS can help physicians choose the right medications for a patient.

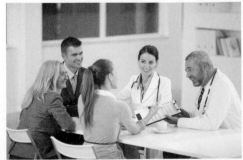
Healthcare organizations work together to improve policies and procedures.

procedures that result in higher quality outcomes. Through data gathering and analysis, EHRs play a significant role in assisting healthcare organizations in these quality improvement activities.

Clinical Decision Support

There are a number of definitions of clinical decision support. The Centers for Medicare & Medicaid Services (CMS) define clinical decision support in relation to the meaningful use standards as "health information technology that builds upon the foundation of an EHR to provide persons involved in care decisions with general and person-specific information, intelligently filtered and organized, at the point of care (POC), to enhance health and health care."

The simplest rendition of a CDSS is any tool that helps healthcare providers make a better clinical decision. Examples of CDSS tools include computerized alerts and reminders, clinical guidelines, standardized order sets, patient data results and reports, documentation templates, diagnostic support, and clinical workflow tools.

There are two basic types of CDSSs, knowledge based and nonknowledge based. Most CDSSs are **knowledge based** and utilize inference software and databases containing the most current medical, scientific, and research information. Nonknowledge-based CDSSs utilize artificial intelligence software to study and learn from data and patterns of medical practice.

CDSSs may also be stand-alone systems or an integrated component of an EHR. For purposes of this discussion, this chapter will focus on the knowledge-based CDSS as an integrated component of an EHR.

A knowledge-based CDSS integrated with an EHR is a good example of semantic interoperability. The data may be shared, exchanged, and interpreted. See Figure 11.1 for an example of a knowledge-based CDSS integrated with an EHR. This figure illustrates how the three components of EHR data, scientific evidence and research, and physician experience work together to make up the CDSS.

Figure 11.1 Knowledge-Based CDSS Integrated with EHR

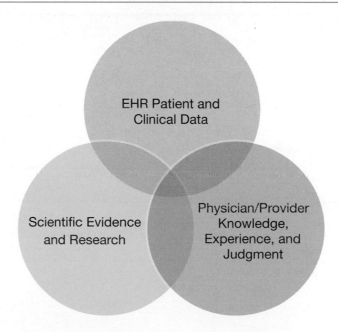

A knowledge-based CDSS integrated with an EHR is effective because it utilizes these three components:

1. Subjective and objective clinical patient data from the EHR
2. State-of-the-art scientific evidence and research
3. Physician knowledge, experience, and judgment

Benefits and Disadvantages of Using a CDSS

Using a CDSS has numerous benefits, the most significant of which improve quality of care and healthcare delivery through the following:

- reduced risk of medication errors
- reduced risk of misdiagnosis
- increased direct patient care time for healthcare providers
- access to state-of-the-art data, research, clinical pathways, and guidelines
- reduction of unnecessary diagnostic tests
- faster diagnoses, resulting in faster treatments
- prescriptions for lower cost medications

However, using a CDSS also has potential disadvantages, including the following:

- high costs of maintaining the CDSS with up-to-date medical research, clinical pathways, guidelines, medication costs, and so forth
- potential overreliance on computer technology
- perception by healthcare providers as a threat to clinical knowledge and skills
- harmful outcomes if software is not thoroughly and continuously updated

CHECKP✚INT 11.1

1. Define a clinical decision support system.

_____

_____

_____

2. List two types of clinical decision support systems.

a. _____

b. _____

3. List three advantages and three potential disadvantages of using a clinical decision support system.

a. _____

b. _____

c. _____

d. _____

e. _____

f. _____

Most Common Uses of a CDSS

The most common uses of a CDSS in health care involve clinical needs such as alerting providers to possible drug interactions, assisting with establishment of correct diagnoses, screening for preventable diseases, and accessing state-of-the-art treatment options. In addition to clinical needs, the CDSS also addresses administrative and financial needs of the healthcare organization by assisting with cost reductions and improving patient satisfaction and provider efficiency. This is accomplished by using CDSS tools to minimize length of hospital stay, alert staff about duplicate testing orders, and increase patient–provider communication. Table 11.1 identifies common uses of a CDSS.

Table 11.1 Common Uses of a Clinical Decision Support System

Use	Examples
Alerts	Drug–drug alerts
	Drug–food interactions
	Duplicate testing alerts
	Abnormal laboratory results
Diagnoses	Suggestions for possible diagnoses that match patient signs and symptoms
Treatment options	Treatment options and guidelines for specific diagnoses
	Medication recommendations
Preventive care	Immunization due-date alerts
	Diagnostic screening
	Disease management/prevention
Hospital/provider efficiency	Care plans and treatment to minimize length of stay
	Standardized order sets
	Suggestions for lower cost medications and testing
Cost reductions and improved patient satisfaction	Duplicate testing alerts
	Drug formulary guidelines
	Faster diagnoses and treatment

Alerts

CDSS components of the EHR Navigator alert the healthcare provider in the following activity in an attempt to place a duplicate order for computed tomography. Although the healthcare provider has an opportunity to place a duplicate order, alerting him or her to the duplication may prevent unnecessary costs.

Tutorial 11.1   **EHR**NAVIGAT⊕R

Adding an Order

Go to Navigator+ to launch Tutorial 11.1. As a physician, practice adding an order using the EHR Navigator.

A common use of a CDSS is to prevent adverse drug interactions. Interoperability of EHR systems can save time, money, and patient lives. For example, a primary care clinic may enter a patient's common prescriptions into the EHR. However, if the patient goes to the hospital and the emergency department does not have access to that list of medications, then the risk for adverse drug interactions increases. The emergency department staff may prescribe a medication that interacts with the patient's regular prescriptions if the staff is unaware of possible interactions. A CDSS component of an EHR compares the list of the patient's prescriptions with the new prescription, alerting the prescriber if there is a potential interaction.

Consider This

A patient enters an emergency department with shoulder pain and is diagnosed with minor inflammation of his shoulder. The healthcare provider prescribes an anti-inflammatory medication to resolve the inflammation, which eliminates his symptoms of pain. Two months later, the patient returns to the emergency department with stomach bleeding and pain. He is diagnosed with a bleeding ulcer caused by an interaction between the anti-inflammatory medication he took for his shoulder and his regular hypertension medicine. Did the emergency department use an EHR with access to a list of the patient's medications? How would a CDSS help to prevent this scenario?

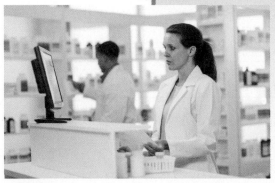

A CDSS alerts prescribers of possible drug interactions.

Alert Fatigue Are more alerts always better? A phenomenon commonly known as *alert fatigue* has become a significant issue for healthcare organizations following CDSS implementation. Healthcare providers may experience **alert fatigue** after encountering excessive numbers of alerts, such as drug–drug, telemetry, and laboratory results outside the normal range, within the EHR system. The provider may ignore such alerts without studying each one because of the large number they encounter in daily practice. The consequences of alert fatigue may be life threatening if a provider inadvertently ignores a serious alert. Therefore, to reduce the chances of alert fatigue, the thresholds of when an alert is triggered in a CDSS must be set at an appropriate level, which can be accomplished by defining policies regarding the types of results (normal, abnormal, and critical) that trigger an alert. Medical staff should be instrumental in determining thresholds to ensure continued buy-in regarding alert delivery from the CDSS. Constant monitoring of these thresholds is imperative to ensure that healthcare providers are alerted when significant or potentially significant care concerns arise. Provider feedback regarding the types of valuable alerts is also important.

Drug–Drug Interaction

Go to Navigator+ to launch Tutorial 11.2. As a physician, experience what happens when a drug–drug alert occurs in the EHR Navigator.

Diagnoses

A CDSS can assist physicians in diagnosing patient conditions based on a variety of factors. For example, a college student may present at the emergency department with a high fever, stomach pain, stomach bleeding, appetite loss, headache, and weakness. Routine laboratory results reveal only an elevated white blood cell count. The patient is then admitted for further testing and diagnosis. The attending physician uses the CDSS integrated with the hospital's EHR system, which searches the patient's EHR, filters the information, and suggests a diagnosis of typhoid fever based on the patient's symptoms and a documented recent trip to Kenya. Based on the suggestion from the CDSS, the attending physician agrees with this possibility and orders a special laboratory study for *Salmonella typhi*. The test result is positive for the bacteria, and the physician begins treatment.

Treatment Options

CDSSs can also monitor treatment options and assist physicians in keeping up with the latest advancements in medicine. For example, an oncologist using the CDSS component of his or her practice's EHR system can review the latest research trials for all types of carcinoma treatments and offer his or her patients choices if traditional treatment options are unsuccessful.

Preventive Care

Good preventive care has a host of benefits. Patients stay healthier when they go to their physicians for routine, preventive care, which in turn can help healthcare facilities save money by catching health issues earlier.

For example, a physician's practice may have a patient population with a high percentage of patients with diabetes. Because of the significant health risks associated with undiagnosed diabetes, a physician's practice may routinely use the preventive screening aspect of the CDSS to identify patients at risk for diabetes. According to the American Diabetes Association, anyone with a body mass index above 25 who has additional risk factors, such as high blood pressure and high cholesterol levels, is at risk for diabetes. Therefore, a physician's practice may routinely run reports to identify at-risk patients, sending alerts via their preferred method of contact to ask these patients to make an appointment for diabetes screening.

Identifying patients who meet the pattern of certain diseases would be far more complicated without the assistance of a CDSS.

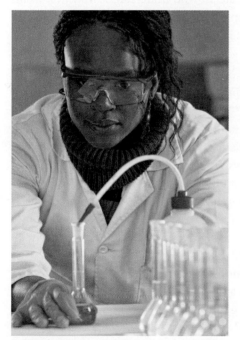

A CDSS allows practitioners to track the latest scientific research.

Preventive Care Report

Go to Navigator+ to launch Tutorial 11.3. As an office manager, practice running a preventive care report using the EHR Navigator.

Provider Efficiency

CDSSs can contribute to greater efficiencies for the providers. The hospital can incorporate the care plans for certain types of diseases in the system, thus making it easier for physicians and other clinicians to follow them and increase compliance with Medicare or accreditation requirements. For example, for patients presenting with a possible diagnosis of pneumonia, the detailed instructions for the care of patients with this diagnosis, also known as the *protocol of care*, includes a chest X-ray and a blood culture within 24 hours of admission to confirm the diagnosis of pneumonia. Such protocols can be programmed in the CDSS, thus contributing to greater compliance with requirements, quicker diagnosis, quicker treatment, and possible decreased length of stay.

Cost Reduction

Another common role a CDSS plays in healthcare support is reducing costs. Patients are becoming increasingly savvier consumers of health care, and often they are invested in keeping costs down. Although many ways exist to help patients and physicians work together to reduce costs, a CDSS plays a key role in achieving cost-effective health care. For example, a family physician who understands how important the cost of medications is to her aging patient population may use the CDSS component of the practice's EHR system to select the best, most cost-effective medications covered by her patients' insurance plans.

Meaningful Use Requirement

As you learned in Chapter 1, the Health Information Technology for Economic and Clinical Health (HITECH) Act specifies criteria for meaningful use of EHRs. Clinical decision support is a requirement of an EHR system that meets specified meaningful use criteria. Each stage (Stage 1, 2, 3) of meaningful use requires an increase in the functionality of the clinical decision support component of the organization's EHR. For example, the Final Rule of Stage 2 requires the CDSS to be used to improve performance on high-priority health conditions by using five CDSS interventions related to four or more clinical quality measures (CQMs).

The Final Rule for Stage 3 requires the demonstrated use of multiple CDSS interventions that apply to quality measures in at least four of the six National Quality Strategy priorities. The National Quality Strategy priorities include:

1. Preventive care

2. Chronic condition management (e.g., diabetes, coronary artery disease)

3. Appropriateness of lab and radiology orders (e.g., medical appropriateness, cost effectiveness)

4. Advanced medication-related decision support (e.g., renal drug dosing, condition-specific recommendations)

5. Improving the accuracy/completeness of the problem list, medication list, drug allergies

6. Drug–drug and drug–allergy interaction checks

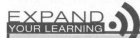

Learn more about the Clinical Decision Support Rule Meaningful Use Requirement by accessing the resources found on the HealthIT.gov website: http://EHR2 .ParadigmEducation .com/CDS.

The National Quality Forum (NQF) is a nonprofit, nonpartisan, membership-based organization that works to bring about improvements in health care. The NQF is responsible for organizing and convening the National Priorities Partnership (NPP). The NPP is a partnership of 52 major national organizations with a shared vision to achieve higher quality health care that is more cost effective and equitable for all individuals. The NPP provides annual input to the secretary of Health and Human Services regarding the National Quality Strategy (NQS) priorities.

Role of EHRs in Quality Improvement Activities

EHRs can play a major role in a healthcare organization's quality improvement activities, but the question remains as to whether the healthcare organization is fully utilizing the data available through the use of EHRs. Reporting capabilities in EHR systems provide healthcare organizations with important statistics and can help identify opportunities to improve patient care. A routine review of clinical and outcome data and statistics can assist healthcare providers and administrators to identify potential quality issues.

Typical subject areas of statistical review and monitoring in an inpatient facility include infection rates, ventilator weaning success rates, lengths of stay, fall rates, morbidity and mortality rates, types and frequency of diagnostic tests per diagnosis-related group (DRG), and medication errors. A CDSS integrated with an EHR can provide statistics on many typical functions of an inpatient facility, so physicians, hospital managers, and other stakeholders can take necessary steps to improve areas in which the inpatient facility falls short.

Typical subject areas of statistical review and monitoring in an outpatient facility or physician practice include mammography, diabetes and colorectal screenings, and routine physical examinations. A CDSS integrated with an outpatient EHR system can provide information on that practice's patient population, allowing healthcare staff to send reminders or schedule follow-up procedures.

In our previous discussion of the CDS requirement in Meaningful Use, we discussed the NQF, a national initiative to improve health care. There are two other major, national initiatives that are important to learn about. These initiatives include the National Quality Measures of the Joint Commission (also known as the Core Measures) and the National Quality Measures Clearinghouse (NQMC), which is sponsored by the Agency for Healthcare Research and Quality (AHRQ).

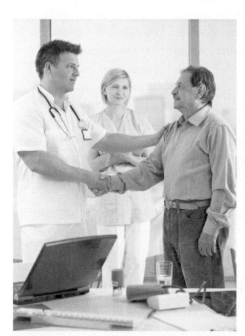

A CDSS integrated with an EHR system can help improve patient care.

National Quality Measures of the Joint Commission

The Joint Commission took a major role in working toward improving health care in US hospitals as early as 1999 and has continued to roll out more standards and requirements for many providers of health care with its biggest focus on inpatient acute care hospitals. The Joint Commission's ORYX Program requires hospitals to gather performance data for the purposes of identifying opportunities for improvement in the services they provide. For accreditation purposes, hospitals are required to demonstrate data gathering, data analysis, and steps to improving quality of care. The Joint Commission has worked with CMS to develop a set of common quality measurements, which has resulted in the Specifications Manual for Hospital Inpatient Quality Measures. This specifications manual contains a data dictionary, measure information forms, algorithms, and other tools to be used by CMS and the Joint Commission. The goal of this common set of quality measures, of course, is to improve quality of care, minimize data collection efforts for these quality measures, and focus efforts on the use of data to improve the delivery and quality of health care in the United States.

For more information regarding the Specifications Manual for Hospital Inpatient Quality Measures, go to: http://EHR2.ParadigmEducation.com/Specifications.

National Quality Measures Clearinghouse

The National Quality Measures Clearinghouse (NQMC) is a resource regarding quality measures reported by all types of healthcare settings. These measures are available to the public by accessing the website www.qualitymeasures.ahrq.gov. The NQMC contains two major categories of measures that include healthcare delivery measures and population health measures. Healthcare delivery measures are measures of care delivered to individuals and populations defined by their relationship to healthcare providers, organizations, or insurance plans. Population health measures are measures that address health issues of individuals or populations defined by geographic area. Using the search criteria found at the AHRQ quality measures website, healthcare delivery measures and population health measures may be found according to the type of healthcare setting—that is, hospital, ambulatory care, long-term care, or a specific organization such as the Joint Commission or the American Medical Association. It is important to note that the NQMC is a repository for quality measures and measure sets that healthcare organizations may choose to use for research, study, and/or reporting. The NQMC does not, however, gather or report on data from healthcare organizations according to these quality measures.

Electronic Clinical Quality Improvement

The implementation of EHRs has significantly affected the processes of data gathering and data analysis with the goals of improving the quality of health care, reducing the costs of health care, and making health care more accessible to all individuals. CMS and the Office of the National Coordinator for Health Information Technology (ONC) are working together to promote electronic clinical quality improvement (eCQI) for the monitoring and analysis of the quality of health care provided to patients and the patient outcomes. The use of electronic clinical quality measures (eCQMs) is the primary focus of eCQI. eCQI looks at patient care and outcomes both retrospectively and concurrently with the use of computerized data. The eCQMs use the data from EHRs to measure healthcare quality both in the provision of healthcare and patient outcomes.

Figure 11.2 demonstrates the process of eCQI. Beginning with the provision of care to patients, patient care and patient outcomes are then measured using eCQMs. These measurements are analyzed, and opportunities for improvement in patient care are identified. Improvements are implemented, patient care is rendered, and the cycle of eCQI is repeated.

Hospitals accredited by the Joint Commission are required to report at least six eCQMs.

Examples of eCQMs include the following:

- Home management plan of care document given to patient/caregiver

- Primary percutaneous coronary intervention (PCI) received within 90 minutes of hospital arrival

- PCI administered to heart attack patient within 90 minutes of hospital arrival

- Wait times from emergency room arrival time to inpatient admission time

Figure 11.2 eCQI Process

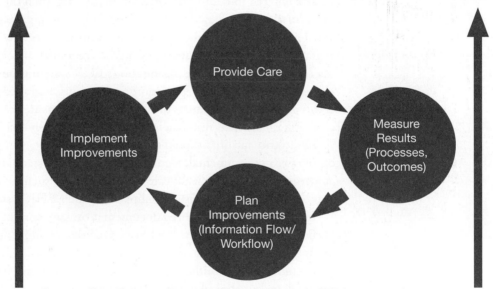

Optimal Care Delivery: Healthcare Transformation Supported by Health IT-Enabled eCQI

Current Care Delivery: Everyone Trying to Improve Efficiency and Outcomes

Future of CDS and eCQI

Future plans by CMS and ONC include the provision of standards that would require CDS systems to use evidence-based medicine and each patient's personal history, preferences, and data to customize a plan of care for each patient. Evidence-based medicine is the practice of medicine in which the physician uses the most up-to-date methods of treating the diagnosis that are based on research. The use of evidence-based medicine ensures that patients are receiving the benefits of medical breakthroughs and best practices, rather than receiving care from a physician that has "always done it this way."

1. Discuss the role of EHRs in the quality improvement activities of a healthcare organization.

_____

_____

_____

2. List two examples of subject areas of statistical review and monitoring for an inpatient healthcare organization and two examples of subject areas of statistical review and monitoring for an outpatient facility or physician practice.

_____

_____

_____

_____

**EXPAND))
YOUR LEARNING**

Learn more about improving health care through the use of data by reviewing the following article:

http://EHR2.Paradigm
Education.com/
MeaningfulUse.

Garbage In, Garbage Out

The term *garbage in, garbage out* is commonly used in the field of computer science, and it refers to computers that produce faulty output when input data is inaccurate. If the data entered into an EHR system is inaccurate, then the output data is also unreliable, unusable, or as stated in the previous expression, garbage.

Members of the healthcare staff must continually review and monitor EHR documentation processes and systems for pertinence and accuracy. Inaccurate and unreliable data residing in a healthcare organization's EHR system is potentially life threatening because healthcare policies, procedures, treatments, and medication decisions are based on this data. Strict procedures must be in place to ensure accurate EHR data and the correction of any incorrect data is completed in a timely fashion.

Healthcare facilities should create strict documentation policies and guidelines to comply with governmental, regulatory, and industry standards. Facilities should use a standardized format for healthcare documentation, such as SNOMED CT to record diagnoses, and create consistent templates in their EHR systems for documentation.

In addition to standardized documentation, any corrections to EHR data should also be handled consistently. Healthcare facilities should establish policies that outline who may amend records and what guidelines should be followed. For example, as a staff member of the healthcare information team, you may be able to change demographic data, but clinical data can be corrected only by the appropriate clinical staff.

Accurate data is important to patient safety, and it plays an important role in a successful CDSS. A CDSS of an EHR system will not properly function if entered data is not accurate. If a patient's medications are not entered into the EHR system, then the CDSS will not detect drug–drug interactions. If the patient's weight and height are not accurate, then the CDSS cannot accurately assess his or her risk for diabetes. It is crucial for healthcare facilities to ensure consistent and accurate documentation if they want a CDSS to provide its many benefits.

Clinical Documentation Improvement

Clinical documentation improvement (CDI) is easily defined because the term describes itself. We know that clinical documentation is the information documented in a health record, and we also know that clinical documentation needs to be accurate, timely, and thorough. A program of CDI is the review and improvement of clinical documentation in a healthcare organization.

Hospitals that implement a formal CDI process typically employ nurses or practitioners certified in documentation improvement (CDI). The CDI staff review health records, identifying areas of documentation that are conflicting or incomplete or that require clarification, and then query the physician or provider for documentation to resolve the conflict or deficiency. Physicians/providers document the health record to answer/resolve the query. This has been and continues to be primarily a retrospective process, which is one of the weaknesses of the current state of CDI programs. The best case scenario, of course, would be for the physicians and providers to document completely at the time services are provided. The next best thing would be to have a CDI program that functions concurrently—in other words, while the patient is still in the hospital. A concurrent CDI program would result in higher quality care, since documentation conflicts would be resolved quickly and hopefully before the patients receive care based on incorrect documentation that could potentially be harmful. A concurrent CDI program would also result in faster coding and billing time frames after the patient is discharged, because coders would have all the information needed to accurately code the episode of care without having to query physicians and wait for responses.

Implementing Clinical Documentation Improvement Processes

CDI is not a new concept, but with the widespread implementation of EHR systems, CDI processes, can be more easily and quickly carried out. For example, with paper health records the time to locate the record alone can cause a significant delay in the review process. Then there is the manual review and querying of the physician, the physician's location of the paper record, his or her subsequent clarification documentation, the rereview of the paper record by the CDI and the coder, and other possible steps. You can probably identify many areas in which using an EHR in the CDI process would streamline the processes significantly. The health record is immediately accessible with the EHR, queries can be sent electronically, the physician/provider can add clarifying documentation into the health record immediately, and the coder can be sent an alert that documentation has been added so the coding function can be completed.

CDI has primarily been a process carried out in the hospital setting; however, more physician practices are realizing the advantages of implementing a CDI program. They reap the same benefits as a hospital with better documentation, timely billing and coding, and higher quality of care.

As discussed in Chapter 10, information governance is not a new concept, because it has been used in many industries. It is, however, a fairly new buzzword in the healthcare industry, arising primarily with the widespread implementation of EHR systems. Healthcare organizations find themselves faced with more information and documentation than they know what to do with. Implementing a well-organized, successful CDI program should be considered a requirement to all healthcare information governance programs.

Clinical decision support systems (CDSSs) play an important role in electronic health record (EHR) systems, elevating the medical record from a stagnant paper chart to an electronic interactive system that assists healthcare organizations with diagnostic decision-making and improves quality of care and healthcare delivery. The benefits of a CDSS include reduced risk of medication errors; reduced risk of misdiagnosis; increased direct patient care time; access to state-of-the-art data, research, clinical pathways, and guidelines; reduction of unnecessary diagnostic tests; faster diagnoses; faster treatments; and prescriptions for less expensive medications.

However, using a CDSS also has potential disadvantages, including high costs of maintaining the CDSS, potential overreliance on computer technology, perception by healthcare providers as a threat to clinical knowledge, and harmful outcomes if software is not thoroughly and continuously updated. A CDSS component of an EHR is required as a part of meaningful use.

Some of the most common uses of a CDSS are alerts, diagnoses, treatment options, preventive care, hospital/provider efficiency, cost reductions, and improved patient satisfaction.

It is imperative that a CDSS is kept up to date with current trends in medical diagnosis and treatment; otherwise, the CDSS may become more of a liability than an asset. EHRs play an important role in a healthcare organization's quality improvement activities, assisting with assessing and monitoring healthcare processes and outcomes. The Joint Commission has required accredited healthcare organizations to participate in quality improvement activities. It has continued working with CMS to develop a set of common quality measurements, which has resulted in the Specifications Manual for Hospital Inpatient Quality Measures. The goal of this common set of quality measures is to improve quality of care, minimize data collection efforts for these quality measures, and focus efforts on the use of data to improve the delivery and quality of health care in the United States.

The implementation of EHRs has significantly affected the processes of data gathering and data analysis, with the goals of improving the quality of health care, reducing the costs of health care, and making health care more accessible to all individuals. The use of eCQMs is the primary focus of eCQI. eCQI looks at both past and current patient care and outcomes with the use of computerized data. The eCQMs use the data from EHRs to measure healthcare quality both in the provision of healthcare and patient outcomes. Future plans by CMS and ONC include the provision of standards that would require CDS systems to use evidence-based medicine and each patient's personal history, preferences, and data to customize a plan of care for each patient.

Clinical documentation improvement (CDI) is not a new concept, but with the widespread implementation of EHR systems, CDI processes can be more easily and quickly carried out. CDI has primarily been a process used in the hospital setting; however, more physician practices are realizing the advantages of implementing a CDI program. They reap the same benefits as a hospital with better documentation, timely billing and coding, and higher quality of care.

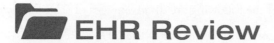

EHR Review

Navigator ⊕ The following EHR Review, EHR Application, and EHR Evaluation activities are also available online in the Navigator+ learning management system. Your instructor may ask you to complete these activities online. Navigator+ also provides access to flash cards, study games, and practice quizzes to help strengthen your understanding of the chapter content.

Acronyms/Initialisms

Study the following acronyms discussed in this chapter. Go to Navigator+ for flash cards of the acronyms and other chapter key terms.

CDSS: clinical decision support system

CMS: Centers for Medicare and Medicaid Services

DRG: diagnosis-related group

HITECH: Health Information Technology for Economic and Clinical Health Act

ONC: Office of the National Coordinator for Health Information Technology

Check Your Understanding

To check your understanding of this chapter's key concepts, answer the following questions.

1. All of the following are examples of clinical decision support system (CDSS) tools *except*

   a. computerized alerts and reminders.

   b. clinical guidelines.

   c. standardized order sets.

   d. email tools.

2. Which of the following is a benefit of using a CDSS?

   a. It helps eliminate the need for medical research.

   b. It may promote an overreliance on computer technology.

   c. It helps reduce the risk of medication errors.

   d. It may produce alert fatigue.

3. The two basic types of CDSS are

   a. knowledge driven and documentation driven.

   b. knowledge based and documentation based.

   c. knowledge driven and nonknowledge driven.

   d. knowledge based and nonknowledge based.

4. All of the following are disadvantages of CDSS *except*

   a. cost of maintenance of the CDSS.

   b. overreliance on computer technology.

   c. perceived threat by healthcare providers to their knowledge and skills.

   d. software that does not need updating.

5. Typical subject areas of statistical review and monitoring in an inpatient facility include all of these, *except*

   a. lengths of stay.

   b. ventilation wean rates.

   c. number of cardiologists on staff.

   d. infection rates.

6. True/False: A 2005 review of 100 studies showed that CDSSs improved practitioner performance in 95% of the studies.

7. True/False: A facility's drug–drug interaction software component meets the requirement for a CDSS as required for meaningful use.

8. True/False: The electronic health record (EHR) can play a major role in a healthcare organization's quality improvement activities.

9. True/False: Corrections to EHR documentation are never allowed.

10. True/False: Clinical decision support does not play a role in cost-effective health care.

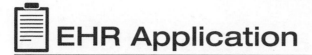

EHR Application

Go on the Record

To build on your understanding of the topics in this chapter, complete the following short-answer activities.

1. Why is the CDSS a necessary component of an EHR system?

2. Describe the two different types of CDSSs.

3. Describe three benefits of CDSSs.

4. List three common uses of CDSSs with examples.

5. Describe Measure 11 of the 14 meaningful use core measures.

Navigate the Field

To gain practice in handling challenging situations in the workplace, consider the following real-world scenarios and describe how you would respond to each.

1. As the information technology manager for Northstar Medical Center, you receive a report that physicians have substantially increased their disregard for the clinical decision support system laboratory result alerts. You take this information to the president of the medical staff of the facility. Do you agree that this was the appropriate action to take? If so, what should the president of the medical staff do? If not, what should the IT manager have done?

2. You are the manager of a hospital that has recently incorporated a CDSS. One of your staff members does not want to use the new system, as he feels it makes him overly reliant on technology and does not use his knowledge and experience as a physician. How would you explain the advantages of a CDSS and persuade him to use it in practice?

🔬 EHR Evaluation

Think Critically

Continue to think critically about challenging concepts and complete the following activities.

1. Identify *Yes* or *No* if the following are examples of clinical decision support:

    _____ a.   Dr. Smith is alerted to a drug–drug interaction.

    _____ b.   The dietician for Northstar Physicians mails out information about diabetes to patients diagnosed with diabetes mellitus.

    _____ c.   Dr. Jones is an orthopedic surgeon who takes a "time-out" for "right patient, right procedure, right site."

    _____ d.   A pharmacist receives an alert regarding a lower-cost medication to be substituted for a patient's current medication.

    _____ e.   A pharmacist looks up a national drug code number to order a medication.

2. Conduct an Internet search to identify the top three clinical decision support systems. Briefly discuss the components of each of these systems and identify the interoperability of each system.

Make Your Case

Consider the scenario and then complete the following project.

You are the office manager for BayView Physician Group and have been asked to prepare a presentation for the staff regarding the CDSS component of the EHR system that its group uses. The physicians would like you to explain to the staff the following items:

- Definition of a CDSS

- Why a CDSS is important

- Whether or not a CDSS is a requirement

- Three examples of how the staff of BayView Physician Group will use the CDSS

Prepare the presentation for the BayView Physician Group staff.

Explore the Technology

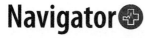

Complete the EHR Navigator practice assessments that align to each tutorial and the assessments that accompany Chapter 11 located on Navigator+.

Are You Ready?

Networking and volunteering can be some of the best ways to get a job, regardless of the field, but it is especially important in the health information industry. Studies show that approximately 85% of jobs are obtained through networking. How can you start developing a network in health information or allied health? Have you looked into volunteer opportunities? Consider asking your professors or mentors. Online networking sites such as LinkedIn can be valuable resources. Professional associations also provide networking opportunities.

Beyond the Record

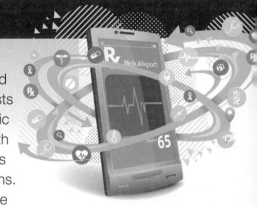

- Approximately 80% of Internet users say that they have conducted an online search to determine what medical condition they or someone they know might have.

- A 2015 study found that there are more than 165,000 health and medical apps. Two-thirds are focused on general wellness topics such as fitness, lifestyle, stress, and diet. The remainder consists of apps focused on specific health conditions (9%), with mental health and diabetes the most popular conditions. Other popular apps include medication information and reminders (6%) and women's health and pregnancy (7%).

Personal Health Record Time Line

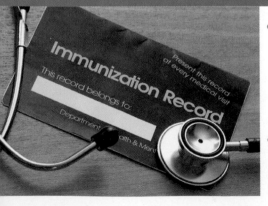

- **1950s**—Patients were encouraged to keep written personal health logs to help track their health information.

- **1978**—The term *personal health record* was first used in an article.

- **2000s**—The idea of storing an electronic personal health record grows in popularity.

- **2012**—A patient portal is part of Meaningful Use Stage 2. Stage 2 encourages the implementation of a secure online website that provides 24-hour access to a patient's health information.

- **2014**—Stage 2 Meaningful Use encourages patients' participation in their health.

The Personal Health Record and the Patient Portal

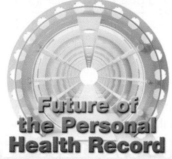

Future of the Personal Health Record

As people do more and more tasks on their smartphones, such as communicating with friends, banking, and shopping, managing health information on a mobile device will likely increase in popularity. The image to the right shows a screen shot of a personal health record on a mobile device.

- **2017**—Stage 3 Meaningful Use gives patients access to self-management tools.

- **2018**—Only one Meaningful Use Attestation Stage is required, which is the combination of Stages 1, 2, and 3.

Field Notes

Electronic prescribing has had a positive effect on the practice of pharmacy and the quality of care of patients. It allows healthcare providers to send prescriptions to the pharmacy more quickly, meaning medications are ready for the patients when they arrive at the pharmacy, reducing their wait time. Electronic prescribing also reduces medication errors, since handwriting is not a factor. Overall, electronic prescribing is improving patients' quality of care as well as their safety.

– *Michelle Watters, PharmD, Pharmacist*

12.1 Explain the personal health record (PHR).

12.2 Identify the characteristics (or content) of the PHR.

12.3 Examine the various types of PHRs.

12.4 Explain the various ways PHRs are stored.

12.5 Explain the ownership of the PHR.

12.6 Identify the advantages of the PHR.

12.7 Identify the challenges to implementing a PHR.

12.8 Explain the connection between the PHR and the electronic health record (EHR).

12.9 Describe the steps in creating a PHR.

12.10 Identify the components of a patient portal.

12.11 Demonstrate use of the Northstar Patient Portal.

Consumers today are faced with many decisions regarding their health care. For that reason, they have become better educated about healthcare costs, treatment options, and preventive care. In addition to becoming more informed, many individuals have taken control of their health care by creating a personal health record or participating in a patient portal. Personal health records and patient portals have two goals: (1) to have health information available at the point of care, and (2) to help foster enhanced communication between the patient and the healthcare provider. This chapter examines these HIM tools and their evolving roles in patient care.

Personal Health Record

A **personal health record (PHR)** is a tool that enables individuals to plan and manage their health information with practitioners to make more informed decisions, which may contribute to better quality of health care. To use this tool, patients gather their demographic information and health data and enter the information into a formatted document or an online template. The result is a record that contains a complete overview of the individual's health history and current health status. Aside from forming a complete summary of an individual's health, a PHR may also be used to do the following:

- Track and update healthcare information from any location via a computer, tablet, or smartphone

- Coordinate care among selected healthcare providers and facilities

- Locate information about diseases and conditions

- Avoid duplication of tests and procedures

- Monitor prescriptions, allergies, wellness, and research

- Share health information with selected providers and healthcare facilities

EXPAND YOUR LEARNING

What does Facebook have to do with your health information? Doctors saved a woman's life by reading some of her health information on her Facebook account. Read the article at http://EHR2.ParadigmEducation.com/Facebook to learn how social media helped save a life. What effect can social media tools such as Facebook have on your health?

Rise of the PHR

As you can see by the time line on pages 312–313, PHRs emerged at the turn of this century. Since 2000, there has been a steady rise in both interest and use of PHRs by individuals who want to take control of their healthcare needs. Because of the relatively recent popularity of PHRs and changes in health care, national organizations have struggled to come up with a common definition of a PHR (see Table 12.1).

Table 12.1 National Organizations and Their Definitions of PHRs

Name of Organization	PHR Definition
National Committee on Vital and Health Statistics (NCVHS)	"The collection of information about an individual's health and health care, stored in electronic format."
American Health Information Management Association (AHIMA)	"An electronic, universally available, lifelong resource of health information needed by individuals to make health decisions. Individuals own and manage the information in the PHR, which comes from healthcare providers and the individual. The PHR is maintained in a secure and private environment, with the individual determining rights of access. The PHR is separate from and does not replace the legal record of any provider."
US Department of Health and Human Services (HHS)	"An electronic file or record of a [patient's] health information and services, such as ... allergies, medications, and doctor or hospital visits that can be stored in one place, and then shared with others, as [the patient] see[s] fit."
Healthcare Information and Management Systems Society (HIMSS)	"A universally accessible, layperson comprehensible, lifelong tool for managing health information, promoting health maintenance and assisting with chronic disease management via an interactive, common data set of electronic health information and e-health tools. An ePHR [PHR] should be owned, managed, and shared by the individual or legal proxy and must be secure to protect the privacy and confidentiality of the health information it contains. It is not a legal record unless so defined and, therefore, is subject to various legal limitations."

However, what these national organizations can agree on are the attributes that a successful PHR should have. PHRs should give patients ownership of their information and be easily accessible, secure, private, and comprehensive.

To that end, in 2002, the Markle Foundation, an organization that promotes the use of technology to improve people's lives, created Markle Connecting for Health, a public–private collaboration focused on improving health through the use of information technology. Representatives from more than 100 collaborating organizations were tasked to develop policies that would be shared among patients and healthcare providers. The outcomes of this working group were as follows:

- Accelerate the development of the PHR

- Increase the patient's relationship with a healthcare provider and involvement in his or her care and safety

- Develop a common data set

- Develop a variety of approaches to creating a PHR

To fulfill these goals, Markle Connecting for Health developed seven best practices for a PHR:

1. Each individual would have his or her own PHR.

2. PHRs are to provide a complete medical history for an individual from birth to death.

3. PHRs are to contain information from healthcare providers.

4. PHRs are to be accessible from any place at any time.

5. PHRs are to be private and secure.

6. PHRs are to be transparent. An individual can see who entered data, when the data was entered, and where data was imported or transferred from as well as who is viewing the data in the PHR.

7. PHRs will permit the seamless exchange of information across healthcare systems.

Contents of a PHR

As mentioned earlier, a PHR contains demographic information and healthcare data, such as the individual's current medications, allergies, past hospitalizations, diagnoses, and more. Table 12.2 lists recommended information for inclusion in a PHR.

Table 12.2 Recommended Information for the PHR

Demographic	Name
	Address
	Telephone
	Email
	Date of birth
Emergency contact	Name
	Address
	Telephone
	Email
Insurance information	Company name
	Address
	Telephone
	Group number
Religious preferences	Name of spiritual leader
	Address
	Telephone
	Email

Table 12.2 Recommended Information for the PHR *(continued)*

Advance directives	Scanned copies of do not resuscitate directive, living will, and healthcare proxy
Providers	Name Address Telephone Email Specialty
Health issues	List health issues providers are addressing
Dentist(s)	Name Address Telephone Email
Dental issues	List dental issues providers are addressing
Pharmacy	Name Address Telephone Email
Optometrist	Name Address Telephone Email
Allergies	List all allergies
Blood type	List blood type
Current medications	Every drug or supplement, including vitamins
Past medications	Every drug or supplement, including vitamins taken in the past
Immunizations, vaccinations	Flu shots and other vaccinations, including dates
Illnesses, conditions, treatments	Diagnoses/treatments/dates of occurrence/failed treatments
Hospitalizations	Inpatient and outpatient services
Pregnancies	All maternity encounters (live, stillbirth, etc.)
Surgeries	All inpatient and outpatient surgeries
Additional medical tests	All medical tests
Permission forms	Release of information and medical procedures
Imaging	X-rays Magnetic resonance imaging Computed tomography scans
Alternative therapies	Alternative therapies or treatments
Correspondence	Correspondence among healthcare providers and facilities

The PHR should be organized so it is easily accessible to the necessary parties and covers all pertinent health information. Depending on the type of PHR selected (paper or electronic), the information would either be keyed or scanned to the PHR. Many health information organizations have created templates for individuals to use. For example, the American Health Information Management Association (AHIMA) created the MyPHR website (www.myphr.com) to inform consumers about PHRs, suggest information for them to gather, and provide them with links to PHR templates. Many insurance companies also provide PHRs, as will be discussed later (see Figure 12.1).

Figure 12.1 Sign-In Screen of a Typical PHR

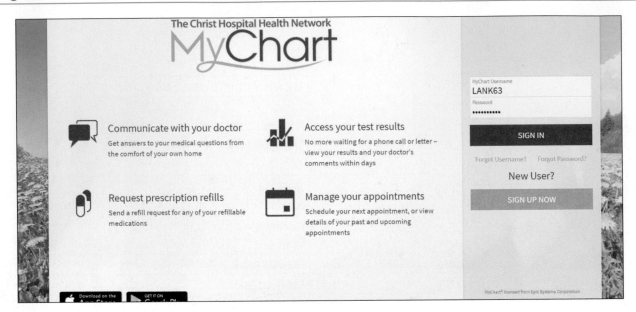

Ownership of a PHR

A patient has complete ownership of a PHR, including the setup and maintenance of the record. In light of this fact, a patient also establishes the parameters for the parties who can view the record and for the data they can access. A patient can limit the type of medical information provided to family, healthcare providers, or healthcare facilities. For example, a patient may choose to have only information about medications and allergies available to family members but may grant a healthcare provider or facility access to the entire health record. Patients should be aware, however, that a PHR is not a substitute for a legal medical record that healthcare providers and facilities maintain.

General Types of PHRs

There are three general types of PHRs: paper, computer based, and web based. Each type of PHR has certain advantages and disadvantages that individuals need to consider.

Paper PHRs

The traditional paper PHR, a collection of medical documents and personal journals of an individual's health history, rose to prominence in the 1950s as families were encouraged to document medical treatments (including drug therapy), procedures, and vaccinations. The goals also included monitoring and improving their overall health status. This type is losing its appeal as electronic record keeping becomes the norm.

Advantages

A paper PHR has the advantage of being a low-cost method of record keeping. Individuals who continue to use a paper health record also like the privacy and security of keeping the record safe at home rather than out in cyberspace. This type of record is portable and can be carried by a patient to a healthcare visit.

Disadvantages

There are many disadvantages associated with a paper PHR. For a patient, a paper health record may be difficult to assemble, organize, and update. Without an established format, a paper PHR may also lack the necessary details to provide a complete picture of the patient's health status. Lastly, in an emergency, a paper record is either unavailable for use or difficult to decipher by an attending healthcare provider or emergency facility. Privacy and security of paper PHRs are also drawbacks to this type of record. Unless placed in a secure location, a paper PHR is accessible to others who may invade the privacy of the record's owner.

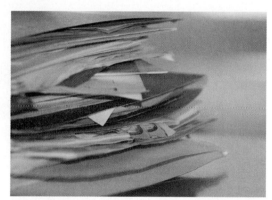

Paper PHR files are difficult to store and organize.

Computer-Based PHRs

Computer- or software-based PHRs are similar to paper PHRs, but they have an electronic format. Patients can purchase or download PHR software and install it on their chosen electronic devices. This type of PHR system is known as a stand-alone or untethered PHR, and it is not designed to share information electronically with other PHR or EHR systems. The patient or his or her designee is responsible for entering the data into the program as well as attaching any documents or images to accompany the data. Therefore, the patient is in control of an untethered PHR. When the patient visits a healthcare provider or facility, he or she can print the health information or transfer it to a portable storage device, such as a flash drive, memory card, or CD, so that the data can be transferred to the legal health record.

Advantages

In addition to the portability feature mentioned earlier, computer- or software-based PHRs are often password protected and are not connected to the Internet, making these health records more secure than paper PHRs. Computer-based PHRs also allow patients to back up their health information, thus helping to prevent a loss of valuable data.

Disadvantages

Of course the data contained in computer-based PHRs is only as accurate as the accuracy of the typist. Patients must exercise caution when inputting information into the health record. Another disadvantage of these records is the lack of Internet connectivity. Although this feature aids security of data, it also makes patients bear the sole responsibility of updating their health records and maintaining their accuracy. Lastly, not all healthcare providers have computer system compatibility that allows them to accept an external media transfer of information into the EHR. If the system is not compatible, then the healthcare provider or facility cannot read or upload the information.

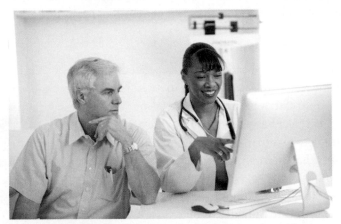

Patients can take their PHRs to their healthcare providers to view.

Web-Based PHRs

To use web-based PHRs, patients must have access to a computer or digital device and have an Internet connection. Web-based PHRs are either tethered or untethered. A **web-based tethered PHR** is health information that is attached to a specific organization's health information system. A **web-based untethered PHR** is not attached to a specific organization's health information system.

Tethered PHRs

This web-based PHR may be provided through a patient's health insurance, employer, healthcare facility, or healthcare provider and is stored on a server owned by a third-party organization. To gain access to health data on a tethered PHR, a patient must use a portal. Once access is granted, a patient may only make limited changes to the record, such a change in insurance coverage. Because the PHR is attached to a covered entity, the patient's health information is protected by the Health Insurance Portability and Accountability Act (HIPAA). However, patients should be aware that this type of PHR does not meet the best practices criteria of the Markle Foundation.

Tethered PHRs may be provided by health insurers, healthcare facilities, and employers, as discussed next.

Health Insurer–Provided PHRs Many health insurers offer subscribers the opportunity to participate in their health care with tethered PHRs known as **health insurer–provided PHRs**. A health insurer often populates information about a subscriber, such as insurance claim information, a list of providers, prescriptions, and benefits coverage. However, a subscriber can also enter his or her own data. Subscribers may also access additional resources, such as wellness information on exercise, nutrition, weight loss, pregnancy, smoking cessation, and other topics that will encourage them to make healthy choices to improve their quality of life as well as reduce costs to the health insurer. Because health insurer–provided PHRs are owned by companies rather than patients, these records are not considered to be "true" PHRs. One advantage of a health insurer–provided PHR is that the health insurer updates the PHR as information becomes available. That way, the patient is not solely responsible for entering the health information updates. Information may be extracted, printed, saved, and sent to various healthcare providers or facilities.

Facility-Provided PHRs Another type of tethered PHR comes from a physician or healthcare facility. This type of PHR, known as a **facility-provided PHR**, links the EHR and the PHR and allows the patient to access the PHR portion online using a username and access code. This type of technology is relatively new and is increasing in popularity. Many of these types of PHRs are static, meaning that the patient may only view the information. There are several features that a tethered PHR from a physician or healthcare facility may include, such as a messaging feature that provides the patient with the opportunity to email a provider, request an appointment, view test results, request a prescription refill, and view reminders. The section titled Patient Portal on page 332 walks you through the features of a facility-provided PHR. See Figures 12.2 and 12.3 to view screenshots from this type of portal.

Figure 12.2 Log-In Screen of a Facility-Provided PHR/Patient Portal

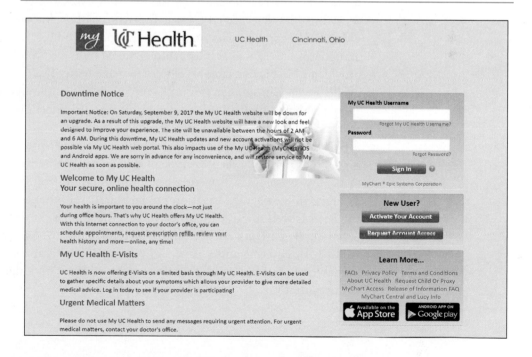

Figure 12.3 Facility-Provided PHR/Patient Portal

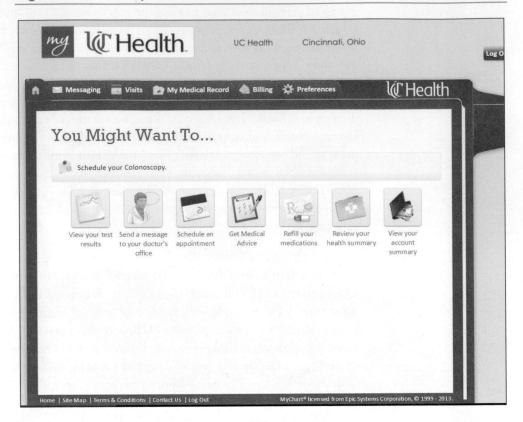

Employer-Provided PHRs Employers are also getting involved in the area of PHRs. In 2006, several companies, including Intel, BP America, Pitney Bowes, and Walmart, formed an organization called Dossia. In 2008, Dossia offered PHRs to employees of the companies that formed Dossia. This type of PHR, known as an **employer-provided PHR**, contains data from hospitals, doctors' offices, health plans, laboratories, and pharmacies as well as information entered by the employee. The goal of employer-provided PHRs is to enable employees to make better health decisions. Achieving this goal is a win–win situation for both employees and employers: employees improve their health and well-being, and employers reap the benefit of decreased insurance costs and employee absenteeism.

There are several advantages to using an employer-provided PHR. One of the biggest advantages is that this type of PHR is not limited to one healthcare provider or facility. Employees may enter health information from all of their providers and can determine what information can be shared. Another advantage is that, because the PHR is web based, patients can access the content anytime and anywhere. So, for example, patients can access their PHRs from providers' offices or healthcare facilities by entering a username and password. Lastly, an employer-provided PHR is available to the employee for life, even if he or she is no longer employed by one of the organizations.

Employer-provided PHRs also have a few disadvantages. One of the disadvantages is that employees are responsible for entering the information and keeping it current. Another potential disadvantage for an employer-provided PHR is that many employees are not comfortable sharing sensitive health information with their employers or have misgivings regarding how their data will be used.

Untethered PHRs

This type of PHR allows the patient to control the information in the record by customizing access rights for family and providers. The patient can create a username and password to ensure the security of his or her health information. Because the PHR is web based, the patient can access the record at any time. Web-based untethered PHRs are available for free or by paying a fee.

Networked PHRs

A web-based, networked PHR is the type Markle Connecting for Health imagined. It can transfer information to and from various healthcare providers and facilities (e.g., doctors, pharmacies, laboratories, and insurance companies) and the patient, thus allowing for continuous updates. This interoperability saves the patient time and ensures that the information in the patient's PHR is accurate and current. For example, when a patient visits a dermatologist, the office staff updates the patient's diagnoses and procedures. Then when that patient goes to the pharmacy to retrieve the prescription the dermatologist just prescribed, the pharmacy staff updates the insurance claim information to the networked PHR.

A networked PHR has several advantages:

- This type of PHR is accessible anytime from anywhere as long as the patient has an Internet connection.

- Information is shared among multiple providers and facilities, unlike the other types of PHRs previously discussed.

- Individuals can select the information that is shared with family, healthcare providers, and facilities.

- The PHR is kept more accurate, up to date, and complete because of the input of healthcare staff.

Although the networked PHR offers several advantages, one disadvantage is the issue of privacy and security. The exchange of information over the Internet and among multiple healthcare providers and facilities opens the PHR for potential compromise of health information.

Because of the fluidity of web-based PHR developers, patients must consider the ramifications of a developer who, for whatever reason, cancels the site. For example, in 2011, Google Health—a free, opt-in, web-based PHR that contained voluntary information by the user—was shut down after three years of operation. To find out more about this occurrence, refer to the Consider This feature box.

CHECKP⊕INT 12.1

1. What are the advantages and disadvantages of a paper PHR?

   _____

   _____

2. What are the advantages and disadvantages of a computer-based PHR?

   _____

   _____

3. List three types of web-based PHRs.

   a. _____

   b. _____

   c. _____

Evaluation of PHRs

Some clear benefits have emerged as PHRs are being increasingly used by consumers. Indeed, many national healthcare organizations have been outspoken advocates of PHRs. They have not only encouraged consumers to use these health records but also created website templates for their use.

There are several issues that a patient should consider when determining the type of PHR to select, including the following:

- Is remote access available?

- Is online storage available?

- If the PHR is web based, how trustworthy is the site?

- How is the information kept private?

- Is the information secure?

Overall Benefits of PHRs

The primary benefit of a PHR is that a patient and his or her healthcare providers can view a complete chronological health history of the patient. Patients can access information about their healthcare providers, treatments, vaccinations, medications, allergies, and other types of health data. Knowing this information allows patients to make informed decisions about their own health and wellness. Healthcare providers can also access the information in a PHR, making all practitioners aware of the patient's past and current health status, test results, medication interactions, overdue preventive tests, and so on. This data access allows providers to work in tandem to provide patients with optimal, safe care. For emergency healthcare providers in particular, a PHR provides them with the necessary information to act quickly and decisively when treating their patients during a critical time.

There are also healthcare cost benefits from the use of PHRs. For patients, PHRs may prevent duplicate tests and treatments and allow them to select lower-cost treatments and medications. For healthcare providers, PHRs allow them to start the correct treatment sooner, which leads to shorter hospital stays and emergency visits.

PHRs that are offered by covered entities, such as healthcare providers and health plans, have the added advantage of being covered under HIPAA. The HIPAA Privacy Rule protects the privacy of the information contained in the PHRs.

The National Committee on Vital and Health Statistics and the Benefits of PHRs

In 2006, the National Committee on Vital and Health Statistics (NCVHS) developed a list of key potential benefits for a variety of users of PHRs. This list was presented in the NCVHS's Personal Health Records and Personal Health Record Systems report and recommendations. Table 12.3 lists the key potential benefits of PHRs and PHR systems for patients, providers, payers, employers, and society as a whole.

Advocates of PHRs

As mentioned earlier, many healthcare organizations have voiced their support for the benefits of PHRs. In 2003, the **Veterans Administration** rolled out the MyHealth*e*Vet website, which is a web-based PHR that veterans can use to maintain and update their health information (see Figure 12.4).

A PHR, like MyHealth*e*Vet, improves the continuity of care for veterans who move often and/or visit a variety of healthcare specialists.

Another outspoken advocate for the use of PHRs is the Centers for Medicare and Medicaid Services (CMS). The CMS encourages the use of PHRs to decrease medical errors and reduce healthcare costs. In 2006, the CMS began several pilot programs to encourage Medicare recipients to use PHRs.

Table 12.3 Key Potential Benefits of PHRs and PHR Systems

Roles	Benefits
Consumers, patients, and caregivers	• Support wellness activities • Improve understanding of health issues • Increase sense of control over health • Increase control over access to personal health information • Support timely, appropriate preventive services • Strengthen communication with providers • Verify accuracy of information in provider records • Support home monitoring for chronic diseases • Support understanding and appropriate use of medications • Support continuity of care across time and providers • Manage insurance benefits and claims • Avoid duplicate tests • Reduce adverse drug interactions and allergic reactions • Reduce hassle through online appointment scheduling and prescription refills • Increase access to providers via e-visits, which are interactions with the healthcare provider via email, phone, or video
Healthcare providers	• Improve access to data from other providers and the patients themselves • Increase knowledge of potential drug interactions and allergies • Avoid duplicate tests • Improve medication compliance • Provide information to patients for both healthcare and patient services purposes • Provide patients with convenient access to specific information or services (e.g., laboratory results, prescription refills, e-visits) • Improve documentation of communication with patients
Payers	• Improve customer service (transactions and information) • Promote portability of patient information across plan • Support wellness and preventive care • Provide information and education to beneficiaries
Employers	• Support wellness and preventive care • Provide convenient service • Improve workforce productivity • Promote empowered healthcare consumers • Use aggregate data to manage employee health
Societal/population health benefits	• Strengthen health promotion and disease prevention • Improve the health of populations • Expand health education opportunities

Figure 12.4 MyHealtheVet Website

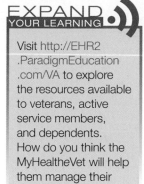

EXPAND YOUR LEARNING

Visit http://EHR2
.ParadigmEducation
.com/VA to explore
the resources available
to veterans, active
service members,
and dependents.
How do you think the
MyHealtheVet will help
them manage their
health information?

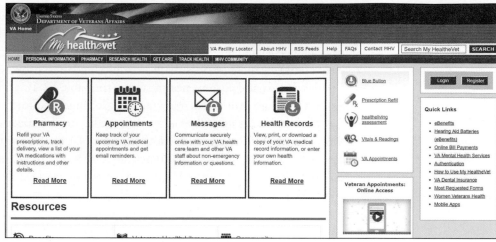

Source: www.myhealth.va.gov

Overall Challenges of PHRs

Similar to the lack of EHR interoperability, PHRs are faced with the same communication challenges. Some networked PHRs can communicate with healthcare provider systems, but most PHRs are not interoperable.

Privacy and security concerns also affect the adoption of PHRs. Those PHRs not offered by HIPAA-covered entities fall under the privacy policies of the PHR vendor, as well as any other applicable laws that govern how information in the PHR is protected. In addition, there is currently no federal law that covers the storage or transmission of PHR content. These privacy and security issues are troubling and must be addressed.

Lastly, depending on the type of PHR, the information in the record may not be accurate, up to date, or both. For PHRs to be effective, patients must assume the responsibility of maintaining the record—a task that can be time consuming.

Consider This

AHIMA prepared an article to help consumers select a PHR to meet their needs. To access this article, go to http://EHR2.Paradigm Education.com/AHIMA-PHR. Read the article and review the questions to ask when choosing a PHR. Consider how you would answer the questions. How would your answers apply to the type of PHR that would fit your situation?

The EHR–PHR Connection

As you have already learned, an EHR system stores information about a patient's health. Depending on the type of PHR a patient establishes, his or her information may be shared and/or integrated. Although an EHR and a PHR have different characteristics, these records share a common goal: to provide a complete picture of a patient's past and current health status (see Table 12.4). To meet this goal, the two entities must be connected, allowing the exchange of information.

Healthcare organizations agree that the key to the effective use of PHRs is the linkage to an EHR system. The Office of the National Coordinator for Health Information Technology (ONC) has determined that a PHR plays an important role in the implementation of the EHR and the Nationwide Health Information Network (NwHIN).

The Institute of Medicine (IOM) also agrees that a PHR can help providers using an EHR system. In its research, the IOM discovered that patients see many different healthcare providers in a variety of healthcare facilities, and often these providers do not have a complete view of the patient's health history because each provider and facility keeps individual records on patients. A networked PHR, discussed earlier, is the tool that allows complete health record access to all parties.

Table 12.4   EHR and PHR Comparison

	EHR	PHR
Purpose	Maintain up-to-date health information	Maintain up-to-date health information
Ownership	Healthcare provider facility	Individual
Updates	Healthcare provider or facility	Individual
Legal	Legal documents created and maintained based on federal and state laws	Not a legal document
Access	Controlled by healthcare provider or facility, requires patient authorization	Controlled by patient
Information	Health information by single provider or facility	Health information from multiple providers or facilities
Use	Healthcare provider or facility	Individual

A Networked PHR and HL7

A networked PHR is the only type of PHR that has the ability to exchange information between the PHR and an EHR system. To that end, Health Level Seven International (HL7) began to address the standard for the EHR in 2007 by developing a model known as the PHR-System Functional Model (PHR-S FM). PHR-S FM identifies the features and functions of a networked PHR. These features and functions are also linked to the functions in an EHR, creating a pathway for providers, facilities, and patients to exchange information (see Figure 12.5).

Figure 12.5 Personal Health Record System

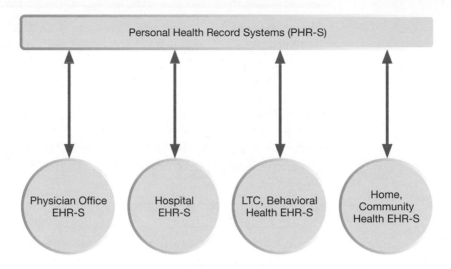

Features of a PHR-S FM

There are three sections of features and functions in a PHR-S FM: personal health, supportive, and information infrastructure. Personal health focuses on patient demographic data, clinical wellness, management of care, decision support, and management of encounters with providers. The supportive section provides administrative and financial information related to patient medical care, including information necessary for processing claims, sharing of information for research, and quality improvement. The last section, information infrastructure, allows the PHR to efficiently and effectively exchange information with the EHR. Table 12.5 describes the three sections of the PHR system functions in more detail.

Table 12.5 HL7 Personal Health Record System Functional Model

Personal health	PH.1 Account holder profile
	PH.2 Manage historical clinical data and current state data
	PH.3 Wellness, preventive medicine, and self care
	PH.4 Manage health education
	PH.5 Account holder decision support
	PH.6 Manage encounters with providers
Supportive	S.1 Provider management
	S.2 Financial management
	S.3 Administrative management
	S.4 Other resource management
Information infrastructure	IN.1 Health record information management
	IN.2 Standards-based interoperability
	IN.3 Security
	IN.4 Auditable records

Creating a PHR

There are several steps an individual must consider before creating a PHR. Individuals should consider what their needs are, how they will organize their PHRs, and what their preferred storage mediums are.

Requesting Records

First, a consumer should request a copy of his or her health records. Requesting health records entails completing a HIPAA-compliant form for a release of records from healthcare providers and facilities. Each provider may require a fee for processing the copies of the records.

Organizing Records

While waiting for the health information, consumers should review the various types of PHRs and select the one that meets their needs. They should then organize their health information in folders or a binder until all the information has been acquired so that the transfer of information from paper to electronic format will be easier. The information received in an electronic format may be copied or transferred into the PHR.

Storing Records

There are several ways to store health information for a PHR, such as on a flash drive, CD, secure digital card, portable hard drive, online cloud storage, computer hard drive, or even a three-ring binder. The selection of a storage device depends on the needs of the owner of the PHR. Several factors to consider include issues of portability, security, maintenance, and accessibility.

Other considerations include whether the owner of the PHR wants to do the following:

- physically transfer data or use a web-based PHR

- store information online or use a physical storage device

- export the health data in a portable document format (PDF) that would be readable in many different programs

See Figure 12.6 for a screen illustrating the options for linking, sharing, and storing PHR data.

Figure 12.6 Linking, Sharing, and Storing PHR Data

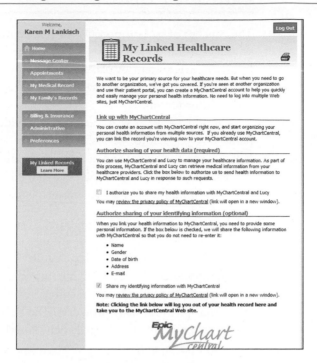

Consider This

Sally was a 70-year-old woman diagnosed with heart failure five years ago. Since then, she had been taking warfarin, an anticoagulant to help reduce the risk of stroke. While attending her water aerobics class, she began to feel light-headed and short of breath. She collapsed and was rushed to the hospital. The aerobics instructor, who was only an acquaintance, knew none of the medications Sally was taking nor how to contact her next of kin. The hospital placed Sally on heparin to reduce her risk of developing blood clots while in the hospital.

Heparin is also an anticoagulant, and, when given with warfarin, increases the risk of bleeding. These medications are sometimes used together but only with special monitoring. Because the staff members at the hospital were unaware that Sally was taking warfarin, they were not monitoring her as closely as they should have been. Sally had internal bleeding and died while in the hospital. How could this tragedy have been prevented if Sally had a personal health record?

CHECKPOINT 12.2

1. List two organizations that advocate for the use of PHRs.

   a. _____

   b. _____

2. List three steps in creating a PHR.

   a. _____

   b. _____

   c. _____

Patient Portal

The concept of patient portals was created out of the growing popularity of PHRs as well as the adoption of EHR technology because it interfaces with the healthcare facility's EHR system. A patient portal provides a patient access to his or her medical records, appointments, messages, billing, connection to family records, and administrative information.

During a patient visit, healthcare providers offering patient portal access will invite patients to register for access, ultimately providing them usernames and access codes. Patients can then create an account and gain access to the portal.

Many facilities have implemented patient portals to help them achieve Stage 2 and 3 meaningful use patient engagement and self-management requirements.

Menu of a Typical Patient Portal

Many patient portal systems have similar characteristics. The menu of a typical portal includes options for messages, appointments, medical records, family records, billing and insurance, administration, and preferences. There is also an option to link records from multiple healthcare providers. The EHR Navigator has a patient portal integrated with its system, the Northstar Patient Portal. Figure 12.7 illustrates the Northstar Patient Portal menu.

Figure 12.7 Northstar Patient Portal Menu Screen

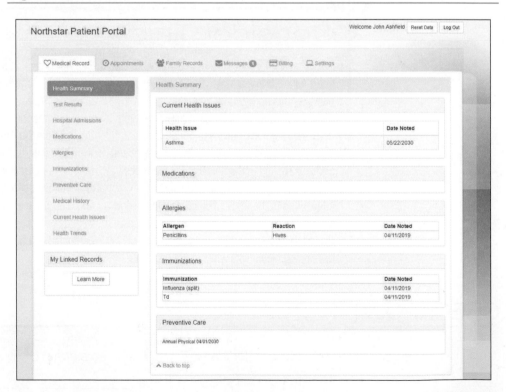

Home

The Home menu of the patient portal provides quick access to the *Medical Record, Appointments, Family Records, Messages, Billing, Settings*, and *Link Medical Records*. The Northstar Patient Portal Home screen is shown in Figure 12.8.

Figure 12.8 Northstar Patient Portal Menu Options

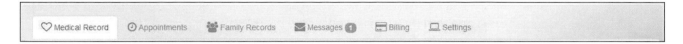

Medical Record

The *Medical Record* allows patients to track their health information, which may include test results, current health issues, medications, allergies, immunizations, preventive care, health summary, medical history, and hospital admissions. As a user of the Northstar Patient Portal, the patient can download a summary of his or her health information that can be shared with someone or simply be available when traveling abroad.

Health Summary

The *Health Summary* feature of the Northstar Patient Portal provides links to current health information, medication, allergies, immunizations, and preventive care information. The *Health Summary* screen is shown in Figure 12.9.

Figure 12.9 Northstar Patient Portal Health Summary

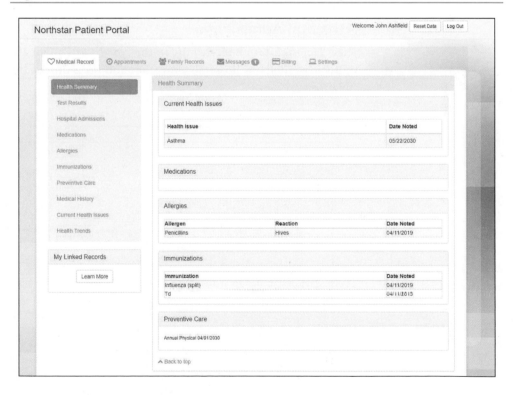

Test Results

The patient can view a list of tests and results. The healthcare provider can contact the patient if there are any issues with the test results. The *Test Results* screen is shown in Figure 12.10.

Figure 12.10   Northstar Patient Portal Test Results

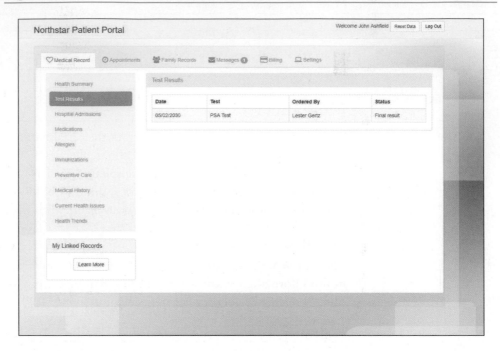

Hospital Admissions

The *Hospital Admissions* feature in the Northstar Patient Portal provides detailed information about hospital admissions and procedures. This screen is illustrated in Figure 12.11.

Figure 12.11   Northstar Patient Portal Hospital Admissions

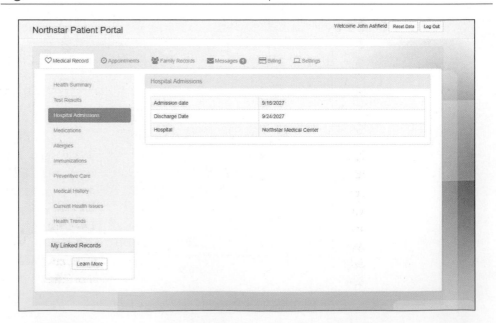

Medications

The Northstar Patient Portal includes a list of the patient's current medications and information regarding the medications, as illustrated in Figure 12.12.

Figure 12.12 Northstar Patient Portal Medications

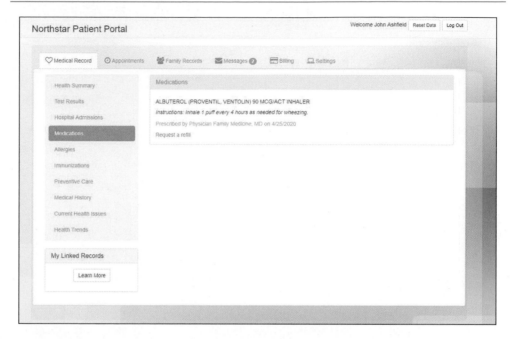

Allergies

Any allergies that affect a patient will be listed in the Northstar Patient Portal. A patient may remove or add allergies in the portal. Figure 12.13 shows the *Allergies* screen.

Figure 12.13 Northstar Patient Portal Allergies

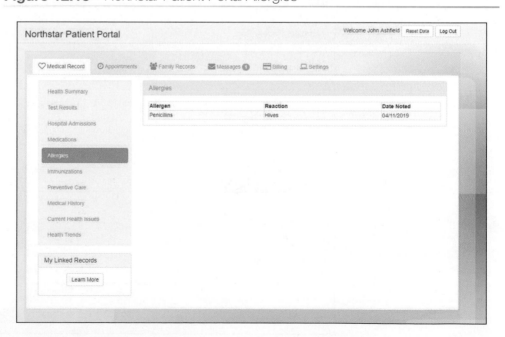

Immunizations

The portal can also track immunization information. Any additional immunizations may be entered by a provider to update the patient's immunization record. Figure 12.14 shows the *Immunizations* screen.

Figure 12.14   Northstar Patient Portal Immunizations

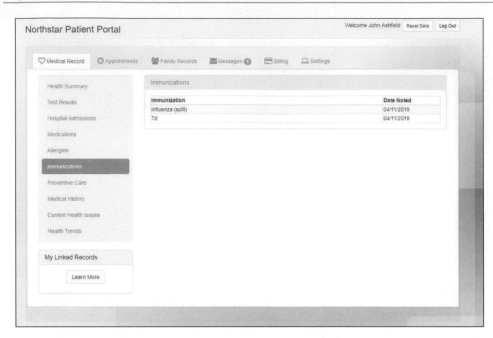

Preventive Care

A patient may view suggestions for preventive care based on age, sex, and medical history. This screen is illustrated in Figure 12.15.

Figure 12.15   Northstar Patient Portal Preventive Care

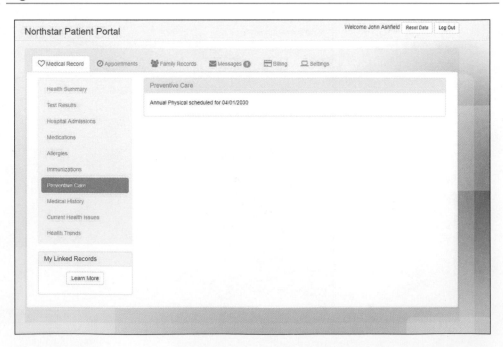

Medical History

A provider may update a patient's medical history, which can include personal notes; procedures; family, medical, and social histories; and family status. Figure 12.16 illustrates the *Medical History* screen.

Figure 12.16 Northstar Patient Portal Medical History

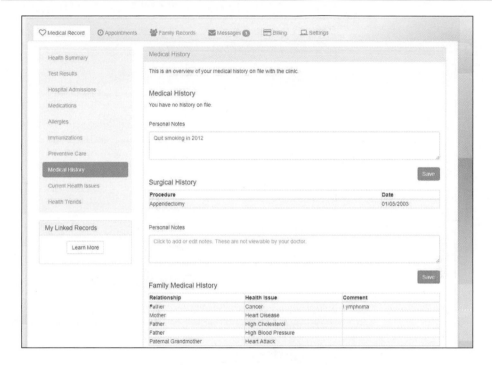

Current Health Issues

A patient's current health issues are listed in the patient portal. Patients may monitor their health issues here. This screen is shown in Figure 12.17.

Figure 12.17 Northstar Patient Portal Current Health Issues

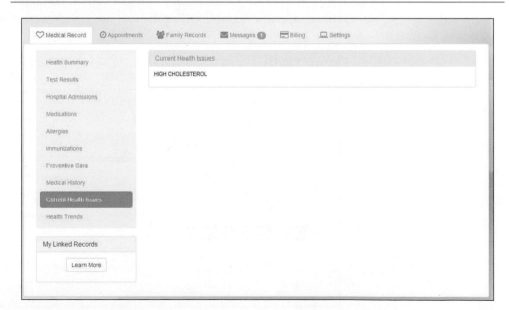

Health Trends

Patients may access their health reports through the *Health Trends* feature of the patient portal, as illustrated in Figure 12.18. Patients may access their health reports, such as a table that details a patient's blood pressure, pulse, respirations, height, weight, and body mass index based on visits to the physician.

Figure 12.18   Northstar Patient Portal Health Trends

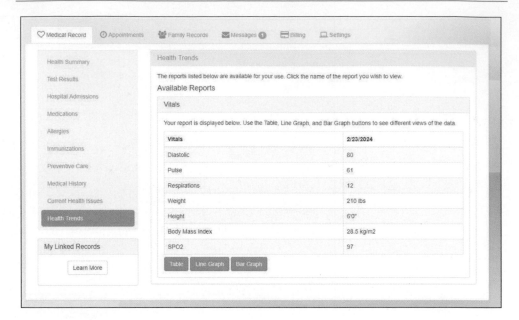

Appointments

The PHR allows a patient to view upcoming appointments, cancel appointments, or request an appointment.

Appointments

The *Appointments* feature in the Northstar Patient Portal provides a list of all the patient's appointments, detailing the day, time, healthcare provider, and location. See Figure 12.19.

Figure 12.19   Northstar Patient Portal Appointments

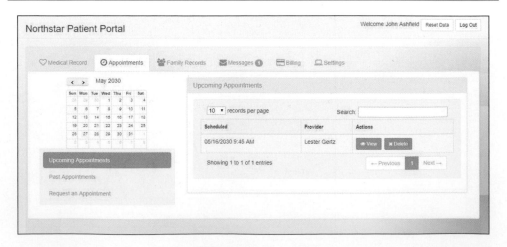

Cancel My Appointments

The portal provides a convenient way for a patient to cancel an appointment. Rather than placing a telephone call, the patient may log in to the patient portal and select the appointment he or she would like to cancel. Figure 12.20 illustrates the cancel appointment feature.

Figure 12.20 Northstar Patient Portal Cancel My Appointments

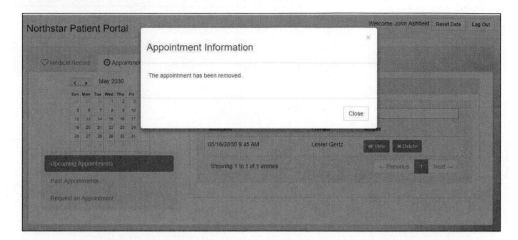

Request My Appointment

The *Request My Appointment* feature permits a patient to request an appointment. The patient may select the healthcare provider he or she would like to see or another provider he or she would be willing to see. In addition, the patient can select the reason and preferred date or days and times. In the *Notes* field, the patient can communicate any specific information necessary for the healthcare provider or facility about the requested appointment. Figure 12.21 shows the *Request My Appointment* dialog box.

Figure 12.21 Northstar Patient Portal Request My Appointment

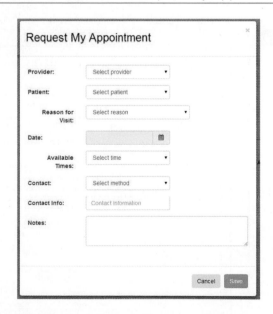

Family Records

There are times when patients may want someone in their families to have access to their health information. The *Family Records* feature allows patients to change the settings in the portal to allow family members access to all or some of their health information. The *Family Records* screen is illustrated in Figure 12.22.

Figure 12.22 Northstar Patient Portal Family Records

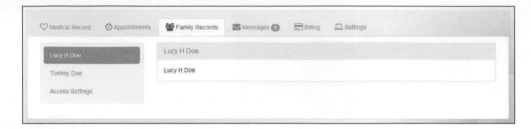

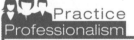
Messages

The *Messages* feature is a communication area that allows the patient and healthcare provider to communicate. Most patient portals have an *Inbox, Sent Message, Get Medical Advice, Request Rx Refill*, and *Request a Referral*.

Get Medical Advice

There are times when a patient has a medical question for his or her healthcare provider. The *Get Medical Advice* option in a patient portal allows the patient to direct a question to a specific provider by selecting a subject line from a drop-down list such as *Non-Urgent Medical Question, Prescription Question, Test Result Question*, or *Visit Follow-Up Question*. Some patient portals are even allowing for telehealth visits, which is when health care is provided remotely via telecommunications technology. The *Get Medical Advice* feature is shown in Figure 12.23.

Figure 12.23 Northstar Patient Portal Get Medical Advice

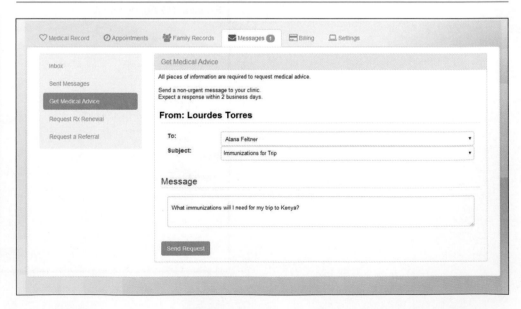

Request Rx Refill

Medications are an important part of an individual's health care. Depending on a prescription, healthcare providers may alter medical treatment. The Northstar Patient Portal provides information on refills and refill history. Patients may also request refills through the patient portal. The *Request Rx Refill* feature is illustrated in Figure 12.24.

Figure 12.24 Northstar Patient Portal Request Rx Refill

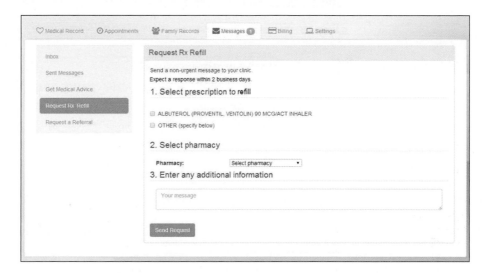

Request a Referral

Sometimes a patient may wish to request a referral to see a specialist or other physician. The Northstar Patient Portal provides an option to request a referral to another physician by filling out a form. The computer program informs the patient that up to two days may be required for a response. Figure 12.25 illustrates the *Request a Referral* feature.

Figure 12.25 Northstar Patient Portal Request a Referral

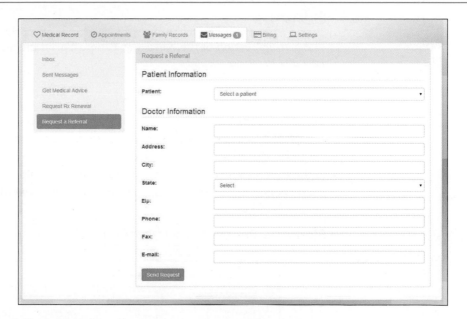

Billing and Insurance

Patients may view their billing and insurance information in the Northstar Patient Portal. The patient may track his or her payments, insurance payments, and outstanding balances.

Billing Account Summary

The *Billing Account Summary* feature provides a list of visits and payments and is illustrated in Figure 12.26.

Figure 12.26   Northstar Patient Portal Billing Account Summary

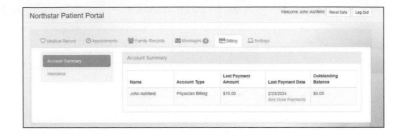

Insurance Summary

A summary of the patient's insurance coverage is listed here in the patient portal, as shown in Figure 12.27.

Figure 12.27   Northstar Patient Portal Insurance Summary

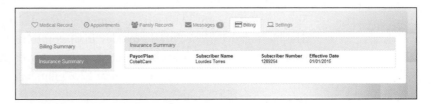

Settings

The *Settings* section of the Northstar Patient Portal includes the patient's *Profile* and *Portable PHR*.

Patient Profile

The *Patient Profile* section includes the patient's address, telephone number, and email address as well as primary care provider and provider location. The patient may find his or her PHR identification, medical record number, or account number for billing purposes in the administrative information. The *Patient Profile* also allows a patient to edit his or her demographic information or change his or her password. Figure 12.28 illustrates the *Patient Profile* section.

Figure 12.28   Northstar Patient Portal Profile

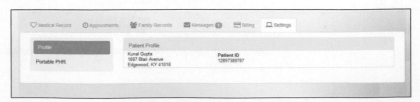

Portable PHR

A patient may print, download, or link his or her health information such as allergies, medications, current health issues, procedures, and test results to share with others. The *Portable PHR* print feature provides a printable summary of a patient's information, medical information, contacts, and insurance information. The *Portable PHR* download option allows a patient to download his or her health information to a flash drive to share with others. The downloaded information may be password protected.

Link Medical Records

The Northstar Patient Portal provides an option to link a patient's health information, which is a useful tool if a patient is seen by another healthcare facility or provider, as the health information may be quickly and easily shared. This allows the patient to manage his or her personal health information from multiple sources. The patient also may authorize a healthcare provider or facility to send health information to other providers and facilities. Linking medical records is important because other providers and facilities may need access to health information such as medications, previous test results, previous procedures, hospital admissions, and any complications experienced. When a healthcare provider has access to this information, thus better knowing a patient's health history, the delivery and quality of care improves.

Tutorial 12.1   **EHR**NAVIGAT✛R

Enrolling a Patient and Exploring the Patient Portal

Go to Navigator+ to launch Tutorial 12.1. As a physician, practice enrolling a patient in the Northstar Patient Portal using the EHR Navigator. Then, explore the Northstar Patient Portal as the patient.

Tutorial 12.2   **EHR**NAVIGAT✛R

Requesting a Refill and an Appointment in the Patient Portal

Go to Navigator+ to launch Tutorial 12.2. As a patient, practice reviewing a record, requesting a prescription refill, and scheduling an appointment in the Northstar Patient Portal.

Tutorial 12.3   **EHR**NAVIGAT✛R

Requesting Medical Advice and Printing Information in the Patient Portal

Go to Navigator+ to launch Tutorial 12.3. As a patient, practice requesting medical advice in the Northstar Patient Portal.

Tutorial 12.4   **EHR**NAVIGAT✛R

Reviewing Test Results and Adding Family History to the Patient Portal

Go to Navigator+ to launch Tutorial 12.4. As a patient, practice viewing test results and adding family history to the Northstar Patient Portal.

CHECKPOINT 12.3

1. Name four features in a patient portal that you would use to improve monitoring your own health care.

    a. _____

    b. _____

    c. _____

    d. _____

2. Why is it important to link medical records together in a patient portal?

    _____

    _____

Chapter Summary

Individuals have started to assemble and maintain their own health information so that they have a complete picture of their health history and current health status. One way patients can accomplish this task is by creating a personal health record (PHR). A PHR allows patients to gather, track, update, and share health information. While the definition of a PHR varies somewhat among healthcare organizations, these organizations do agree that a PHR should be a collection of an individual's health information, electronically or on paper, securely accessed by an individual patient. To that end, in 2002, the Markle Foundation created a working group to develop best practices for patients and healthcare providers using PHRs.

PHRs may be one of three types: paper, computer based, or web based. In addition to the format of PHRs, they can be classified as tethered and untethered. Tethered PHRs are linked to a healthcare provider, facility, or third-party payer. Untethered PHRs are those in which the creator of the PHR enters the health information, and the record is not associated with a healthcare provider, facility, or third-party payer. Many different parties play an important role in keeping the PHR up to date, and patients and providers use PHRs to help them make better medical decisions, avoid duplicate tests, reduce adverse drug interactions, and support wellness and preventive care.

Aside from maintaining a complete health history of a patient, a PHR also provides additional benefits to patients and healthcare providers such as improved communication between the patient and his or her caregivers, increased patient safety, and significant cost savings for patients and providers. These benefits have not been overlooked by several healthcare organizations who endorse the use of PHRs, including the Centers for Medicare and Medicaid Services, the Veterans Health Administration, and the Office of the National Coordinator for Health Information Technology. The latter organization has determined that PHRs are key components of the electronic health record (EHR).

As PHRs have grown in popularity, many healthcare providers have created their own patient portals as part of the EHR technology. A typical patient portal includes messaging, scheduling, medical history, billing and insurance, and administrative features. The patient portal, along with the PHR, improves the delivery and quality of health care.

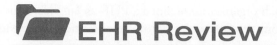

EHR Review

Navigator ⊕ The following EHR Review, EHR Application, and EHR Evaluation activities are also available online in the Navigator+ learning management system. Your instructor may ask you to complete these activities online. Navigator+ also provides access to flash cards, study games, and practice quizzes to help strengthen your understanding of the chapter content.

Acronyms/Initialisms

Study the following acronyms discussed in this chapter. Go to Navigator+ for flash cards of the acronyms and other chapter key terms.

AHIMA: American Health Information Management Association

CMS: Centers for Medicare and Medicaid Services

HHS: Department of Health and Human Services

HIMSS: Health Information and Management Systems Society

HL7: Health Level 7 International

IOM: Institute of Medicine

NwHIN: Nationwide Health Information Network

ONC: The Office of the National Coordinator of Health Information Technology

PHR: personal health record

Check Your Understanding

To check your understanding of this chapter's key concepts, answer the following questions.

1. The acronym PHR stands for
   a. protected health record.
   b. personal health report.
   c. personal health record.
   d. protected health report.

2. The primary goal of the PHR is to
   a. act as a substitute for the legal medical record.
   b. develop a common data set.
   c. have health information available at the point of care.
   d. foster communication between providers and healthcare facilities.

3. Which organization defined a PHR as "an electronic universally available lifelong resource of health information needed by individuals to make health decisions. Individuals own and manage the information in the PHR, which comes from the healthcare providers and the individual. The PHR is maintained in a secure and private environment, with the individual determining rights of access."?

   a. US Department of Health and Human Services

   b. Healthcare Information and Management Systems Society

   c. National Committee on Vital and Health Statistics

   d. American Health Information Management Association

4. A tethered PHR is

   a. personal health information attached to a specific organization's health information system.

   b. personal health information not attached to a specific organization's health information system.

   c. personal health information the patient enters into the health information system.

   d. protected health information not attached to a specific provider's health information system.

5. Which of the following is a key benefit of the PHR for healthcare providers?

   a. an increased sense of control over health

   b. supports understanding and appropriate use of medications

   c. improved access to data from other providers and patients

   d. use of aggregate data to manage employee health

6. True/False: One of several issues patients need to consider when determining the type of PHR is remote access.

7. True/False: Google Health is a PHR currently used by many patients.

8. True/False: In 2010, the Markle Foundation created Connecting for Health.

9. True/False: PHRs may be paper-, computer-, or web-based.

10. True/False: A typical patient portal includes messaging, scheduling, billing, and record linking features.

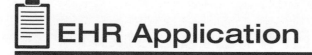

EHR Application

Go on the Record

To build on your understanding of the topics in this chapter, complete the following short-answer activities.

1. What are the benefits of having a personal health record (PHR)?

2. What are the challenges with using a PHR?

3. How do you see the future of the PHR?

4. What are the seven best practices for a PHR as described by Markle Connecting for Health?

5. Explain the difference between tethered and untethered PHR systems.

Navigate the Field

To gain practice in handling challenging situations in the workplace, consider the following real-world scenarios and identify how you would respond to each.

1. You are a patient who wants to begin using a PHR. Using a search engine of your choice, research the various PHRs available from both free and subscription services. Compare and contrast the various PHRs for their features and ease of use. Select three PHRs and write a three- to four-page paper comparing the selections. After careful analysis, make a recommendation of a PHR that best fits your needs.

2. Your employer is going to begin offering a PHR. Many of your coworkers are signing up, whereas others have misgivings about their privacy. Would you be likely to use a PHR offered by an employer? Why or why not?

EHR Evaluation

Think Critically

Continue to think critically about challenging concepts and complete the following activities.

1. Prepare a pamphlet for patients of South Community Hospital on how to use and access the patient portal. The pamphlet should include information about the definition of a patient portal, advantages of using a patient portal, features of a patient portal, and methods of using and accessing the patient portal.

2. Investigate the patient portal system that accompanies this textbook, and complete a scavenger hunt by answering questions from your instructor.

Make Your Case

Consider the scenario and then complete the following project.

You are a member of the CobaltCare insurance company, which is promoting personal health records (PHRs) for all of its insured members. You are hosting a session on how to begin a PHR, exploring what information should be included and how to keep the PHR current. Prepare the presentation you will share with the enrollees that attend the information session.

Explore the Technology

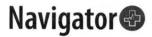

Complete the EHR Navigator practice assessments that align to each tutorial and the assessments that accompany Chapter 12 located on Navigator+.

Are You Ready?

Mastering an EHR system and demonstrating knowledge of why EHRs are important will help you in any healthcare career you choose. As you continue your education and training, you may wish to refer back to this text and the tutorials in the EHR Navigator.

Beyond the Record

- As of May 2017, more than $36.5 million in Medicare and Medicaid EHR Incentive payments had been paid to providers.

- In a 2017 KPMG survey, 38% of CIOs planned to invest in EHR system optimization because many healthcare organizations have been unable to optimize their EHR systems to realize the value.

- South Dakota, Massachusetts, Colorado, North Carolina, Minnesota, Indiana, and Wyoming lead the office-based physicians in the use of certified EHRs.

- As of July 2017, 684 health IT developers supplied certified health IT to 354,395 ambulatory care specialists participating in the Medicare EHR Incentive program. Epic Systems, Allscripts, eClinicalWorks, and athenahealth supply certified technology to 60% of all providers.

Chart Migration Checklist

The Health Information Technology Research Center (HITRC) developed a Chart Migration and Scanning Checklist to help healthcare providers implement an EHR system. The full document is provided by the National Learning Consortium and can be found at www.healthit.gov.

The Chart Migration and Scanning Checklist provides guidance on what information is needed to import into the EHR. The checklist gives the healthcare organization consideration as to what information will be migrated from the paper record system to the EHR.

13

Implementation and Evaluation of an EHR System

To ensure it attracts creative programmers, Epic Systems, one of the largest EHR providers, has a two-story spiral slide and a statue of the Cat in the Hat in its Wisconsin office building. Workers also hold meetings in an on-site tree house.

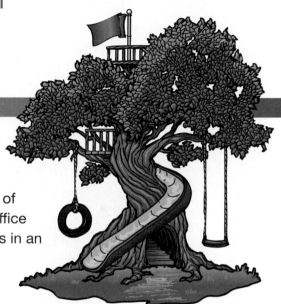

National Learning Consortium

1   Scanning and Preload Checklist

To use this checklist, follow the steps below:

1. Identify who will complete the worksheet based on knowledge of chart scanning
2. Complete w
3. Review the
4. Formulate t
5. Build in che
6. Communica
7. Initiate plan

1.1   ADMINIS

1. What is you

2. Will scannin

| Yes |
| No, if no th |

3. What is the

   Scannin

   Manuall

4. How many

5. How many
   Click here t

6. How many

7. How soon a
   in the EHR?

8. Who will be
   Click here to

National Learning Consortium

9. What are the practice's goals for EHR implementation? Check all that apply to practice.

Exhibit 1 Goals

Goal	Check if 'Yes'
2.1 Become a paperless office	☐
2.2 Become an office with less paper	☐
2.3 Move paper charts off site (storage)	☐
2.4 Eliminate chart pulls for visits	☐
2.5 Eliminate chart pulls for messages	☐
2.6 Reduce document filing time	☐
2.7 Implement a document imaging management system	☐
2.8 Interface with lab	☐
2.9 Interface with hospital	☐
2.10 Interface with radiology	☐
2.11 Redesign current systems	☐

1.2   CHART SPECIFICS

1. Which paper charts will be scanned (Check one)?

Exhibit 2 Scanned Charts

Charts	Check if 'Yes'
All	☐
Patients seen in past five years	

13.1 Explain the role of the Office of the National Coordinator for Health Information Technology in certifying EHR systems.

13.2 Describe how to assess a healthcare facility's readiness for the implementation of an EHR system.

13.3 Examine the importance of creating goals for a healthcare facility's EHR system.

13.4 Explain the importance of establishing a steering committee.

13.5 Examine the role of a project manager.

13.6 Describe the EHR migration plan.

13.7 Explain how workflow analysis affects the EHR implementation.

13.8 Describe the evaluation process of EHR systems.

13.9 Explain the meaning of total cost of ownership.

13.10 Examine the EHR implementation plan.

13.11 Describe the stages of meaningful use.

As discussed throughout this textbook, the 2009 Health Information Technology for Economic and Clinical Health (HITECH) Act has accelerated the adoption of electronic health record (EHR) systems in US healthcare facilities. As of 2017, 67.4% of physicians are using a certified EHR, and this number is expected to grow. The previous chapters discussed the advantages of EHRs, such as access to data, improved patient care, and monetary incentives for the implementation of a certified EHR system. However, system selection may be challenging because so many types of EHR systems are available.

Centers for Medicare and Medicaid Services (CMS) and the Office of the National Coordinator for Health Information Technology (ONC) have established standards and other criteria for structured data that EHRs must meet to be considered a certified electronic health record. Certification indicates that an EHR system offers the necessary technological capability, functionality, and security to help providers meet meaningful use criteria. Certification also indicates that the EHR system is secure, maintains confidentiality, and has interoperability.

As of the writing of this text, all providers participating in the Medicare and Medicaid programs must attest to meeting meaningful use criteria, using EHR technology certified to the 2014 edition of EHR certification criteria. The 2015 version of EHR certification criteria has been published in the Federal Register and is optional at this time.

There are different levels of certification based on the complexity of the EHR system. Table 13.1 demonstrates the three levels of EHR certification complexity.

MAKE AN IMPACT!

Ninety-six percent of all nonfederal acute care hospitals use certified health IT. Small rural and small urban acute care facilities had the lowest rates at 94%, while 96% of critical access hospitals use certified health IT. The highest rates of use came from large hospitals, at 98%.

Table 13.1 Levels of EHR Certification

EHR Functions Required	Basic EHR without Clinician Notes	Basic EHR with Clinician Notes	Comprehensive EHR
Electronic Clinical Information			
Patient demographics	•	•	•
Physician notes		•	•
Nursing assessments		•	•
Problem lists	•	•	•
Medication lists	•	•	•
Discharge summaries	•	•	•
Advance directives			•
Computerized Provider Order Entry			
Lab reports			•
Radiology tests			•
Medications	•	•	•
Consultation requests			•
Nursing orders			•
Results Management			
View lab reports	•	•	•
View radiology reports	•	•	•
View radiology images			•
View diagnostic test results	•	•	•
View diagnostic test images			•
View consultant report			•
Decision Support			
Clinical guidelines			•
Clinical reminders			•
Drug allergy results			•
Drug-drug interactions			•
Drug-lab interactions			•
Drug dosing support			•
NOTES: Basic EHR adoption requires each function to be implemented in at least one clinical unit, and Comprehensive EHR adoption requires each function to be implemented in all clinical units			

Initial Steps in Implementing an EHR System

Implementing an EHR system is a time-consuming, labor-intensive project that, with proper planning, may be implemented with few disruptions. If the planning is not started long in advance of the implementation date, then the process may be challenging.

The planning stages of EHR implementation involve a series of initial steps. The first step is determining a facility's readiness to change from paper records to electronic records. Once that factor is determined, a facility needs to set goals and establish a steering committee to lay the groundwork and move the EHR planning process forward.

Assessing Readiness

Before acquiring an EHR system, it is essential to assess the readiness of the healthcare organization or facility to undergo this transition. Organizations should be advised to analyze their clinical, financial, and administrative computer applications; their technical capabilities; and their staffing resources. They should also examine their reporting needs, such as hospital utilization, gross patient revenue, and emergency visits. Several other factors, such as current technology, technical support, and facility operations must also be considered. Lastly, the organization's culture of change management and process improvement must be reviewed. This factor is critical to a facility's successful EHR adoption. To that end, a facility must understand the distinction between implementation and adoption. The installation of an EHR system is one thing; the willingness of staff members to embrace the technology and use its applications to the fullest extent is another thing. Consequently, adoption may take more time and effort than all of the other elements of implementation.

Setting Goals

Once the readiness of a facility to implement EHR technology has been assessed, the organization must establish goals. Although these goals may differ among healthcare facilities, many organizations share some key objectives in common:

- Reduced medical errors

- Increased revenue

- Improved operational efficiency

- Supervised compliance

- Improved reporting

Establishing a Steering Committee

To move the EHR implementation process forward, a healthcare facility must create a cross-disciplinary steering committee whose members represent groups with a direct role or involvement in the proposed EHR system. A typical steering committee is composed of healthcare providers, nurses, health information professionals, administrators, financial staff, and staff members of other integral departments. The committee is led by a chair or cochairs (commonly clinicians) and is tasked with examining factors such as operational issues with the current technology infrastructure. The members then come to a consensus as to what changes need to be made to the infrastructure and draw up a plan that outlines the steps needed for successful migration to an EHR system. The committee also examines policies and procedures in support of EHR staff and resources with regard to implementation and maintenance.

The steering committee should plan to attend regularly scheduled meetings during the vendor selection process to make decisions and recommendations, as well as evaluate short- and long-term goals. During the implementation process, the committee should meet weekly to address implementation issues or challenges.

Assigning a Project Manager

It is highly recommended that, starting early in the vendor selection process, a healthcare facility hires or assigns a project manager to help implement the EHR system. The project manager may be an internal employee of the healthcare facility or an external or contracted staff person. Both types of project managers offer advantages and disadvantages.

Internal Project Manager

Hiring an internal project manager has several advantages. This individual is familiar with the culture and structure of the facility, thus allowing a better transition to an EHR system. As a permanent employee of the facility, he or she also has a vested interest in the success of the adoption process. Finally, an internal project manager is on site and available to manage any issues that arise once implementation takes place. One disadvantage of hiring an internal person is his or her possible lack of objectivity in the decision-making processes.

External Project Manager

Hiring an external project manager also offers several advantages and disadvantages. This type of project manager or contractor is a neutral party and can therefore provide objectivity in implementing the migration plan. However, he or she must spend a significant portion of time learning about the organization's standards, culture, and employees—a task that certainly decelerates the EHR implementation process. In addition, an external project manager is typically hired to complete the migration process and is unavailable after that time to manage any adoption issues.

Qualities of a Project Manager

When selecting a project manager, an organization must evaluate a potential candidate for skills in communication, facilitation, negotiation, leadership delegation, and follow-up. Although he or she does not have to be a clinician, the project manager should have a good understanding of health care and clinical information.

Responsibilities of a Project Manager

The project manager handles all issues related to the selection and implementation of the EHR system. The issues may be the transition from paper to electronic records,

A project manager will spend time getting to know the employees and culture of an organization.

a change from one EHR system to another, different approaches to performing a job, or the frustration that stems from lack of technical skills by employees or patients. The project manager should be able to visualize the end results of an organization's goals, be detailed at task monitoring, and have working knowledge of what can and cannot be accomplished. He or she will work closely with the information technology department and the vendor implementation team. Lastly, the project manager along with the vendor implementation team must identify the roles of the healthcare facility employees, create a training schedule, and monitor the training progress of the staff.

Migration Plan

In addition to the preliminary analysis, the healthcare facility should create a migration plan. A **migration plan** provides the framework to identify the basic steps that must be completed during the transition from paper health records or an existing electronic system to EHRs.

Basic Steps in a Migration Plan

A migration plan must direct a healthcare facility through these six key steps:

1. Identify requirements

2. Create a design

3. Analyze current systems

4. Test the functionality

5. Create a time line for implementation

6. Provide ongoing maintenance

The first step, identifying **requirements**, asks a facility to identify the scope of the project and user needs. Creating a **design**, which is the second step, provides a blueprint that illustrates the transition process from paper health records to the new EHR system. The third step is to analyze the current systems and processes in place. This **analysis** step will examine how the healthcare facility currently uses its healthcare records and performs tasks. A workflow analysis (described in a later section) will be useful during this step. An **environmental analysis** is the process of evaluating the people and process of workflow in a healthcare organization and is part of the analysis step. The fourth step is to **test** the functionality of the new EHR system. This type of testing focuses on several aspects such as the way system modules work, the system load, or reliability of the system. The fifth step of a migration plan is to create a time line for **implementation**. The time line, which is often created to look like a **Gantt chart** (a graphic representation of a project schedule), may include **schedules**, **resources**, and **dependencies**. Project managers schedule tasks for implementation, allocate resources (such as equipment and staff), and create dependencies (tasks that must occur before the next tasks can take place). Project managers often use programs like Microsoft Project to create a time line (see Figure 13.1). Finally, ongoing maintenance on the new EHR system must be considered and planned for.

Figure 13.1 Sample Time Line

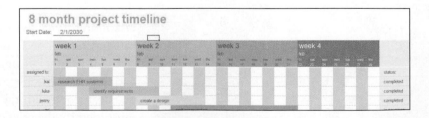

Key Considerations of a Migration Plan

Organizations that invest the appropriate amount of time and effort into a viable and sustainable migration plan will reap the rewards of successful EHR implementation. A facility's migration plan must also be fluid. There will be additional specialty software applications, such as those used by pharmacy, rehabilitation, or occupational therapy departments that require integration into the EHR system. Healthcare providers and staff must assess and add these applications to the implementation plan as needed.

CHECKPOINT 13.1

1. Describe the purpose of the ONC certification of electronic health records.

   _____

   _____

   _____

2. Name the five key steps to electronic health record migration.

   a. _____

   b. _____

   c. _____

   d. _____

   e. _____

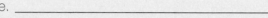

Consider This

When preparing to evaluate and implement an electronic health record (EHR) system, one aspect of the migration plan is an environmental analysis. A key part of the environmental analysis is identifying barriers to the EHR implementation. One barrier may be the employees of the healthcare facility. For example, at Jackson Family Practice, many of the office and medical staff members are not technically savvy. Although the staff members are skilled in working with patients, some are not fond of change and are accustomed to certain processes that have historically been in place. Some were resistant to a previous migration from paper calendars to electronic scheduling. The staff eventually learned the new system, but it was a difficult process. Now that the practice is considering moving from paper health records to EHRs, staff members are concerned that learning a new technology will take time away from their patients. These are common barriers that healthcare facilities face. Employees may not be confident in their technology skills, be resistant to change, or be concerned about increased time to complete tasks. If you were serving on the team assigned to complete the environmental analysis of Jackson Family Practice, how would you suggest the healthcare organization address these barriers?

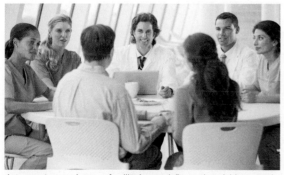

A team to analyze a facility's workflow should be made up of employees from many different departments.

Analyzing Workflow

A **workflow analysis** is an important assessment to conduct when selecting an EHR system. A workflow analysis reviews how the organization currently functions and how the paper records are used to care for patients. Workflow analysis should be considered for all back office, front office, health information management, and provider processes. Multiple stakeholders will be engaged in this process, and key internal stakeholders that comprehensively understand the flow of information in the facility are essential to an accurate analysis. Stakeholders may vary by facility but generally include health information managers, physicians, nurses, IT, and other department managers.

Use of a Flowchart

A **flowchart** showing all of the necessary steps in a particular procedure is an effective tool for understanding workflow analysis. Figure 13.2 depicts a flowchart mapping the emergency room workflow process. The chart helps identify locations of break-downs, insufficiencies, or bottlenecks. Armed with the knowledge that a flowchart provides, an organization or facility may be able to isolate the challenges to the flow of patient information and find a vendor that can address these workflow problems before final implementation of the EHR system.

Figure 13.2   Emergency Room Workflow Process

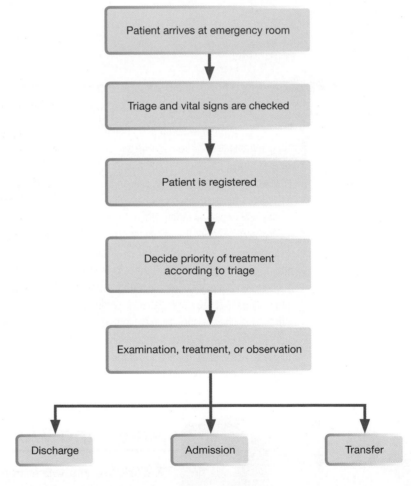

Collection of Information

Before a facility can begin the task of gathering data for a workflow analysis, it must determine its approach. The organization may implement one of the following directives:

- Put together a cross-disciplinary team
- Assign staff members to perform their job requirements and analyze how work is completed

- Conduct an internal analysis rather than working through a vendor

- Assign overall responsibility to a project manager or internal staff person

Another approach that some facilities use to collect data is to ask departments or staff members to review how a patient is treated by "stepping into the patient's shoes." This role reversal helps them analyze the interaction between the patient and healthcare facility from the moment he or she checks in to the moment he or she leaves the facility.

Still another technique for collecting information for a workflow analysis is to ask staff members to write detailed descriptions of their tasks, actions, and sequences. Some questions may include the following:

- What are the tasks or steps involved in the process?

- Are there variations to these processes?

- Are there acceptable reasons for process variations by your department?

- Who completes the process?

- How long does the process take?

- Where are the bottlenecks where the process gets interrupted or slows down?

- Do some tasks need to be completed more than once in a given process?

Collection of Forms

During the workflow analysis process, it is also vital to gather all the paper forms used by healthcare facility employees, because these forms will now be entered electronically in an EHR system. Understanding where and how the forms are used, as well as what information is collected and communicated, is an integral part of the EHR workflow analysis.

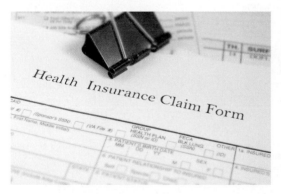

Healthcare facilities need to gather all of the paper forms they use to perform workflow analysis.

Desired Outcome of Workflow Analysis

A workflow analysis provides an integrated framework that coordinates the processes of several departments in a healthcare facility. This workflow sequence serves:

- the facility by setting realistic expectations for the software functions

- the staff by streamlining processes and improving communication

- the patient by coordinating treatment and improving the overall quality of administered health care.

The workflow analysis should also reflect a sequence that aligns with the organization's goals regarding the EHR. Figures 13.3 and 13.4 show a workflow process for a medication refill—both before and after EHR system implementation.

Figure 13.3 Medication Refill Workflow Process Before EHR Implementation

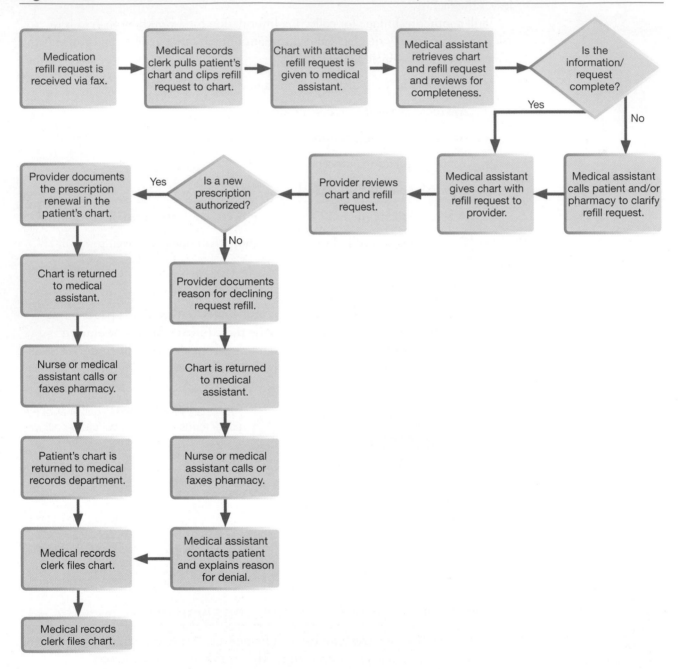

Chapter 13 Implementation and Evaluation of an EHR System

Figure 13.4 Medication Refill Workflow Process After EHR Implementation

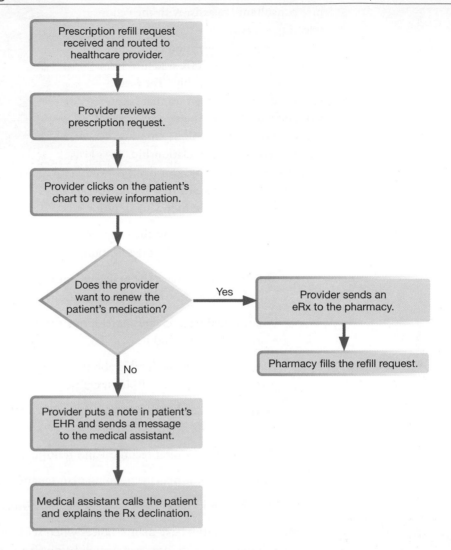

Evaluation of EHR Systems

Once a facility decides to purchase an EHR system, the organization's steering committee begins the vendor selection process. This process can be challenging and requires the input of employee representatives from several key departments of the healthcare facility. These department representatives may include management, health information staff, administrative staff, clinical staff, healthcare providers, and information technology staff. Making such an important decision regarding the EHR system should involve representatives from the entire organization. Depending

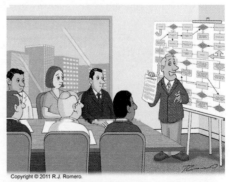

Copyright © 2011 R.J. Romero.

"Our new Electronic Health Record system is so easy to use and dependable that we don't even provide training or tech support. Just sign here and it's all yours."

on size, some facilities may choose to hire consultants to assist with the vendor selection process.

One helpful suggestion is to think of working with an EHR system vendor as a long-term relationship. The healthcare facility must be certain that it can work effectively with the selected vendor because both parties will be entering a closely collaborative relationship. To determine if an EHR vendor fits the needs of a facility, the steering committee should consider the following questions:

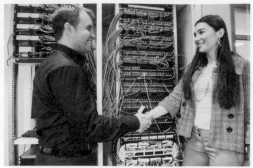

Positive support from an EHR system vendor is an important part of a collaborative relationship.

- Does the vendor have the support staff, financial resources, and capabilities to meet the needs of the organization?

- Does the vendor have the management expertise to ensure the completion of all tasks related to EHR implementation?

- Is continued research and development in technology and health information a priority for the vendor?

- Is the vendor knowledgeable about the requirements for government certification and regulations of EHR systems?

- Does the vendor have a functional product with the ability to adapt to changes required by the healthcare industry?

- Does the vendor offer technical and training support for healthcare personnel?

- Does the vendor manage ongoing maintenance and updates?

- Has the vendor received positive reviews by other healthcare organizations?

EXPAND)))
YOUR LEARNING

You may view a full list of certified EHR systems on the HealthIT.gov website at http://EHR2 .ParadigmEducation .com/CertifiedList.

Healthcare facilities have many choices when selecting an EHR system. They may choose to build their own, use several applications from a variety of vendors, or choose an **integrated system**. No matter which option a facility pursues, the organization must select a certified EHR system to receive federal incentives. A **best-of-breed** EHR system is when the healthcare organization goes to market to find a vendor or vendors to supply the clinical applications needed. The healthcare facility then chooses various vendors evaluated to be the best in the particular area of health care and integrates them into an entire EHR system.

Features of an Effective EHR System

Selecting an EHR system is a difficult task, with significant pressure on the steering committee to choose a system that demonstrates profitability and improved clinical quality. Essential features of an effective EHR system include the following:

- ONC certification
- Operating system
- Web-based or on-site server

- Backup, downtime, and disaster recovery
- Data management and reporting systems

- Meaningful Use Attestation
- Functionality
- Security
- Interoperability

- Payer interface
- License agreement
- Maintenance and support

Tutorial 13.1

EHRNAVIGAT✚R

Generating an Attestation Report

Go to Navigator+ to launch Tutorial 13.1. As an IT manager, practice generating an attestation report.

Meaningful Use

As you learned in Chapter 1, the adoption of EHR systems is based on the idea of meaningful use, which connects all parts of the EHR into a system that can effectively communicate and deliver electronic healthcare services. To qualify a system as succeeding in this standard, a practitioner must demonstrate that the EHR system is used in a significant and measurable manner by attesting to meeting meaningful use.

Vendor Evauation

As part of the vendor evaluation process, the steering committee should request an onsite or online demonstration. After the demonstration, the committee should evaluate the EHR system based on a previously developed assessment tool. See Figure 13.5 for a sample demonstration request and evaluation tool. The evaluation tool should include the essential features similar to the list provided in Figure 13.6.

Once the steering committee narrows down the short list of potential EHR systems, the committee should request a quote from the vendor. This quote is often referred to as a **request for proposal (RFP)**, which is typically executed near the end of the vendor selection process. The RFP includes requirements, services, vendor information, and a bid or quote for the EHR system. For example, after the committee recommends the top three EHR systems, an RFP is sent to each of those vendors. The facility and its committee receive system requirements and services along with bids or quotes from the vendors and compare each of them. After the committee selects the EHR system, the healthcare facility enters an agreement with the chosen vendor.

Consider This

You are a member of the steering committee at Cincinnati Grace Physicians. Your committee has developed an electronic health records (EHR) checklist and has requested demonstrations from four different EHR vendors. However, one of the committee members has a relative who works for one of the proposed vendors. Several members of the committee are concerned that the member will try to persuade the rest of the committee to select the vendor where the relative is employed. What measures should the committee implement to ensure an objective evaluation of all four EHR vendors?

National Learning Consortium
HealthIT.gov
Advancing America's Health Care

Vendor Meaningful Use Compare Tool

Instructions: Score each vendor on a scale from 1 (poor) to 5 (excellent) on each item. Total up your ratings for each vendor to help make your comparisons. Write the names of the vendors you are comparing in the watermark space provided in vendor columns. Use the blank rows at the end of the worksheet to ask your own questions.

	Vendor	Vendor 1	Vendor 2	Vendor 3	etc.			
1	**Demographics / Care Management**							
1.1	The system has the capability to record demographics including: Preferred language, insurance type, gender, race, ethnicity, and date of birth.							
2	**Patient History**							
2.1	The system has the capability to import patient health history data from an existing system.							
2.2	The system presents a chronological, filterable, and comprehensive review of patient's EHR, which may be summarized and printed, subject to privacy and confidentiality requirements.							
3	**Current Health Data, Encounters, Health Risk Appraisal, and Coordination of Care**							
3.1	The system can exchange key clinical information among providers of care and patient authorized entities electronically.							
3.2	The system obtains test results via standard HL7 interface from: laboratory.							
3.2.1	The system obtains test results via standard HL7 interface from: radiology/imaging.							
3.2.2	The system obtains test results via standard HL7 interface from: other equipment such as Vitals, ECG, Holter, Glucometer.							
3.3	The system can record and chart changes in vital signs including: heights, weight, blood pressure, calculate and display BMI, plot and display growth charts for children 2-20 years including BMI.							
3.4	The system provides a flexible, user modifiable, search mechanism for retrieval of information captured during encounter documentation.							
3.5	The system provides a mechanism to capture, review, or amend history of current illness.							
3.6	The system enables the origination, documentation, and tracking of referrals between care providers or healthcare organizations, including clinical and administrative details of the referral.							
3.7	The system can track and provide a summary care record for each transition of care and referral visit.							
4	**Encounter – Progress Notes**							
4.1	The system records progress notes utilizing a combination of system default, provider-defined templates.							
4.2	The system includes a progress note template that is problem oriented and can, at the user's option be linked to either a diagnosis or problem number.							
5	**Problem Lists**							
5.1	The system creates and maintains patient-specific problem lists of current and active diagnoses based on ICD9/10 CM or SNOMED CT.							
5.2	For each problem, the systems has the capability to create, review, or amend information regarding a change on the status of a problem to include, but not be limited to, the date the change was first noticed or diagnosed.							
5.3	The system can record smoking status for patient 13 years or older.							
6	**Care Plans**							
6.1	The system provides administrative tools for organizations to build care plans, guidelines, and protocols for use during patient care planning and care.							
6.2	The system generates and automatically records in the care plan document, patient-specific instructions related to pre- and post-procedural and post-discharge requirements. The instructions must be simple to access.							
7	**Prevention**							
7.1	The system has the capability to display health prevention prompts on the summary display. The prompts must be dynamic and take into account sex, age, and chronic conditions.							
7.2	The system includes user-modifiable health maintenance templates.							
7.3	The system includes a patient tracking and reminder capability (patient follow-up) updatable by the user at the time an event is set or complied with.							
7.4	The system has the capability to send reminders to patients per patient preference for preventive/follow up care.							
8	**Patient Access to Personal Health Information/Patient Education**							
8.1	The system can provide patients with an electronic copy of their health information.							
8.2	The system can provide patients with timely electronic access to their health information.							
8.3	The system can provide clinical summaries to patients for each visit							
8.4	The system has the capability to create, review, update, or delete patient education materials. The materials must originate from a credible source and be maintained by the vendor as frequently as necessary.							
8.5	The system has the capability of providing printed patient education materials in culturally appropriate languages on demand or automatically at the end of the encounter. Please provide current list of available languages.							
9	**Alerts / Reminders**							

Vendor MU Compare   1   October 21, 2011

15.4.1	Allowing patient tracking and follow-up based on user defined diagnoses.							
15.4.2	Providing a longitudinal view of the patient medical history.							
15.4.3	Providing intuitive access to patient treatments and outcomes.							
15.5	What reporting engine is utilized within the software?(ex. Crystal Reports, Excel, proprietary).							
15.5.1	If utilizing Crystal Reports do you provide a listing of all reportable data elements?							
15.6	Does the end user have the ability to create custom reports?							
15.7	Can reports be run on-demand during the course of the day?							
15.8	Can reports be set up to run automatically as well as routed to a specific person with in the office?							
16	**Cost Measuring/Quality Assurance**							
16.1	The system has built-in mechanism/access to other systems to capture cost information.							

Vendor MU Compare   2   October 21, 2011

Vendor MU Compare   3   October 21, 2011

VENDOR EVALUATION MATRIX

Before evaluating vendors, categorize each function or usability characteristic as a HP (high priority), MP (medium priority) or LP (low priority). During demonstrations and interviews, make sure you get answers from each vendor to your high priority questions. Score each vendor on a scale from 1 (poor) to 5 (excellent).

Vendor name: _____

Date: _____

Vendor contact information: _____

ISSUE	PRIORITY	COMMENTS
Charting the visit		
Method of data entry/documentation – Forms, drop-down lists, templates, hybrids.		
Does the system contain templates for the conditions my clinic treats?		
Can templates be customized?		
Are templates easily customized?		
When is it necessary to insert free text into the note/template?		
Is it easy to insert free text?		
Describe how voice recognition works.		
How easy is it to use voice activation?		
Is it easy to move through the process of creating a note?		
Are notes flexible?		
Does the system alert about unfinished portions of documentation?		
Can the alert system be bypassed		

Total Cost of Ownership

Total cost of ownership is more than just the price of purchasing an EHR system. A healthcare organization must examine all relevant costs to make an informed decision, including accounting, opportunity, and economic costs. A facility will also incur many additional expenditures associated with EHR implementation.

Accounting Costs

An **accounting cost** is the total amount of money paid out for products, goods, or services. The accounting costs of an EHR system include the hardware, software, productivity loss, implementation, ongoing technical support, and software licenses. Hence, the accounting cost is the direct cost of the EHR system.

Opportunity Costs

An **opportunity cost** is the value of a decision. Something must be given up for the benefit of something else. For instance, an opportunity cost could include the consequence of not implementing an EHR system and losing patients to healthcare facilities that have one. Accounting worksheets do not show opportunity costs.

Economic Costs

An **economic cost** is the combination of accounting and opportunity costs. It includes the cash outlays related to the implementation of the EHR and is what is given up following the EHR implementation decision.

Additional Financial Considerations

Healthcare providers interested in purchasing an EHR system must understand that, in addition to accounting and opportunity costs, there are additional financial expenditures that must be considered:

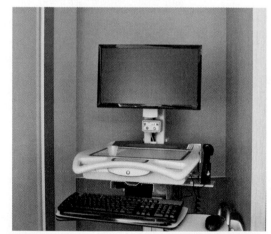

Hardware such as computer stations are part of the cost of implementing an EHR.

- The healthcare facility may have to hire additional staff trained in health informatics.

- The technical support staff may need to hire additional employees or outsource the job functions.

- The healthcare facility must conduct and assess workflow analysis.

- The healthcare facility must provide training and ongoing support for all healthcare employees.

- Data dictionaries and templates must be created, developed, and reviewed.

Other factors that must be considered are as follows:

- Hardware—initial cost, maintenance, and other ongoing expenses

- Software—license fees, electronic claims and remittance, and electronic prescribing costs

- Implementation and training—cost of installing, building, testing, and training

- Maintenance—annual fees for upgrades, support, training, and customization

- Downtime and recovery—depending on the type of EHR system (web-based or on-site server), the vendor should communicate its plans for downtime and data backup and storage (such as cloud, online, disk, or tape)

Once an EHR system has been purchased, installed, and implemented, the healthcare facility continues to perform regular maintenance on the system. For example, the software must be continually updated with information on the latest evidence-based medicine, new and recalled drugs, new disease terminology, and new processes and workflows of external factors such as reimbursement or patient needs.

CHECKP⊕INT 13.2

1. Name four financial considerations when purchasing an electronic health records (EHR) system.

   a. _____

   b. _____

   c. _____

   d. _____

2. Name the three costs included in the total cost of EHR ownership.

   a. _____

   b. _____

   c. _____

Return on Investment

When preparing to make a decision about implementing an EHR system, a healthcare facility may perform a **cost–benefit analysis** to determine the return on investment. **Return on investment (ROI)** is a performance measurement that calculates the benefit or gain of an investment. The healthcare facility will need to pinpoint the payback period by comparing the cash flow (cash inflow minus cash outflow) with the cost of the investment to determine how long it takes to achieve a positive difference. If the payback period is longer than five years, the investment may not be worth it. Therefore, the healthcare organization may look at a less expensive EHR system to achieve a payback period of two to five years.

Internal rate of return (IRR) and net present value (NPV) should also be calculated. The **internal rate of return (IRR)** is a calculation used to measure the profitability of an investment—in this case, the EHR system. The **net present value (NPV)** is the present value of future cash flows minus the purchase price of goods or services. The NPV measures the excess or shortfall of cash flows once the financial obligations are met. If the IRR or NPV for an EHR system is greater than the IRR or NPV of other EHR systems considered, then the EHR system is considered a good investment. Many healthcare organizations are recognizing that an EHR system must not be considered as a cost of doing business but rather as a necessary component of healthcare delivery.

Most vendors provide an ROI analysis; however, this analysis requires a careful interpretation of the results. Typically, a vendor assigns a monetary value to every benefit, whether or not actual savings will result, so it is important for the steering commitee of the facility to scrutinize these numbers.

Consider This

Many times, healthcare organizations state that the implementation of an EHR system had a significant return on investment (ROI). To view one perspective on this issue, go to http://EHR2 .ParadigmEducation.com/ROIarticle. Read the following case about Centura Health, the 2015 HIMSS Enterprise Davies Award of Excellence, and its view of ROI and EHR implementation. What did the article say were the key areas that benefited from implementing an EHR system?

Costs versus Benefits of EHR Implementation

The costs and benefits associated with EHR implementation depend on a number of factors. To meet the meaningful use provision of EHRs required by the US Department of Health and Human Services (HHS), a healthcare facility must make such an investment, and, depending on the type of healthcare facility, the total cost will vary. For example, a small community hospital working with a single vendor may spend $3 million, a medium-sized hospital that selects a best-of-breed system may spend $10 million to $15 million, and a large hospital may spend up to $100 million.

The size of the facility, complexity of the practice, implementation strategy, and types of services offered or performed factor in to the total cost of EHR implementation.

The benefits of EHR use depend on a variety of factors in the areas of efficiency, finance, quality, and compliance. The benefits in these areas are listed here:

- Efficiency
  - Reduces duplication of tests
  - Increases accuracy in patient information
  - Allows healthcare providers and services to view automated transfers

- Financial
  - Offers internal and external savings
  - Decreases malpractice insurance costs
- Quality
  - Provides reminders about preventive care
  - Eliminates illegible medication prescriptions
  - Standardizes data and improves quality of patient care

- Compliance
  - Creates reports
  - Complies with requirements from The Joint Commission and the Centers for Medicare and Medicaid Services (CMS)
  - Determines eligibility for Medicaid and Medicare programs

A healthcare facility must determine the overall costs and benefits to justify the investment. The real key, after all the numbers have been crunched, is the level of acceptance from a facility's staff. If its employees do not embrace the EHR system, then the facility will find its path to implementation difficult.

EHR Implementation

Implementation is as important as the selection of the EHR system. One of the factors that often contributes to implementation failure is fear and a lack of support from management; therefore, leadership is an essential aspect of implementation. The steering committee of the facility must identify leaders in each department who will champion the EHR system. These leaders should encourage adaptability and flexibility in their discussions with coworkers and act as a link between the departments and steering committee to provide staff feedback and suggestions for implementation.

The steering committee must devise a plan to train and manage the healthcare facility staff and to create security levels for staff members. The plan should contain the time line of when to begin training, how the training will take place, and how quickly the healthcare facility will be ready to switch over to the EHR system. As discussed in Chapter 3, the security level assigned to each healthcare facility staff member is based on the job requirements. Employees of the healthcare facility can access only portions of the EHR system directly related to their positions.

Rollout Process

With the EHR system selected, the project manager in place, and the implementation plan created, the **rollout** process can begin. The rollout process occurs in three phases: organizational, training, and operational.

Organizational Phase

The first phase is organizational, which entails the plan for installation of the EHR system. This phase is usually complete once the rollout begins. The healthcare organization selects a cut-off date, which determines how many years the healthcare organization will go back and convert paper records. For example, the facility may choose to go back five years, and all those records will be digitally converted to the EHR. The remaining records will most likely be scanned and stored electronically. As healthcare delivery systems begin the conversion process, there may be portions of patient records on paper and other portions stored electronically. As you learned in Chapter 2, this type of record is known as a hybrid health record. Healthcare providers with a small patient population may convert to an EHR system in a shorter time frame. However, a provider with a larger patient population, such as a major hospital, may take longer to fully convert to an EHR system; therefore, larger organizations may use a hybrid health record for a considerably longer period than their smaller counterparts.

Training Phase

The second phase is training and heavily emphasizes learning, fine tuning, customizing, and testing of the EHR system.

Operational Phase

The rollout process ends with the operational phase, which includes the launch of the EHR system and continual training while maintenance begins. A successful EHR launch depends on the efforts put into the other phases. Prior to the "go-live" date, the EHR system must be tested many times, including its hardware, software, backup, networking, connectivity, and recovery components. Most healthcare organizations choose to complete pilots prior to going live. A **pilot** is a test run of the EHR system. In addition, during the pilot, users can identify issues or problems that they encounter.

Preparation Phase

A few weeks prior to the go-live date, all staff members should be trained for the required functionalities and assessed for mastery. **Functionality testing** often requires a facility to use a test environment before implementing the EHR system facility-wide. Key users, who are selected because of their expertise and knowledge, run the system to ensure it works as described and meets the needs of the facility. Lastly, the healthcare facility should notify its patients that its facility is implementing an EHR system and inform them of the go-live date. This notification prepares patients for upcoming changes, including any potential delays in scheduling, billing, or wait times.

Go-Live Date

Healthcare organizations have different approaches to going live. Some facilities choose a phased implementation in which one function of the EHR system is made available at a time. This staggered approach allows for the organization to resolve issues and receive feedback on individual features or applications. Alternatively, an organization can choose a "big bang" approach, making all EHR functions immediately available to all users. This approach speeds up implementation but runs the risk of creating multiple problems or delays.

It is important that every member of the organization be prepared for the go-live date of the EHR system. If a healthcare facility is using a commercial product, then the vendor usually provides a customized checklist. The checklist may include determining healthcare provider schedules, planning downtime to catch up, informing users where they can go to receive help, informing third parties in case there is a delay or need to provide additional support to the healthcare facility, and planning for end-of-day debriefing.

Consider This

One aspect of electronic health record (EHR) implementation is to plan for an information technology (IT) outage. Boulder Community Hospital in Boulder, CO, learned this lesson when it experienced a computer system outage, leaving patients frustrated. To learn more about this incident and the measures taken to rectify the situation, go to http://EHR2 .ParadigmEducation.com/Outage

How would you handle an IT outage that meant the EHR system would be unavailable?

Chapter Summary

The transition from paper health records to electronic health records (EHRs) can be a challenge. Each organization must be thoughtful as it determines how to initiate this process.

A healthcare organization must first assess its readiness to adopt an EHR system before it selects a system to meet its needs. The organization should form a steering committee, set goals, and create a migration plan. A migration plan should identify the EHR requirements, create a design, analyze current systems, test the new system, and set an implementation date for the EHR system. The committee should also conduct a workflow analysis for each area of the organization and prepare a cost–benefit analysis to present to the administration. The return on investment (ROI) should be calculated to determine the benefit or gain of the investment in the EHR system.

Once these initial steps have been taken, the steering committee should then review potential vendors based on the organization's criteria. These vendors should be selected by reviewing a list of EHR systems that have been certified for functionality, interoperability, and security by the Office of the National Coordinator for Health Information Technology (ONC). They may use vendor demonstrations and issue proposal requests to help them select an EHR system.

Upon system selection, it is necessary to establish a rollout process and a go-live date. Internal leaders from all areas of the organization are necessary to champion the newly selected system and enhance buy-in. A healthcare organization that follows this process enhances the probability of successful EHR implementation.

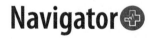 **Navigator** The following EHR Review, EHR Application, and EHR Evaluation activities are also available online in the Navigator+ learning management system. Your instructor may ask you to complete these activities online. Navigator+ also provides access to flash cards, study games, and practice quizzes to help strengthen your understanding of the chapter content.

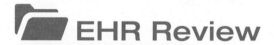 EHR Review

Acronyms/Initialisms

Study the following acronyms discussed in this chapter. Go to Navigator+ for flash cards of the acronyms and other chapter key terms.

AHRQ: Agency for Healthcare Research and Quality

ASHIM: American Society of Health Informatics Managers

CMS: Centers for Medicare and Medicaid Services

HHS: US Department of Health and Human Services

HITECH Act: Health Information Technology for Economic and Clinical Health Act

HITRC: Health Information Technology Research Center

ONC: Office of National Coordinator for Health Information Technology

IRR: internal rate of return

RFP: request for proposal

IT: information technology

ROI: return on investment

NPV: net present value

Check Your Understanding

To check your understanding of this chapter's key concepts, answer the following questions.

1. For a healthcare organization to receive stimulus funds, the electronic health record (EHR) system must be certified by the

    a. Office of the National Coordinator-Authorized Testing and Certification Bodies (ONC-ATCB).

    b. American Health Information Management Association.

    c. American Medical Association.

    d. Centers for Medicare and Medicaid Services.

2. The first step in selecting an EHR system is to

    a. establish goals.

    b. assess readiness.

    c. form a steering committee.

    d. create a budget.

3. The accounting costs of an EHR system may include any of the following *except*

    a. hardware, software, vendor support, and software licenses.

    b. software, productivity loss, implementation, and vendor support.

    c. hardware, software, technical support, and project management.

    d. productivity loss, implementation, technical support, and software license.

4. Return on investment is a/an

    a. formula that calculates the cost of the EHR system.

    b. analysis of the cost–benefit of an EHR system.

    c. performance measurement that calculates the expense of an investment.

    d. performance measurement that calculates the benefit of an investment.

5. Benefits of adopting an EHR system include all of the following *except*

    a. financial.

    b. analysis.

    c. quality.

    d. compliance.

6. True/False: The five key steps of a migration plan are: identify the requirements, create a design, analyze current systems, test functionality, and create a time line for implementation.

7. True/False: A workflow analysis reviews how an organization will function in the future and how EHRs are used.

8. True/False: A facility that selects an EHR vendor or vendors from the market to meet its need is adopting a "best-of-breed" system.

9. True/False: A request for proposal (RFP) is a request for demonstration by an EHR vendor.

10. True/False: The rollout process is the planning phase of the EHR system selection.

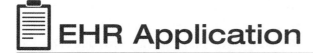
EHR Application

Go on the Record

To build on your understanding of the topics in this chapter, complete the following short-answer activities.

1. Describe the importance of selecting an EHR system certified by the Office of National Coordinator for Health Information Technology (ONC).

2. Explain how an organization may assess its readiness to move to an EHR system.

3. Describe the key areas of a workflow analysis.

4. Discuss the key players on an EHR selection committee and how their roles affect EHR selection.

5. Compare three areas (accounting, opportunity, and economic costs) of the total cost of ownership and how those areas may affect EHR selection.

Navigate the Field

To gain practice in handling challenging situations in the workplace, consider the following real-world scenarios and identify how you would respond to each.

1. You are testing HealthWest Physician Practice's EHR system. Suddenly, the computer screen goes blank. You now realize you should have had an EHR system downtime plan to continue so the practice may keep operating. Go to http://EHR2.ParadigmEducation.com/DowntimePlan and review the article. Then prepare a plan for HealthWest Physician Practice. After reviewing the article, prepare the appropriate guidelines for your healthcare facility to implement during this EHR system downtime.

2. You work for St. Stephen's Hospital and are leading the EHR steering committee. The committee has met and is in the RFP preparation phase. Your task is to write the introduction of the RFP. Be sure to include an overview of the healthcare organization, the opportunity, and the facility's goals in this introduction.

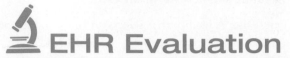 **EHR Evaluation**

Think Critically

Continue to think critically about challenging concepts and complete the following activities.

1. You are the EHR Implementation Specialist at Northstar Physicians. You are assigned the task of migrating the paper records to the EHR Navigator. Research migration plans for converting paper records to electronic records. Create a checklist that identifies which documents and information will need to be migrated to EHR Navigator.

2. As part of the EHR selection team, you have been given the task to research three certified complete Inpatient EHR Systems. You may use http://EHR2 .ParadigmEducation.com/CertifiedList as one source to locate certified EHR systems. You are to prepare a report comparing and contrasting the three systems. Write a two- to three-page report that would be submitted to the EHR selection committee making a recommendation based on your analysis of the three products.

Make Your Case

Consider the scenario and then complete the following project.

You are the chair of the EHR system steering committee. Your team has met and reviewed the entire vendor selection process. Now you must present your findings and a recommendation to the administrators of your healthcare facility. Include the team's process in contacting vendors and examining the EHR systems, its recommendation, and the time line for implementation.

Explore the Technology

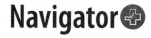

Complete the EHR Navigator practice assessments that align to each tutorial and the assessments that accompany Chapter 13 located on Navigator+.

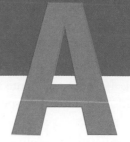

Checkpoint Answer Keys

Checkpoint 1.1

1. An electronic version of patient files within a single organization that allows healthcare providers to place orders, document results, and store patient information for one facility.

2. The patient health information gathered from the EMRs of multiple healthcare delivery organizations that is electronically stored and accessed.

3. a. EMR belongs to a single healthcare provider or organization whereas EHR integrates EMRs from multiple providers.

   b. EHRs contain subsets of patient information from each visit that a patient has experienced.

   c. EHRs are interactive and can share information among multiple healthcare providers.

Checkpoint 1.2

1. The ability of one computer system to communicate with another computer system.

2. Level 3: Semantic interoperability level.

3. Health Level 7 (HL7).

Checkpoint 1.3

1. a. Improved documentation.

   b. Streamlined and rapid communication.

   c. Immediate and improved access to patient information

2. a. High cost.

   b. Privacy and security.

   c. Inexperience in implementation and training.

   d. Significant daily process changes.

Checkpoint 2.1

1. Data includes the descriptive or numeric attributes of one or more variables. Data collected and analyzed becomes information. A record is a collection, usually in writing of an account or an occurrence.

2. Administrative data includes demographic information; clinical data is information such as admission dates, office visits, laboratory test results, evaluations, or emergency visits; legal data is composed of consents for treatments and authorizations for the release of information; financial data includes the patient's insurance and payment information.

Checkpoint 2.2

1. The source-oriented record is the most common used by healthcare facilities. It organizes the health documents into sections that contain information from a specified department or type of service.

2. S(subjective) O (objective) A (assessment) P (plan).

Checkpoint 2.3

1. Answers may vary, and could include five of the following: admission record, history and physical, progress notes, laboratory tests, diagnostic tests, operative notes, pathology reports, physician orders, consents, consultations, emergency department encounters, and discharge summary.

2. Answers may vary, and could include five of the following: demographic information, contact information, history and physical, immunization records, problem lists, allergy lists, prescription lists, progress notes, assessment, consultations, referrals, treatment plans, patient instructions, laboratory tests and results, consents, communication, external correspondence, and financial information.

Checkpoint 3.1

1. a. input

   b. processing

   c. output

   d. storage

2. A LAN is a group of computers connected through a network confined to a single area or small geographic area. The network is secure and reliable. The networked computer system allows computer workstations to work and communicate together.

Checkpoint 3.2

1. The messages feature allows you to communicate with other system users in your organizations using a HIPAA-compliant feature. It improves the collaboration and continuity of patient care.

2. a. Schedules view

   b. Read-only Calendar

Checkpoint 3.3

1. Answers may vary, and could include four of the following: medical diagnoses, treatments, procedures, allergies, medical history, medications, test results, and reports.

2. An integrated laboratory feature enables healthcare facilities and providers to connect with national and regional laboratories or to maintain an existing laboratory partner. Integrating laboratories into an EHR system gives you the ability to create laboratory orders and view results from any computer at any time, with abnormal results flagged and organized for easy review.

Checkpoint 4.1

1. Answers may vary, and could include four of the following: acute care setting such as a hospital; ambulatory care settings such as surgery centers, physician offices, clinics, group practices, emergency departments, therapeutic services, dialysis clinics, birthing centers, cancer treatment centers, home care, correctional facilities, and dentist offices; other healthcare settings, such as long-term care facilities, behavioral health settings, rehabilitation facilities, and hospice care.

2. If a patient goes to an ambulatory care facility for a procedure and complications occur, requiring the patient to be admitted to an acute care facility.

Checkpoint 4.2

1. a. Personal/Family

   b. Workers' Compensation

   c. Third-Party Liability

   d. Corporate

   e. Research

2. If two insurance plans cover a child, then the birthday rule is applied. The birthday rule specifies that the insurance of the parent whose birthday falls first in a calendar year will be the primary insurance. It helps to determine which insurance should be used as the primary insurance.

Checkpoint 5.1

1. Meetings, holidays, lunch hours, surgical schedules, physician rounds, or emergencies.

2. a. Open Hours
   b. Time Specified
   c. Wave
   d. Modified Wave
   e. Cluster

Checkpoint 5.2

1. Patient portals are available 24-hours a day and allow the patient to view a provider's calendar. The portal allows patients to enter demographic, insurance, medical history, and current health information prior to the first appointment, reducing the resources necessary from the healthcare facility.

2. a. Select Schedule an Appointment
   b. Select Add Appointment

Checkpoint 5.3

1. a. Change in patient condition
   b. Change in isolation status
   c. Patient preference

2. The patient tracker offers a real-time, at-a-glance view of a patient's current status and location. It improves the healthcare facility's work flow and increases patient satisfaction.

Checkpoint 6.1

1. True
2. False
3. Covered entities

Checkpoint 6.2

1. Answers may vary, and could include three of the following: impermissible uses and disclosures of PHI, lack of safeguards of PHI, lack of patient access to his or her PHI, uses or disclosures of more than the minimum necessary PHI, lack of administrative safeguards of electronic PHI.

2. A civil violation is when a person mistakenly obtains or discloses individually identifiable health information in violation of HIPAA. A criminal violation is when a person knowingly obtains or discloses individually identifiable health information in violation of HIPAA.

Checkpoint 6.3

1. a. General Rules
   b. Administrative Safeguards
   c. Physical Safeguards
   d. Technical Safeguards
   e. Organization Requirements
   f. Policies and Procedures and Documentation Requirements

2. Technical Safeguards
3. Administrative Safeguards

Checkpoint 7.1

1. Because it requires less personnel time, avoids repetitive request of information from patients, and may allow for more consistent data entry.

2. The history is the subjective element and has the following components: history of present illness, past medical history, allergies, medications currently prescribed, family and social histories. The physical examination is the objective element of the H&P, and consists of a physical examination of body systems, an assessment of the patient and his or her condition, and a treatment plan.

Checkpoint 7.2

1. Answers may vary, but could include three of the following: improved prescribing accuracy and efficiency; a decreased potential for medication errors and prescription forgeries; improved billing; less risk for potential medication errors due to a healthcare provider's handwriting, illegible faxes, or misinterpretation of prescription abbreviations.

2. The ability to order controlled substances electronically.

Checkpoint 8.1

1. Answers may vary, and could include three of the following: reimbursement, research, decision making, public health, quality improvement, resource utilization, and healthcare policy and payment.
2. October 1, 2015
3. 2020

Checkpoint 8.2

1. a. Efficient concurrent and final coding

   b. Accuracy in code assignments

   c. Improved access to health records
2. False. Upcoding is illegal. Unintentional upcoding is considered abuse, and intentional upcoding is considered fraud.

Checkpoint 9.1

1. Health Maintenance Organization (HMO)
2. Preferred Provider Organization (PPO)
3. Consolidated Omnibus Budget Reconciliation Act of 1985 (COBRA)

Checkpoint 9.2

1. Medicare, Medicaid, TRICARE, CHAMPVA, workers' compensation
2. Medicare
3. Income replacement benefits, healthcare treatment, mileage reimbursement, and burial and death benefits

Checkpoint 9.3

1. Day-to-day operations of a medical practice
2. CMS-1500
3. The 837 claim is also known as the HIPAA form. HIPAA regulations require that most claims be processed electronically using the 837 form.

Checkpoint 9.4

1. A billing/status report is generated to determine if the practice is receiving the correct monies owed.
2. A Production Report (Production by Procedure, Production by Insurance, Production by Provider)

3. A Production by Provider Report may be used for a variety of reasons including: calculating provider salaries based on the number of patients treated; calculating the number of appointment slots for each provider; scheduling staff and ordering supplies.

Checkpoint 10.1

1. Four of the following: date of birth, race, ethnicity, gender, and laboratory test results
2. Primary data is the original collection or original data found in the health record. Secondary data sources are data that is collected by someone else or data that already exists.

Checkpoint 10.2

1. Together, policies and procedures provide an explanation to employees of the healthcare organization about how to handle data operations. Policies and procedures provide a framework to identify the data standards for a healthcare organization. Policies and procedures also detail the use of data, such as the policies and procedures of using data in relation to privacy and confidentiality.
2. A data dictionary is important to data standards because it provides a way to prevent inconsistencies, define elements and their meaning, and also provide consistency and enforce data standards.
3. Data mapping is a method that is used to connect data from one system to data of another system. Data is analyzed in the original or source system to match data in the other or target system.

Checkpoint 10.3

1. A data set is a structured collection of related data elements. These data elements have standard definitions to provide consistent data for all users. A database is a collection of data that is organized in rows, columns, and tables. The data is indexed. A registry uses clinical information that focuses on the outcomes of data before it is analyzed. A registry is a database focused on a collection of information about a specific condition or disease. Indexes in a database are used to find data without searching every row.

2. Accountability; Transparency; Integrity; Protection; Compliance; Availability; Retention; Disposition

Checkpoint 11.1

1. Health information technology that integrates with the EHR and assists healthcare providers with decision-making tasks such as determining diagnoses, choosing the best medications for the patient, and selecting proper diagnostic tests.

2. a. Knowledge-based

   b. Non-knowledge-based

3. Answers may vary and may include three of the following advantages: reduced risk of medication errors; reduced risk of misdiagnosis, increased direct patient care time for healthcare providers; access to state-of-the-art data, research, clinical pathways, and guidelines; reduction of unnecessary diagnostic tests; faster diagnoses, resulting in faster treatments; and prescriptions for lower cost medications. The potential disadvantages may include three of the following: costs of maintaining the CDSS with up-to-date medical research, clinical pathways, guidelines, and medication costs; potential over-reliance on computer technology; perception by healthcare providers as a threat to clinical knowledge and skills; and harmful outcomes if software is not thoroughly and continuously updated.

Checkpoint 11.2

1. EHRs play a major role in quality improvement activities. Reporting capabilities in EHR systems provide healthcare organizations with important statistics and can identify opportunities to improve patient care.

2. Answers may vary, but could include three of the following for inpatient facilities: infection rates; ventilation wean success rates; lengths of stay; fall rates; morbidity and mortality rates; types and frequency of diagnostic tests per diagnosis-related group; and medication errors. The examples for outpatient facilities may include three of the following: mammography, diabetes, and colorectal screenings; and routine physical examinations.

Checkpoint 12.1

1. The advantages may vary, but could include: low cost, private, secure, and safe at home rather than in cyberspace. The disadvantages may vary, but could include difficulty in assembling, organizing, and updating. There is no established format, and a paper PHR may lack the necessary details to provide a complete picture of a patient's health status. Security may also be an issue. Finally, in an emergency, a paper record may be unavailable or difficult to decipher.

2. The advantages may vary, but could include: portable, password-protected but not connected to the Internet, so therefore more secure. They allow backup of data, which helps prevent a loss of valuable data. The disadvantages may vary, but could include: inaccurate, lack of Internet connectivity, incompatibility with healthcare provider's computer systems.

3. a. Health-insurer-provided

   b. Facility-provided

   c. Employer-provided

Checkpoint 12.2

1. a. The Veterans Administration

   b. The Centers for Medicare & Medicaid Services (CMS)

2. a. Request a copy of your health records.

   b. Review the various types of PHRs and select one that meets your needs.

   c. Organize your health information.

Checkpoint 12.3

1. Answers may vary, but could include four of the following: Medical Record, Health Summary, Test Results, Hospital Admission, Medications, Allergies, Immunizations, Preventive Care, Medical History, Current Health Issues, Health Trends, View My Appointments, Cancel My Appointments, Request My Appointment, My Family Records, Message Center, Get Medical Advice, Request Rx Refill, Request a Referral, Billing and Insurance, Billing Account Summary, Insurance Summary, Settings, or Portable PHR.

2. Linking medical records is important because other providers and facilities may need access to health information such as medications, previous test results, previous procedures, hospital admissions, and any complications experienced. When a healthcare provider has access to this information, thus better knowing a patient's health history, the delivery and quality of care may improve.

Chapter 13.1

1. CCHIT developed a rigorous process to examine EHR systems for functionality, interoperability, and security. CCHIT also provides resources to help healthcare facilities select an appropriate EHR system.

2. a. Identify requirements

   b. Create design

   c. Analyze current systems

   d. Create a timeline for implementation

Checkpoint 13.2

1. Answers may vary, but could include four of the following: the healthcare facility may have to hire additional staff trained in health informatics; the technical support staff may need to hire additional employees or outsource the job functions; the healthcare facility must conduct and assess workflow analysis; the healthcare facility must provide training for all healthcare employees; data dictionaries and templates must be created, developed, and reviewed.

2. a. Accounting costs

   b. Opportunity costs

   c. Economic costs

Sample Paper Medical Record

A medical record, in any form, is the legal record of the care and treatment provided to a patient. In this textbook, *Exploring Electronic Health Records*, Second Edition, you have read about and have experienced hands-on activities using the EHR. In these hands-on activities you accessed the EHR Navigator as many different healthcare professionals including a physician, nurse, IT administrator, admissions clerk, front desk clerk, health information management professional, etc.

Now that you have experienced an EHR, perhaps you would benefit from a review of a sample paper medical record. As you have read in this textbook, paper records are being phased out. However, you may still experience patient's historical information in paper form in the workplace. The average medical record is generally more than 200 pages long. The sample paper medical record included in this appendix is significantly smaller and is meant to provide you with exposure to a paper medical record. The dates within this sample record reflect a time period when paper records were more common.

The paper medical record in this appendix includes:

- Facesheet
- Consent to Treat
- Informed Consent for Invasive, Diagnostic, Medical & Surgical Procedures
- Notice of Acknowledgment of Advance Directive
- Discharge Summary
- Consultation Report
- History and Physical
- Operative Report

- Physician's Orders
- Progress Notes
- Lab Results
- Radiology Report
- Nurse's Notes
- Physical Therapy Evaluation
- Speech Evaluation
- Patient Continuum of Care Transfer Form
- Medication Administration Record

The health care providers involved in the completion of this paper medical record include:

- Admission Clerk
- Attending Physician
- Consulting Physician
- Surgeon
- Laboratory Technician
- Radiologist
- Nurses

- Physical Therapist
- Speech Therapist

NORTHSTAR MEDICAL CENTER

NORTHSTAR
Medical Center

Facesheet

PATIENT INFORMATION

Patient's Last Name	First	Middle Initial	Type of Care: ☒ In Patient ☐ Same Day Surgery
Walker	Marjorie	R	☐ Maternity ☐ Surgery ☐ Outpatient

Race	Marital Status	Religion	Primary Language	Date of Birth (mm/dd/yyyy)	Date of Scheduled Visit
Caucasian	M	Mormon	English	06/03/1956	

Physician's Last Name	First Name	☒ Female	Social Security No.
Chaplin	Patrick	☐ Male	000-00-0000

Patient's Street Address	Apt. No.	City	State	Zip
3370 Oakwood Ave		Cincinnati	OH	45203

Home Phone	Work Phone	Cell Phone	Visit Reason or Diagnosis	Admission Date
(513) 555-1632	(513) 555-1818	(513) 555-0823	Left Leg Wound	03/18/2012

Temporary Address	Apt. No.	City	State	Zip

Patient's Current Employer Name	Employer Address	City	State	Zip
Rapid Printing	6240 Parkland Drive	Cincinnati	OH	45201

Employer Phone	Patient's Occupation	Employment Status: ☐ Not Employed ☒ Full Time
(513) 555-1818	Pre-Press Operator	☐ Part Time ☐ Student ☐ Retired and Date:

Full Name of Emergency Contact	Relationship	Home Phone	Work Phone
Fulton Walker	Husband	(513) 555-1632	(513) 555-1471

Have you ever been a patient at Northstar Medical Center? ☒ Yes ☐ No	If yes, when was your last visit? 02/06/1980	Under what name? Buehler

Guarantor

Last Name	First	Middle Initial	Relationship	Date of Birth (mm/dd/yyyy)
Walker	Marjorie	R	Self	06/03/1956

Street Address	Apt. No.	☐ Female	Marital Status	Social Security No.
3370 Oakwood Ave		☐ Male	M	000-00-0000

City	State	Zip	Home Phone	Work Phone	Cell Phone
Cincinnati	OH	45203	(513) 555-1632	(513) 555-1818	(513) 555-0823

Employer Name	Employer Address	City	State	Zip
Rapid Printing	6240 Parkland Drive	Cincinnati	OH	45201

Employer Phone	Occupation	Employment Status: ☐ Not Employed ☒ Full Time
(513) 555-1818	Pre-Press Operator	☐ Part Time ☐ Student ☐ Retired and Date:

Insurance Information

Primary Insurance Name	Name of Insured exactly as appears on card
Cobalt Blue	Marjorie Ruth Walker

Insurance Billing Address	City	State	Zip	Phone No.
PO Box 690	Seattle	WA	98119	(800) 475-755X

Policy No.	Group No.	Plan Code	State	Effective Date	Expiration Date
189624733	9985	3	OH	01/01/2012	12/31/2012

Subscriber's Full Name	Subscriber's Soc. Sec. No.	Subscriber's Date of Birth	☒ Female
Marjorie Ruth Walker	000-00-0000	06/03/1956	☐ Male

Subscriber's Employer name (if self-employed, company name)	Relation to Insured	Subscriber's Employment Status: ☐ Not Employed
Rapid Printing	Self	☒ Full Time ☐ Part Time ☐ Student ☐ Retired and Date:

Subscriber's Employer Address	City	State	Zip	Phone No.
6240 Parkland Drive	Cincinnati	OH	45201	(513) 555-1818

<table>
<tr><td rowspan="8">Insurance Information</td><td colspan="3">Medicare Number</td><td colspan="2">Patient's name as appears on card</td><td colspan="3">Effective Date (mm/dd/yyyy)

_____

_____</td><td colspan="2">□ Part A (Hospital Benefit)

□ Part B (Medical Benefit)</td></tr>
<tr><td colspan="3">Medicaid Number</td><td colspan="2">Patient's name as appears on card</td><td colspan="2">Effective Date</td><td colspan="3">State</td></tr>
<tr><td colspan="5">Secondary Insurance Name
NA</td><td colspan="5">Name of Insured exactly as appears on card</td></tr>
<tr><td colspan="3">Insurance Billing Address</td><td colspan="2">City</td><td>State</td><td>Zip</td><td colspan="3">Phone No.

(   )</td></tr>
<tr><td colspan="2">Policy No. (for BCBS, include 3 letter prefix)</td><td>Group No.</td><td colspan="2">Plan Code</td><td>State</td><td>Effective Date</td><td colspan="3">Expiration Date</td></tr>
<tr><td colspan="3">Subscriber's Full Name</td><td colspan="2">Subscriber's Soc. Sec. No.</td><td colspan="2">Subscriber's Date of Birth (mm/dd/yyyy)</td><td colspan="3">□ Female

□ Male</td></tr>
<tr><td colspan="3">Subscriber's Employer name (if self-employed, company name)</td><td colspan="2">Relation to Insured</td><td colspan="5">Subscriber's Employment Status: □ Not Employed

□ Full Time □ Part Time □ Student □ Retired and Date:</td></tr>
<tr><td colspan="3">Subscriber's Employer Address</td><td colspan="2">City</td><td>State</td><td>Zip</td><td colspan="3">Phone No.

(   )</td></tr>
<tr><td rowspan="3">Worker's Compensation</td><td colspan="3">Is this visit the result of an accident?

□ Yes   □ No</td><td colspan="2">□ Employment
□ Automobile
□ Other</td><td colspan="2">Date of Accident: (mm/dd/yyyy)</td><td colspan="3">Claim No.</td></tr>
<tr><td colspan="3">Letter of Authorization

□ Yes   □ No</td><td colspan="2">Claim Adjuster / Contact Name</td><td colspan="2">Phone No.

(   )</td><td colspan="3">Insurance Name</td></tr>
<tr><td colspan="3">Insurance Address</td><td colspan="2">City</td><td>State</td><td>Zip</td><td colspan="3">Phone No.

(   )</td></tr>
</table>

Advance Directive

Do you have an Advance Directive, such as a Living Will or Durable Power of Attorney for Health Care?   ☒ Yes   □ No
Please specify the type: ___Living Will_____
*** *If yes, please bring a copy at the time of your admission****

Self-Pay

* If insured but your procedure is not covered or verified by your plan, a deposit is required at the time of admission.

* If you do not have insurance, please call our *Northstar Financial Services at 513-555-122X* before your scheduled arrival date to discuss financial arrangements.

Additional Information

Do you need special accommodations, such as Translation, Visual Aid, etc.?   □ Yes   □ No

*** If yes, please specify so that prior arrangements can be made for the day of your visit. ***

□ Language Interpreter _____   □ Sign Language Interpreter   □ Visual aid   □ Other: _____

NORTHSTAR MEDICAL CENTER

NORTHSTAR
Medical Center

Walker, Marjorie
PT#1772571 MRN#585120
DOB: 06/03/1956 Age: 56   Sex: F
Physician: Chaplin, Patrick
Admit: 03/18/2012

CONSENT TO TREAT

Thank you for selecting Northstar Medical Center to provide for your healthcare needs. We are committed o providing exceptional healthcare. The first step pin this process is to provide information regarding patient rights, risks and responsibilities. The second step is to obtain your consent to treat the patient. The admitting staff can answer any questions you may have in regards to the following agreement.

I agree to the following

1. **Consent to Treat**: I consent to the treatment or admission of ___3/18/12___ at Northstar Medical Center for services or supplies that have been or may be ordered by a licensed professional healthcare provider. I understand that treatment may include but is not limited to: radiological examinations, laboratory procedures, physical therapy, anesthesia, nursing care or medical and surgical treatment. Your case may be attended by vendors and clinical students. I understand that all licensed professional healthcare providers that render service to the patient are responsible and liable for their own acts, orders and omissions. I acknowledge that the hospital has not made nor can it make a guarantee of the outcome of treatment.

2. **Financial Agreement**: I agree to pay for all services and supplies rendered to the patient in accordance with the rates and financial policies in effect at the time of service. I agree to pay interest fees on any unpaid balance after 30 days of discharge or date of service.

3. **Assignment of Insurance Benefits**: I assign and authorize payment directly to Northstar Medical Center of any healthcare benefits that the patient is entitled to receive. This assignment will not be withdrawn or voided at any time unless I pay the account in full. I understand that I am responsible for any and all charges not covered by my insurance policy(s).

4. **Assignment of Physician Benefits**: I am aware that physician services by Radiologist, Pathologist, Anesthesiologist, as well as medical, surgical and emergency care are not billed by the hospital but are billed separately. I understand that I am under the same obligation to those providers as stated in this agreement unless otherwise agreed to in writing with those providers. I authorize payment of any medical benefits for such claims to the appropriate provider.

5. **Release of Medical Information**: I authorize the hospital or any professional healthcare provider who rendered services to the patient to release any medical or other information necessary to process claims.
    - ☑ I acknowledge that I have received a copy of the Privacy Notice
    - ☐ I decline to accept a copy of the Privacy Notice

6. **Personal Valuables and Belongings**: I understand that the hospital maintains a safe for the protection of valuables. I agree that the hospital is not responsible for the loss or damage of any article or personal property unless they are deposited in the safe.

7. **Advance Directive/Living Will**: Northstar Medical Center honors the patient's right to formulate, review or revise their Advance Directives or Living Will and can refer you to resources for assistance if necessary
    - ☑ I have provided a copy of my Advance Directive or Living Will and request that it be put in my chart as part of my Medical Record
    - ☐ I have received information with regard to my right to make Advance Healthcare Directives
    - ☐ My Advance Directive or Living Will is suspended for this elective procedure
    - ☐ I have not provided nor do I have an Advance directive or Living Will and I decline information on Advance Directives
    - ☐ I understand if my Advance Directive or Living is not present in my medical record its directives will not be followed.

    Action taken by registrar _____

8. **Right to Donate Organs**: The patient understand that they have a right to donate organs and they have discussed their decision with their family. Should circumstances arise please do the following:
    - ☐ Speak with the family regarding the matter
    - ☐ The patient does NOT wish to donate. Please DO NOT speak to the family in regards to the matter.
    - ☑ I wish to donate my organs.

I understand and accept the terms of this agreement and certify that I am duly authorized by the patient or by law to execute the above agreement in their behalf

Patient _Marjorie Walker_ Date _3/18/12_ Time _6:32_

_____   _____   _____
Patient's Guardian or Representative   Relationship   Witness

Northstar Medical Center
Informed Consent for Invasive, Diagnostic, Medical & Surgical Procedures

Patient Name __Walker, Marjorie__

Date of Birth __6/3/56__

Medical Record # __585120__

I hereby authorize __Dr. Stillwater__ and/or ___—___ and/or such assistants and associates as may be selected by him/her/they to perform the following procedure(s)/treatment(s) upon myself/the patient
Procedure(s)/Treatment(s) __Excisional debridement, Lft leg__

The procedure has been explained to me and I have been told the reasons why I need the procedure. The risks of the procedure have also been explained to me. In addition, I have been told that the procedure may not have the result that I expect. I have also been told about other possible treatments for my condition and what might happen if no treatment is received.

I understand that in addition to the risks describe to me and about this procedure there are risks that may occur with any surgical or medical procedure. I am aware that the practice of medicine and surgery is not an exact science, and that I have not been given any guarantees about the results of this procedure.

I have had enough time to discuss my condition and treatment with my health care providers and all of my questions have been answered to my satisfaction. I believe I have enough information to make an informed decision and I agree to have the procedure. If something unexpected happens and I need additional or different treatment(s) from the treatment I expect, I agree to accept any treatment which is necessary.

I agree to have transfusion of blood and other blood products that may be necessary along with the procedure I am having. The risks, benefits and alternatives have been explained to me and all of my questions have been answered to my satisfaction. If I refuse to have transfusions I will cross out and initial this section and sign a Refusal of Treatment form.

I agree to allow this facility to keep, use or properly dispose of, tissue, and parts of organs that are removed during this procedure.

__Marjorie Walker__   __3/18/12__
Signature of Patient or Parent/Legal Guardian of Minor Patient   Date

---

If the patient cannot consent for him/herself, the signature of either the health care agent or legal guardian who is acting on behalf of the patient, or the patient's next of kin who is asserting to the treatment for the patient, must be obtained.

_____   _____
Signature of Patient or Parent/Legal Guardian of Minor Patient   Date

_____   _____
Signature and Relationship of Next of Kin   Date

Witness:
I, _____, am a facility employee who is not the patient's physician or authorized health care provider named above and I have witnessed the patient or other appropriate person voluntarily sign this form

_____
Signature and Title of Witness

NORTHSTAR MEDICAL CENTER

NORTHSTAR
Medical Center

NOTICE OF ACKNOWLEDGEMENT ADVANCE DIRECTIVE

PATIENT NAME: _Walker, Marjorie_   DOB: _6/3/56_

An Advance Directive is a legal document allowing a person to give directions about future medical care or to designate another person(s) to make medical decisions if he or she should lose decision making capacity. Advance Directives are the following written instruments: The Living Will and The Durable Power of Attorney for Heath Care. The instrument may be revoked and a notation of the date and time must be made to the patient's medical record.

Do you have an Advance Directive?

A. Directive to Physicians (Living Will)   Yes __✓__ No _____

B. Durable Power of Attorney for Health Care   Yes __✓__ No _____

Is it up to Date?	Yes __✓__ No _____
Where is a copy located?	_With me_
Principal Agent:	_Fulton Walker_
Address:	_3370 Oakwood_
Phone #:	_513-555-1632_
Alternate Agent:	_Anne Walker_
Address:	_1530 Eastland_
Phone #:	_513-555-4445_

Marjorie Walker   _3/18/12_
Signature of Patient or Representative   Date

NORTHSTAR MEDICAL CENTER

NORTHSTAR

Medical Center

Walker, Marjorie
PT#1772571   MRN#585120
DOB: 06/03/1956   Age: 56   Sex: F
Physician: Chaplin, Patrick
Admit: 03/18/2012

Discharge Summary

Date of Discharge: 3/27/2012

Discharge Diagnosis:

1. Left leg wound, S/P MVA, left shin degloving injury
2. Anxiety
3. Hematoma, right thigh
4. Paroxysmal atrial fibrillation

History of Present Illness: This is a 56-year-old white female who on 2/23/12 was involved in a motor vehicle accident when she was driving from Florida to Cincinnati. She was admitted to a Chattanooga, Tennessee hospital and she had suffered multiple rib fractures and also suffered a left nondisplaced fibular fracture and an avulsion and degloving injury on the left shin. She also had possible suprapubic ramus fracture and a fracture of the sternum and a slight laceration of the liver and spleen and she was transfused 19 units of packed red blood cells for acute blood loss anemia. The patient was on Coumadin at the time for atrial fibrillation and she had to be reversed. She also went into a-fib with rapid rate needing Cardizem to reverse it.

She was then transferred to Northstar Medical Center and was pretty stable at the time. She had a lot of pain and then she was seen by Orthopedics for that left tib fib fracture and they said she was okay for weight-bearing and she was see by wound care, physical therapy and occupational therapy. The patient stayed in sinus rhythm throughout. She was maintained on Coumadin and her hemoglobin stayed in the 9 and 10 range and she had later complained of a lot of pain in the right leg and a Doppler had shown some small hematomas, however, the pain and hematomas resolved on their own.

The large wound on her left shin was treated by Dr. Stillwater, Plastic Surgeon. She underwent several debridements of this area and will later likely undergo a skin graft after the wound has healed more.

On the day of discharge, 31 minutes was spent on discharge planning and all medications were discussed with her in detail. Patient is discharged to home with home health care.

Dictated by: Patrick Chaplin, MD

NG
D: 3/27/12 1535
T: 03/28/2012 1124

NORTHSTAR MEDICAL CENTER

NORTHSTAR

Medical Center

Walker, Marjorie
PT#1772571   MRN#585120
DOB: 06/03/1956   Age: 56   Sex: F
Physician: Chaplin, Patrick
Admit: 03/18/2012

CONSULTATION REPORT
PLASTICS AND RECONSTRUCTIVE SURGERY

CHIEF COMPLAINT: Left leg wound

HISTORY OF PRESENT ILLNESS: This is a 56-year-old white female who on 2/23/12 was involved in a motor vehicle accident when she was driving from Florida to Cincinnati. She was admitted to a Chattanooga, Tennessee hospital and she had suffered multiple rib fractures and also suffered a left nondisplaced fibular fracture and an avulsion and degloving injury on the left shin. She also had possible suprapubic ramus fracture and a fracture of the sternum and a slight laceration of the liver and spleen and she was transfused 19 units of packed red blood cells for acute blood loss anemia. The patient was on Coumadin at the time for atrial fibrillation and she had to be reversed. She also went into a-fib with rapid rate needing Cardizem to reverse it.

PAST MEDICAL/SURGICAL HISTORY:
Significant for:
1. Hypertension
2. Rheumatoid arthritis
3. Depression
4. Osteopenia
5. Hyperlipidemia
6. History of perforated diverticulum, for which she required surgery and had a colostomy, and it was reversed.
7. History of hysterectomy
8. Hypothyroidism
9. Bilateral knee replacements
10. The patient does not report that she has congestive heart failure.
11. She does report that she had an angiogram for evaluation of atrial fibrillation, and she does not have any coronary artery disease.

ALLERGIES:
None

MEDICATIONS:

Prior to this accident included:

1. Methotrexate.
2. Misoprostol
3. Remicade
4. Methimazole

CURRENT MEDICATIONS:

That she was on when transferred from a Chattanooga, Tennessee hospital are as follows:

1. Keflex 500 mg every 8 hours for 5 days
2. Ipratropium as needed
3. Coumadin per pharmacy protocol
4. Lovenox 110 mg subcutaneously every twelve hours, to discontinue when INR is more than 2
5. Atenolol 50 mg every 12 hours
6. Vicodin 5/325 mg every four hours as needed for pain.
7. Paxil 20 mg daily

FAMILY HISTORY:

Positive for father dying of leukocytosis at age of 54. Mother had myocardial infarction at the age of 67. Sister has Parkinson disease and another sister died of colon cancer.

PHYSICAL EXAMINATION:

GENERAL:

She is awake, alert and oriented, in no acute distress.

VITAL SIGNS:

Stable. Her blood pressure this morning is 126/64, temperature 98.6, pulse 72.

HEAD, EYES, EARS, NOSE AND THROAT:

Shows pupils equal, round, and reactive to light and accommodation. Mucous membranes are moist.

NECK:

Shows no thyromegaly.

LUNGS:

Clear to auscultation.

HEART:

Regular rate and rhythm, a few missed beats.

ABDOMEN:

Shows no organomegaly.

EXTREMITIES:

Dorsalis pedis pulses bilaterally are 2+. There is a vacuum-assisted closure on the left upper skin extending to the knee. Large left lower leg wound with fairly well vascularized red granulation tissue in the bulk of the wound. There is a deep cavity on the medial aspect in the area of the recently evacuated hematoma. There are sutures in place which the patient was unaware and fibrin covering necrotic tissue on the lateral aspect of the wound space. There is no purulent discharge or evidence of infection. Remainder of the left lower extremity shows no other clinically significant lesions.

LABORATORY DATA:

From 3/17/12, her albumin was 2.4, total protein was 5.2. Her CBC from 3/16/12 shows a white cell count of 9.6, hemoglogin 9.7, platelets 252,000. INR was 1.4.

ASSESSMENT AND PLAN:

The patient needs protein repletion. She will ultimately need the sutures removed and the fibrinous exudate debrided from the lateral aspect of the wound. Would recommend resuming negative pressure wound therapy including packing, black GranuFoam dressing into the current hematoma cavity. The patient will ultimately require skin graft reconstruction.

It is always a pleasure seeing and treating your patients. We look forward to seeing and treating other patients in the future.

Dictated by Frank Stillwater, MD

KR
D: 03/20/12 1904
T: 03/20/12 23:50

NORTHSTAR MEDICAL CENTER

NORTHSTAR

Medical Center

Walker, Marjorie	
PT#1772571	MRN#585120
DOB: 06/03/1956 Age: 56	Sex: F
Physician: Chaplin, Patrick	
Admit: 03/18/2012	

HISTORY AND PHYSICAL

HISTORY OF PRESENT ILLNESS:

History of Present Illness: This is a 56-year-old white female who on 2/23/12 was involved in a motor vehicle accident when she was driving from Florida to Cincinnati. She was admitted to a Chattanooga, Tennessee hospital and she had suffered multiple rib fractures and also suffered a left nondisplaced fibular fracture and an avulsion and degloving injury on the left shin. She also had possible suprapubic ramus fracture and a fracture of the sternum and a slight laceration of the liver and spleen and she was transfused 19 units of packed red blood cells for acute blood loss anemia. The patient was on Coumadin at the time for atrial fibrillation and she had to be reversed. She also went into a-fib with rapid rate needing Cardizem to reverse it.

She has been transferred to Northstar Medical Center and is stable at this time. Dr. Stillwater from Plastics will be consulted to address her wound on her left shin. PT, OT and Wound Care will be ordered. We will monitor her atrial fibrillation and labs for anemia.

PAST MEDICAL/SURGICAL HISTORY:

Significant for:

1. Hypertension
2. Rheumatoid arthritis
3. Depression
4. Osteopenia
5. Hyperlipidemia
6. History of perforated diverticulum, for which she required surgery and had a colostomy, and it was reversed.
7. History of hysterectomy
8. Hypothyroidism
9. Bilateral knee replacements
10. The patient does not report that she has congestive heart failure.
11. She does report that she had an angiogram for evaluation of atrial fibrillation, and she does not have any coronary artery disease.

ALLERGIES:

None

MEDICATIONS:

Prior to this accident included:

1. Methotrexate.
2. Misoprostol
3. Remicade
4. Methimazole

CURRENT MEDICATIONS:

That she was on when transferred from a Chattanooga, Tennessee hospital are as follows:

1. Keflex 500 mg every 8 hours for 5 days
2. Ipratropium as needed
3. Coumadin per pharmacy protocol
4. Lovenox 110 mg subcutaneously every twelve hours, to discontinue when INR is more than 2
5. Atenolol 50 mg every 12 hours
6. Vicodin 5/325 mg every four hours as needed for pain.
7. Paxil 20 mg daily

FAMILY HISTORY:

Positive for father dying of leukocytosis at age of 54. Mother had myocardial infarction at the age of 67. Sister has Parkinson disease and another sister died of colon cancer.

PHYSICAL EXAMINATION:

GENERAL:
She is awake, alert and oriented, in no acute distress.

VITAL SIGNS:
Stable. Her blood pressure this morning is 126/64, temperature 98.6, pulse 72.

HEAD, EYES, EARS, NOSE AND THROAT:
Sclerae are anicteric. Mucous membranes are moist.

NECK:
There is no carotid bruit.

LUNGS:
Clear to auscultation.

HEART:
Regular rate and rhythm, a few missed beats.

ABDOMEN:
Soft, nontender.

EXTREMITIES:
Dorsalis pedis pulses bilaterally are 2+. There is a vacuum-assisted closure on the left upper skin extending to the knee.

LABORATORY DATA:
From 3/17/12, her albumin was 2.4, total protein was 5.2. Her CBC from 3/16/12 shows a white cell count of 9.6, hemoglogin 9.7, platelets 252,000. INR was 1.4.

ASSESSMENT AND PLAN:
1. Status post MVA with multiple injuries. Pain control is an issue. Patient will be scheduled for PT and OT Therapy
2. Avulsion/degloving injury of the left shin with large wound. Plastic surgery will be consulted.
3. History of paroxysmal atrial fibrillation. Will follow and monitor.

_____
Patrick Chaplin, MD

KK
Dictated: 3/18/12 14:45
Trans: 3/18/12 18:30

NORTHSTAR MEDICAL CENTER

NORTHSTAR

Medical Center

Walker, Marjorie
PT#1772571   MRN#585120
DOB: 06/03/1956   Age: 56   Sex: F
Physician: Chaplin, Patrick
Admit: 03/18/2012

OPERATIVE REPORT

DATE OF OPERATION: 03/23/12

PREOPERATIVE DIAGNOSIS: Left leg wound

POSTOPERATIVE DIAGNOSIS: Left leg wound

PROCEDURE PERFORMED: Excision, necrotic tissue, left leg wound, 3.0 cm in length. Application of a Kerlix stack and less than 50 sq. cm negative pressure wound therapy dressing.

SURGEON: Frank Stillwater, MD

ASSISTANT: Karen Tweedle, MD

OPERATIVE PROCEDURE: The patient was properly prepped and draped under local sedation. A 0.25% Marcaine was injected circumferentially around the necrotic wound. A wide excision and debridement of the necrotic tissue taken down to the presacral fascia and all necrotic tissue was electrocauterized and removed. All bleeding was cauterized with electrocautery and then a Kerlix stack was then placed and a pressure dressing applied. The patient was sent to recovery in satisfactory condition.

Dictated by Frank Stillwater, MD

GR
D: 3/23/12 11:14
T: 3/23/12 15:10

NORTHSTAR MEDICAL CENTER

NORTHSTAR
Medical Center

Walker, Marjorie
PT#1772571   MRN#585120
DOB: 06/03/1956   Age: 56   Sex: F
Physician: Chaplin, Patrick
Admit: 03/18/2012

|||||||||||||||||||||||||||||||||||||||||||||||||

PHYSICIAN"S ORDERS

Date/Time		Nurse's Initials
3/18/12 930AM	CBC, BMP in am PT/INR c̄ a.m. labs *Patrick Chaplin MD*	
3/19/12 8AM	U/A, c+s today *Patrick Chaplin MD*	
3/19/12 9AM	D/c oxycontin Vicodin 5/500 g i po q 4-6° prn pain. *Patrick Chaplin MD*	

NORTHSTAR MEDICAL CENTER

NORTHSTAR
Medical Center

Date/Time	Progress Notes
3/18/12 9:15 AM	FP Feels better today less N/V. Appetite better. Up to hallway c̄ assistance. VSS AF Lys - CTAB heart - reg rate no murg. Abd - soft NT NABS Ext - ø c c e wound vac in place ① leg. labs pending A/P - ① wound left leg consult surgery ② PAF coumadin / PT protocol ③ High protein diet _Ann Turrell M_

NORTHSTAR MEDICAL CENTER

NORTHSTAR

Medical Center

Walker, Marjorie		
PT#1772571	MRN#585120	
DOB: 06/03/1956	Age: 56	Sex: F
Physician: Chaplin, Patrick		
Admit: 03/18/2012		

*******************************COMPLETE BLOOD COUNT***************************************

TEST:	WBC	WBC	HGB	HBG	HCT	HCT	PLATELET	PLT	RBC
UNITS:	THOU/mcL	THOU/mcL	g/dl	g/dl	%	%	THOU/mcL	THOU/mcL	THOU/mcL
REF RANGE:	3.9-10.5	3.6-10.5	12.0-15.5	12.0-15.2	36-47	36-46	140-375	140-375	3.80-5.20

03/25/2012

0530		6.0		9.7L		29L		302	
		CBCR		[NS]		[NS]		[NS]	
		[NS]							

03/24/2012

1115		7.4		9.9L		30L		323	
		CBCR		[NS]		[NS]		[NS}	
		[NS]							

03/23/2012		7.8		10.1L		30L		311	
		CBCR		[NS]		[NS]		[NS]	
		[NS}							

03/22/2012		7.1		8.4L		27L		331	
		[NS]		[NS]		[NS]		[NS]	

03/21/2012	9.4		9.8L		31L		370		3.32L
	[NS]		[NS]		[NS]		[NS]		[NS]

03/20/2012	7.9		10.0L		32L		397H		3.32L
	[NS]		[NS]		[NS]		[NS]		[NS]

---FOOTNOTES---

[NS]   Tested at Northstar Medical Center

End of Report

NORTHSTAR MEDICAL CENTER

NORTHSTAR

Medical Center

Walker, Marjorie
PT#1772571 MRN#585120
DOB: 06/03/1956 Age: 56 Sex: F
Physician: Chaplin, Patrick
Admit: 03/18/2012

*****************************COAGULATION***

TEST:	PROTIME	INR
UNITS:	Seconds	
REF RANGE:	9.0-11.4	0.8-1.2

03/18/2012

+ 0615   16.9 H 1.6   H
            [NS]   (a)
                (b)
                (c)
             [NS]

---FOOTNOTES---

(a)   INR Therapeutic Ranges:
(b)   Routine Anticoagulation: 2.0 to 3.0
(c)   Aggressive Anticoagulation: 2.5 to 3.5
[NS]   Tested at Northstar Medical Center

End of Report

NORTHSTAR MEDICAL CENTER

NORTHSTAR

Medical Center

Walker, Marjorie
PT#1772571   MRN#585120
DOB: 06/03/1956   Age: 56   Sex: F
Physician: Chaplin, Patrick
Admit: 03/18/2012

Ordered by: Patrick Chaplin, MD
*All clinical times shown on this page are in
Knee 2 Views – Right 32017251
Site: Northstar Medical Center Radiology
Rad# X081134773
Unit# M000048880
Location: NSMC14CD
Account#: V1030767632B
Req#11-4104931
Order# RAD20120318-0349
Primary Insurance:
Procedure: Knee 2 views – Right 32017251
Admitting Diagnosis: Left Lower Extremity Wound
Reason for exam: Change in Status
Impression
Impression/Conclusion below

Report
Two Views Right Knee 3/20/12

Indication: Motor Vehicle Accident

Comparison: None

Findings: Right total knee arthroplasty is in place. The lateral view was somewhat oblique. No large joint effusion or fracture. There is mild soft tissue swelling

Impression:

No evidence of fracture or gross complication with right total knee arthroplasty in place

Dictated by: Michael Zuckerman MD
Signed by: Michael Zuckerman MD 3/21/2012

End of Report

NORTHSTAR MEDICAL CENTER

NORTHSTAR
Medical Center

Walker, Marjorie
PT#1772571   MRN#585120
DOB: 06/03/1956   Age: 56 Sex: F
Physician: Chaplin, Patrick
Admit: 03/18/2012

Nurse's Notes (Include observations, medications, and treatment when indicated.)

Date/Time	
3/19/12 0816	Assessment complete as noted, sitting up in bed, IVPB infusing s̄ difficulty, dsg dry and intact, foley draining clear yellow urine, denies pain or SOB @ this time will continue to monitor wound care — B. Cullars, RN —
3/19/12 1930	pt resting in bed. A+O x3 VSS LSCTA per nurse assess. Foley draining clear yellow urine. Denies any further issues @ this time. SOB noted previously currently subsided - will cont to monitor. Call light in reach ————— [signature]
3/20/12 0730	VSS. Denies any pain or discomfort at this time. Assessment completed per flow sheet - no changes noted from previous shift. Able to make needs known. Call light in reach. Will monitor ————— [signature]

NORTHSTAR MEDICAL CENTER

NORTHSTAR
Medical Center

Walker, Marjorie
PT#1772571   MRN#585120
DOB: 06/03/1956   Age: 56 Sex: F
Physician: Chaplin, Patrick
Admit: 03/18/2012

Nurse's Notes (Include observations, medications, and treatment when indicated.)

Date/Time	
3/18/2012 @ 1300	Received pt via ACLS transport. Pt transferred from stretcher to bed. Pt did not bring any personal belongings. Admission assessment completed. VSS & WNL. Dr. Chaplin notified of pt's arrival – orders received. Pt informed of POC & instructed on safety. To include use of call light & bed side controls. Will continue to Monitor. B. Schmidt RN.
3/18/2012 2015	Assessment complete & charted. Pt is A+O×4, lungs CTA, +BS ×4, no noted edema, heart sounds regular in rhythm. Pt has #20 @ FA dated 3/17 c̄ a dsg that is CD+I. VSS & hardly unchanged from admit. Pt has no needs or questions at this time & denies any pain. Call light left within reach, will continue to monitor. ———————— J. Salatin RN

NORTHSTAR MEDICAL CENTER

NORTHSTAR
Medical Center

Walker, Marjorie
PT#1772571 MRN#585120
DOB: 06/03/1956 Age: 56   Sex: F
Physician: Chaplin, Patrick
Admit: 03/18/2012

Physical Therapy Ankle Evaluation

DX ⓛ leg wound, s/p mva, wound care Date 3|19|12

PMH Rib fx, fibular fx, degloving injury ⓛ shin, sternum fx, anemia, anxiety, paroxysmal A Fib,

Physician Patrick Chaplin   Onset 2|23|12

Initial Evaluation X   Re-Evaluation____   Pain Rating_____   Funct. Rating_____   Involved: R L

SUBJECTIVE: Pain with X squatting X walking____ sitting NA running NA stairs
Pt reports 5/10 ⓛ leg pain. Pt reports ↑ pain 7/10 č amb č RW č squatting. Pt states she lives č husband & receives his help to get in & out of care. Currently able to live on 1st floor. Reports she is unable to climb 10 steps č 1HR upstairs to her bedroom. Currently has transport w/c, RW, cane (SPC).

Occupation/Social Hx: Pt is a 3rd grade math teacher

Work Duties: standing, walking, bending, squatting, sitting on floor,

Pt. Goals: Pt reports she would like to amb ↑↓ 10 steps 1HR to bedroom, & be able to
squat down to floor for return to work

OBJECTIVE:
Gait: ____antalgic Trendelenburg R L ____Crutches X Walker____Cane____No AD ☐
____FWB____PWB____TTWB____NWB X WBAT
Other_____

Observation: (In Standing)   Ⓦ̶N̶D̶ R L
Knee: _____
Effusion: **R** none X̶ min ☐ mod ☐ severe ☐   **L** none X̶ min ☐ mod ☐ severe ☐
Foot: Pes Cavus R L   Pes Planus Ⓡ Ⓛ   Hallux Valgus R L

Other_____

ROM/ Strength:

	Active				Passive			Strength	
	R		L		R	L		R	L
DF.	4|5	P	3+|5	P	WFL P	WFL P		___ P	___ P
PF	4|5	P	4|5	P	P	P		___ P	___ P
INV	NT	P	NT	P	P	P		___ P	___ P
EV		P		P	P	P		___ P	___ P
1st MTP Ext		P		P	P	P		___ P	___ P
					P	P			

Girth Measurements: (From mid-patella)   WNL   B̶r̶u̶i̶s̶i̶n̶g̶   Temp. Ⓦ̶N̶D̶ Warm

	R	L	
Around Malleoli	NT	NT	Ⓛ leg
Figure 8			Ⓡ thigh

1

Palpation: (R) thigh tenderness anterior (L) anterior shin tenderness

Resting BP: 124 / 76 Resting HR: 71

Name: Marjorie, Walker   DOB: 6/3/56

Flexibility: (NT= normal, T= tight, VT= very tight): very tight BLE hamstring

Special Tests: (+ or —)

	R	L		R	L
Anterior Drawer	NT	NT	Eversion Stress Test	NT	NT
Spring Test	+	+	Inversion Stress Test	+	+

Unilateral Stance Time: R _3_ Sec. L _0_ Sec.

Unilat. Heel
Raise X 5:   R WNL ☐ painful ☐ weakness/↓ control ☒ Unable to perform ☐
               L WNL ☐ painful ☒ weakness/↓ control ☐ Unable to perform ☒
6" step test: R WNL ☐ painful ☐ weakness/↓ control ☐ Unable to perform ☒
               L WNL ☐ painful ☐ weakness/↓ control ☐ Unable to perform ☒
Single leg squat: R WNL ☐ painful ☐ weakness/↓ control ☐ Unable to perform ☒
               L WNL ☐ painful ☐ weakness/↓ control ☐ Unable to perform ☒

Treatment: Pt perf BLE therex SLR, ABD/ADD, heel slide 2×15. amb 100' ×2 c̄ RW ↓ stance time LLE. Pt amb ↑↓ 1 6" step BHR RLE lead c̄ minA.

ASSESSMENT: _____ See Initial Eval Summary/ Plan of Care
Pt demo ↓ BLE strength, ↓ balance ↓ safety awareness. Pt demo ↓ (I) c̄ amb ↓ step length RLE, ↓ stance time LLE, forward head & shoulders. Pt reports ↑ pain c̄ squatting & walking. Pt will benefit from skilled PT to ↓ pain ↑ ability to squat to floor (I) ↑ amb ↑↓ 10 steps LTLR to bedroom.

Rehabilitation Potential: (Excellent) Good Fair Poor

STG/LTG: ✗ See Initial Eval Summary/ Plan of Care

PLAN: (Circle) # Rx/ wk_____ ~ # wks_____

☒ Strengthening   ☒ Stretching   ☐ Joint Mobs   ☒ Moist Heat/ Cold Pack
☐ Bracing/ Taping ☐ Ultrasound ☐ EStim   ☐ PROM   ☒ Gait Training
☒ Other: _neuro re-ed_

Avg. Pain Rating 6/10   Self Reported Functional Rating _____   Foot Function Index: _____

Therapist Signature: _Josie Thomas PT_   Date: 3/19/12 Time: 4:05pm
Allim Summary PT

2

NORTHSTAR MEDICAL CENTER

NORTHSTAR
Medical Center

SPEECH EVALUATION FORM

Nature of the communication problem: _Speech consulted 2° "slurred speech"_
per RN report

Speech/language therapy in the past?   YES___   NO _✓_

Where? _N/A_   For what reason? _N/A_

Brief description of problem:
Pt initially admitted to OSH 3-9-12 following MVA, transferred to Northstar
Medical Center for continued wound care, nutritional support and therapy

Any pain associated with this problem? YES___NO _✓_
Description:
Pt denies pain.

Was this onset gradual or sudden? Describe:
Sudden, following brain trauma sustained in MVA

Mental Status (check all that apply):
    _✓_ alert
    _✓_ responsive
    _✓_ cooperative
    _✓_ confused
    ____ lethargic
    _✓_ impulsive
    ____ uncooperative
    ____ combative
    ____ unresponsive

Oral Motor, Respiration, and Phonation
Lips
    WNL, mild, mode severe impairment
    Observation at rest (WNL, Edema, Erythema, Lesion): _®-droop, drooling_
    Symmetry, range, speed, strength, tone:
        Pucker   _reduced_
        Retraction   _reduced_
        Alternating pucker/retraction _reduced speed/coordination_

Involuntary movement (e.g., chorea, dystonia, fasciculation, myoclonus, spasms, tremor):

not observed

Tongue
    WNL, mild, mode severe impairment
    Observation at rest (WNL, Edema, Erythema, Lesion): lingual fasciculations
    Symmetry, range, speed, strength, tone:
        Protrusion   reduced range + strength
        Retraction   reduced strength
        Lateralization   reduced range + speed
    Involuntary movement   as noted above

Jaw
    WNL, mild, mode severe impairment
    Observation at rest: rests in slightly open position
        Symmetry, range, speed, strength, tone:
        Opening   reduced oral aperture
        Closing   reduced strength
        Lateralization   reduced ROM
        Protrusion   NT
        Retraction   NT
    Involuntary movement   not observed

Soft Palate
    WNL, mild, mode severe impairment
    Observation at rest (WNL, Edema, Erythema, Lesion): WNL
    Symmetry, range, speed, strength, tone: ↓ speed, Ø asymmetry
    Elevation   reduced upon phonation
    Sustained elevation   reduced upon phonation
    Alternating elevation/relaxation reduced range + speed
    Involuntary movement   not present

Respiration/Phonation
Observations/formal measures administered: _____

Activity	Stimulus	Quality	Duration	Loudness	Steadiness
Phonation		WNL (Breathy) Hoarse Harsh Strained-Strangled	_2_ secs WNL Mildly impaired Moderately impaired (Severely impaired)	WNL (Monoloudness) Excessive loudness Variable loudness	
Oral reading		WNL (Breathy) Hoarse Harsh Strained-Strangled	WNL Mildly impaired Moderately impaired (Severely impaired)	WNL (Monoloudness) Excessive loudness Variable loudness	
Conversation		WNL (Breathy) Hoarse Harsh Strained-Strangled	WNL Mildly impaired Moderately impaired (Severely impaired)	WNL (Monoloudness) Excessive loudness Variable loudness	

Findings

_____ Motor speech within normal limits

_____ (Mild, mild-moderate, moderate, moderate-severe, severe) apraxia characterized by:

_____

__✓__ (Mild, mild-moderate, (moderate), moderate-severe, severe) dysarthria characterized by:

_____ moderate dysarthria 2° breathy vocal quality (suspect vocal cord involvement), reduced strength + range of motion for oral structures, and hypernasality during all speech tasks.

Recommendations: (check all that apply)
   __✓__ Speech-language pathology treatment
      Frequency: 3-5 x/week Duration: 4 weeks
   _____ Augmentative-Alternative Communication or Speech Generating Device evaluation
   _____ Other suggested referrals:
      _____ Neurology
      __✓__ Otolaryngology
      _____ Pulmonology
      _____ Other

X _Allison Binny_ MA. CCC-SLP

NORTHSTAR MEDICAL CENTER

Patient Continuum of Care Transfer Form

Walker, Marjorie
PT#1772571   MRN#585120
DOB: 06/03/1956   Age: 56   Sex: F
Physician: Chaplin, Patrick
Admit: 03/18/2012

|||||||| ||| |||||| ||||||| ||| ||||| |||

Patient Last Name: Walker | Patient First Name: Marjorie

Transfer to: Spring Care | Attending Physician: Chaplin

Reason for Transfer: Wound Care | DATE/TIME: 3/18/12 650

❏ Attempted Treatment in SNF unsuccessful?

☒ Please list ALLERGIES (meds, dyes, food): Latex, Demerol

❏ NKA

Relative / Guardian Notified: Yes ☒   No ❏   Phone Number:

Name of Relative Notified: Jennifer DeCapua

Transfer Ambulance: Life Care

VITAL SIGNS TAKEN   Yes ☒ No ❏   Time Taken: 1230 AM ❏ PM ☒

Respirations: 24	Blood glucose: 118 Time: 1210
O2 Sat: 96%	VRE: Yes ❏ No ☒ Hx of ❏
Pulse: 84	MRSA: Yes ❏ No ☒ Hx of ❏
BP: 118/82	C. Diff: Yes ❏ No ☒ Hx of ❏
Temp: 99 2 (A)	ANY pending cultures? Yes ❏ No ☒
Height: 5' 10"	If Yes, what?
Weight: 163 Lbs ☒ Kg ❏	MDRO?

ATTACHMENTS (Please check)

☒ Face Sheet
☒ History & Physical
❏ Discharge Summary
☒ MAR
❏ Wound Assessment & Tx Sheet
☒ Labs
❏ Code Status
❏ MD Orders
☒ X-rays
❏ MD Progress Notes
❏ Nurse's Notes (last 5 days)
❏ Other:
❏ Other:

ISOLATION PRECAUTIONS? Yes ❏ No ☒ | **TYPE:** Contact ❏ Droplet ❏ Airborne ❏ Other: ❏

VACCINATION HISTORY	SKIN OR PRESSURE ULCER CONCERNS
Pneumococcal Vaccine: Yes ☒ DATE: 3-16-12 Refused ❏	**HIGH risk for skin breakdown****PLEASE TURN** Yes ❏ No ❏
Flu Vaccine: Yes ☒ DATE: 11-7-10 Refused ❏	Current Skin Breakdown: Yes ❏ No ❏
Tetanus: Yes ❏ DATE: Refused ❏	Most Recent Treatment Time: AM ❏ PM ❏
TB Skin Test: Negative ❏ Positive ❏ DATE:	Please Treat at (time): AM ❏ PM ❏
OR Chest X-ray ☒ Result Date:	Treat with (product name): Dakins Solution Irrig BID
Comments:	To (what area): (P) LE

MEDICATION INFORMATION	SAFETY CONCERNS
See Attached Medication Reconciliation	History of Falls Yes ❏ No ☒	Risk for Falls Yes ❏ No ☒
Prefers meds with: applesauce	Behavior Issues Yes ❏ No ☒	Explain:
Pain Meds in past 24 hours Yes ☒ No ❏	RESTRAINT Use: Yes ❏ No ☒
Level on **Pain Scale** at time of transfer :	Type of Restraint Used:
(Please circle level) 1 2 3 (4) 5 6 7 8 9 10	When Used:

DIET & FEEDING	ELIMINATION
Current Diet: Diabetic 2000 kcal ADA	Bladder Incontinence ❏ DATE of UTI (within 14 days):
Needs Assistance ❏	Feeds Self ❏	Feeding Tube ❏	Catheter: Yes ❏ No ❏	Date Inserted or Last Changed:
Thickened Liquid ❏ Consistency?	Bowel Incontinence: Yes ❏ No ❏	Colostomy: Yes ❏ No ❏
Supplement ❏ If so, name:	Date of Last BM:

IMPAIRMENTS/DISABILITIES: (Please check all that apply)	PATIENT EQUIPMENT/BELONGINGS: (Check all sent with resident)
Speech ❏ Contractures ❏ Mental Confusion ❏ Vision ☒ Hearing ❏ Amputation ❏ Paralysis ❏ Language Barrier ❏	None ❏ Right Hearing Aid ❏ Left Hearing Aid ❏ Glasses ❏ Upper Denture ❏ Lower Denture ❏
COMMENTS: wears glasses	Jewelry ❏ Please list:
Report Called to: Jane Elson RN	Other (i.e., prosthesis):

| Nurse Name (Print): Karen Scheitlin RN | Nurse Signature: Karen Scheitlin RN | Phone #: 862-4444 | Date/Time: 3/18/12 7:00 |

NORTHSTAR MEDICAL CENTER

NORTHSTAR
Medical Center

Walker, Marjorie
PT#1772571   MRN#585120
DOB: 06/03/1956   Age: 56   Sex: F
Physician: Chaplin, Patrick
Admit: 03/18/2012
Allergies: No Know Drug Allergy

Medication Administration Record

No:	Medication	Start/Stop	Adm	07:00 to 18:59	19:00 to 6:69	00:00 to 00:00
0286618	ATENOLOL 50 MILLIGRAM PO EVERY 12 HOURS ONE DOSE= 50 MILLIGRAM = 1 TABLETS TENORMIN (Atenolol Tab 50 MG) ****FLOOR STOCK****	03/18/2012 at 2200 03/27/2012 at 1000		1000	2200 vy	
0286621	COZAAR 50 MILLIGRAM PO ONCE DAILY ONE DOSE= 50 MILLIGRAM = 1 TABLETS LOSARTAN (COZAAR) (Losartan Potassium Tab 50 MG) ****FLOOR STOCK****	03/18/2012 at 2200 03/27/2012 at 1000		1000		
0286631	DOCUSATE SODIUM 100 MILLIGRAM PO TWICE DAILY ONE DOSE= 100 MILLIGRAM = 1 CAPSULE USED FOR COLACE (Docusate Sodium Cap 100 MG) ****FLOOR STOCK****	03/18/2012 at 2200 03/27/2012 at 1000		1000	2200 vy	
0286619	FLECAINIDE ACETATE 100 MILLIGRAM PO EVERY 12 HOURS ONE DOSE= 100 MILLIGRAM = 1 TABLETS USED FOR TAMBOCOR (Flecainide Acetate Tab 100 MG)	03/18/2012 at 2200 03/27/2012 at 1000		1000	2200 vy	
0286630	LORazepam 0.5 MILLIGRAM PO TWICE DAILY ONE DOSE= 0.5 MILLIGRAM = 1 TABLETS ATIVAN (Lorazepam Tab 0.5 MG) ****FLOOR STOCK****	03/18/2012 at 2200 03/27/2012 at 1000		1000		
0286629	KLOR-CON M10 10 MILLIEQUIV PO ONCE DAILY ONE DOSE= 10 MILLIEQUIV = 1 TABLETS (Potassium Chloride Microencapsulated Crys CR Tab 10 mEq) ****FLOOR STOCK****	03/18/2012 at 2200 03/27/2012 at 1000		1000	2200 my	
0286628	FUROSEMIDE 40 MILLIGRAM PO ONCE DAILY ONE DOSE= 40 MILLIGRAM = 1 TABLETS LASIX 40MG TAB (Furosemide Tab 40 MG) ****FLOOR STOCK****	03/18/2012 at 2200 03/27/2012 at 1000		1000		
0286970	OXYCONTIN 10 MILLIGRAM PO EVERY EVENING ONE DOSE= 10 MILLIGRAM = 1 TABLETS (Oxycodone HCl Tab SR 12HR 10 MG) ****FLOOR STOCK****	03/18/2012 at 2200 03/27/2012 at 2200			2200 vy	
0286627	PARoxetine HCL 20 MILLIGRAM PO ONCE DAILY ONE DOSE= 20 MILLIGRAM = 1 TABLETS PAXIL 20 MG TAB (Paroxetine HCl Tab 20 MG) ****FLOOR STOCK****	03/18/2012 at 2200 03/27/2012 at 1000		1000		

Signatures		Init	Shift	Signatures	Init	Shift
				Ryan Goldman RN		
				Sylvia Yang RN		

A

abuse unintentional upcoding

accounting cost the total amount of money paid out for products, goods, or services

Accreditation Association for Ambulatory Health Care (AAAHC) a specialty accrediting organization

addressable standard should be met if it is a reasonable and appropriate safeguard in the entity's environment

addressable the portions of the privacy and security standards that the covered entities must address to determine if it is a reasonable and appropriate safeguard in the entity's environment

administrative data includes demographic information about the patient such as the patient's name, address, date of birth, race, primary language, religion, and marital status

admission date the day and time the patient is admitted to the acute care facility

admission/registration clerks a staff member generally responsible for entering insurance information into the EHR system at the time the patient is admitted to an inpatient hospital or scheduled for treatment at an outpatient facility or physician's office; also known as *patient access specialists*

advance directive a document that provides information about how the patient would like to be treated if he or she is no longer able to make his or her own medical decisions

Affordable care Act (ACA) enacted in March 2010 with the goal of providing quality, affordable health care for all Americans

alert fatigue a condition that arises when too many alerts cause physicians to disregard them

allowed amount the average or maximum amount that may be reimbursed per service, procedure, or item to the provider from the insurance payer

American College of Surgeons (ACS) an organization that developed a hospital standardization program establishing the minimum standards for reporting care and treatment

American Health Information Management Association (AHIMA) a professional organization that provides resources, education, and networking with other professionals, focusing on the quality of health information used in the delivery of healthcare

American Recovery and Reinvestment Act of 2009 (ARRA) an economic stimulus package signed into law by President Barack Obama

analysis the third step in the migration plan; this step examines how the healthcare facility currently uses its healthcare records and performs tasks

annual limit a cap on the benefits the insurance company will pay in a year

assignment of benefits a patient authorization form that allows his or her health insurance or third-party provider to reimburse the healthcare provider or facility directly

Association for Healthcare Documentation Integrity (AHDI) a professional organization that sets and upholds standards for education and practice in the field of clinical documentation that ensure the highest level of accuracy, privacy, and security for the US healthcare systems to protect public health, increase patient safety, and improve quality of care for healthcare consumers

automated data collection when the data from the initial patient encounter is automatically copied over to each new patient encounter

automatic method the entry of results that allows those results to be immediately available

B

behavioral health setting a facility that provides care to patients with psychiatric diagnoses

benefit year the year of insurance benefits coverage under an individual health insurance plan

best-of-breed an EHR system provided by a vendor or vendors that supplies the clinical applications needed

big data large data sets that are analyzed to reveal trends and patterns

billing/payment status report lists the status of every patient account, allowing the billing staff to identify claims that need to be billed or rebilled and insurance payers that need to be contacted regarding lack of payment

birthday rule a rule which specifies that the insurance of the parent whose birthday falls first in a calendar year will be the primary insurance for a child

breach an impermissible use or disclosure under the Privacy Rule that compromises the security or privacy of PHI such that the use or disclosure poses a significant risk of financial, reputational, or other harm to the affected individual

burial and death benefits used to replace a portion of the employee's lost income due to the work-related illness or injury

C

cancer registry a collection of data focusing on cancer and tumor diseases

Centers for Medicare & Medicaid Services (CMS) a federal agency that oversees federal healthcare programs, including Medicare Conditions of Participation (CoPs)

Certified Healthcare Technology Specialist (CHTS) certification that denotes proficiency in certain health IT roles and is intended for professionals with various education backgrounds who are interested in working with EHRs

CHAMPVA a comprehensive healthcare benefits program in which the Department of Veterans Affairs shares the cost of covered healthcare services and supplies with eligible beneficiaries

charge entry the process of entering medical codes into the billing system

checking out the procedure for a patient leaving an outpatient facility

chief complaint a narrative articulated by the patient as his or her reason for seeking health services

claim scrubbing the process of checking claims for errors prior to transmitting them to insurance companies

classification system a standardized coding method that organizes diagnoses and procedures into related groups to facilitate reimbursement, reporting, and clinical research

clean claims claims without errors

clearinghouse a company that accepts electronic claims from healthcare providers, scrubs the claims, transmits the clean claims to the appropriate payer and returns the claims that have errors to the healthcare provider

clinical coders people who assign or validate diagnostic and procedural codes to represent the patient's diseases or conditions and the treatment rendered

clinical data information such as admission dates, office visits, laboratory test results, evaluations, or emergency visits

clinical decision support system (CDSS) a computer system, usually integrated with the EHR system, that assists healthcare providers with decision-making tasks such as determining diagnoses, choosing the best medications to order for a patient, and selecting proper diagnostic tests

Clinical documentation also known as *clinical inputs*, contains data related to the patient's clinical status that is entered into the patient's EHR or paper record

clinical encoder a software program that helps coding professionals navigate coding pathways with the end result of assigning codes

clinical inputs the data entered into the patient record related to the patient's clinical status, whether they are in an EHR or a paper record clinical outputs clinical data that can be extracted from a patient record and compiled in a meaningful way

clinical reporting also known as *clinical outputs*, contains data that can be extracted from a patient record and compiled in a meaningful way

clinical results reporting an EHR function that allows healthcare providers to view laboratory and diagnostic test results immediately, as long as there is an interface between the clinical results system and the EHR

ClinicalTrials.gov a registry that provides access to information on publicly and privately funded clinical studies

cloned progress notes identical notes resulting from copying and pasting from one encounter or visit to another; also known as cloned progress notes or copycat charting

cloud storage data stored on virtual servers

cluster type of schedule in which similar appointments are scheduled together at specific times of the day

CMS Medicare Physician Fee Schedule (MPFS) standardized fee-paying schedule

CMS-1500 a universal claim form accepted by Medicare, Medicaid, and most insurance payers

Coinsurance the insured person's share of the costs of a covered healthcare service, calculated as a percentage (for example, 20%) of the allowed amount for the service

Commission for Accreditation of Rehabilitation Facilities (CARF) an independent, nonprofit organization that focuses on aging services, behavioral health, child and youth services, employment and community services, medical rehabilitation, and opioid treatment programs

Community Health Accreditation Program (CHAP) a specialty accrediting organization

computer protocol a standardized method of communicating or transmitting data between two computer systems

computer-assisted coding (CAC) programs that automatically assign diagnosis and procedure codes based on electronic documentation, which can increase the productivity of a coder by up to 20%

concurrent coding the process of coding while a patient is still receiving treatment in a hospital

Consolidated Omnibus Budget Reconciliation Act (COBRA) a federal law that may allow individuals to temporarily keep health coverage after their employment ends, they lose coverage as a dependent of the covered employee, or another qualifying event occurs

controlled substance a drug declared by US federal or state law to be illegal for sale or use but may be dispensed under a healthcare provider's prescription

Controlled Substances Act of 1970 legislation that placed tight controls on the pharmaceutical and healthcare industries and outlined the five schedules of controlled substances based on potential for harm

conversion factor (CF) a fiscal-year monetary amount arrived at by a formula set by US Congress, to convert the GPCI into a dollar amount that reflects several elements

copayment the amount that an insured individual must pay for healthcare services received, typically office visits, urgent care visits, or emergency department encounters

core data elements the data elements that are necessary for the master patient index and include patient identification number, patient name, date of birth, Social Security number, address, etc.

cost–benefit analysis a process of looking at the costs and benefits and determining the return on investment of implementing an EHR system

covered entities entities that have to comply with HIPAA Privacy and Security Rules; include healthcare providers, health plans, and healthcare clearinghouses transmitting health information in an electronic format

crosswalking the act of translating a code in one code set to a code in another code set

Current Dental Terminology (CDT®) a classification system used to code dental procedures

Current Procedural Terminology (CPT®) one of the most widely used classification systems in the United States used to code outpatient procedures for facility coding, as well as all physician services rendered

D

data collection both manual and automated data collection

data descriptive or numeric attributes of one or more variables

data dictionary a document that describes the content, format, and structure of data elements within a database

Data Elements for Emergency Department Systems (DEEDS) uniform specifications for data entered into emergency department (ED) patient records

data integrity the accuracy, completeness, and reliability of data in the EHR

data mapping a special type of data dictionary; a method that is used to connect data from one system to data of another system

data mining the process of searching and examining data to organize and reorganize it into useful information, patterns, and trends

data set a structured collection of related data elements

data sort arranging data in a particular sequence, from high to low or low to high

data standards agreed upon definitions and formats of data

data stewardship the authority and responsibility associated with collecting, using, and disclosing health information in its identifiable and aggregate forms

data the descriptive or numeric attributes of one or more variables

data warehouse a database that accesses data from multiple databases that are integrated in order to be used for analytic purposes

database a collection of data that is organized in rows, columns, and tables

day sheet a report of practice activity for a 24-hour period that is used to reconcile patient accounts on a daily basis to ensure that no fraud, abuse, or theft is occurring

deductible the amount an insured individual must pay out of pocket before the insurance will pay

deidentified health information health information that neither identifies an individual nor provides a reasonable basis to identify an individual

demographic information information provided by the patient that includes name, date of birth, address, phone number, email address, etc

dependencies tasks that must occur before the next tasks can take place

deposit reports generated daily, weekly, monthly, and yearly for the deposits made from insurance payers and from patient payments

design the second step in the migration plan; this step creates a blueprint for how the healthcare facility will transition from paper-based records to the new EHR system

diagnosis a statement or conclusion that describes a patient's illness, disease, or health problem

Diagnostic and Statistical Manual of Mental Disorders, Fifth Edition (DSM-5) a classification system used to classify psychiatric disorders

diagnostic-related groups (DRGs) a patient classification system that groups hospital patients of similar age, sex, diagnoses, and treatments

discharge date the day and time the patient leaves the facility

discharge disposition the patient's destination following a stay in the hospital

discharge the procedure for a patient leaving an inpatient facility

Discharged Not Final Billed (DNFB) patient accounts that are not able to be final billed to the insurance company or responsible party due to a lack of final coding, insurance verification, or other data errors

E

e-prescribing a process that allows a physician, nurse practitioner, or physician assistant to electronically transmit a new prescription or renewal authorization to a pharmacy; also known as *electronic prescribing*

economic cost the combination of accounting and opportunity costs

electronic health records (EHRs) a computer system used to improve healthcare delivery; EHRs replace traditional paper medical records and make health information accessible to healthcare providers across the world with only a few keystrokes

electronic medical record (EMR) an electronic version of patient files within a single organization

electronic patient tracking (EPT) tracks a patient's location from the time of their arrival at the healthcare organization to their discharge (for inpatients) or checkout (for outpatients)

electronic protected health information (ePHI) protected health information in electronic format

electronic superbill an itemized form that allows charges to be captured from a patient visit

employer-provided PHR a PHR offered by an employer containing data from hospitals, doctors' offices, health plans, laboratories, and pharmacies as well as information entered by the employee meant to enable employees to make better health decisions

encounter form where physician offices incorporate their most common procedure and diagnosis codes

enterprise data storage a centralized system (online or offline) that businesses use for managing and protecting data

enterprise identification number (EIN) an identifier used by an organization to identify a patient across various healthcare settings

enterprise master patient index (EMPI) a system wide database that maintains patient identifier information across an EHR system for all healthcare settings, allowing a healthcare organization to compile the patient's information into one index using registration, scheduling, financial, and clinical information

environmental analysis process of evaluating the people and process of workflow in a healthcare organization

established patient a patient who has received professional services from a healthcare provider or a provider in the same group and/or specialty within the past three years

external data data that comes from outside the organization

F

facility identifier an identifier that indicates the healthcare setting where the patient is seeking care

facility-provided PHR a type of tethered PHR that comes from a physician or healthcare facility

fee for service a reimbursement method that requests payment for each service or procedure

fee schedule a price list of services and procedures

financial data information that includes the patient's insurance and payment information for healthcare services

flow chart a document that demonstrates a workflow process

fraud intentional upcoding

functionality testing a process that requires a facility to use a test environment before implementing the EHR system facility-wide

functionality the ability to create and manage EHRs for all patients in a healthcare facility

G

Gantt chart a graphic representation of a project schedule

general consent for treatment a form used in acute care facilities that gives the healthcare provider the right to treat a patient

geographic practice cost indices (GPCI) adjustments applied to the RVU values to account for variations in the costs of practicing medicine in specific geographic regions

group health insurance plan an insurance plan that provides healthcare coverage to a specific group of people, typically based on an employer

guarantor account a record that saves the information about the guarantor, including the guarantor's name and address

guarantor the person or financial entity that guarantees payment on any unpaid balances on the account

H

Health Care and Education Reconciliation Act amendment to the Affordable Care Act

health coverage legal entitlement to payment or reimbursement for healthcare costs, generally under a contract with a health insurance company, a group health plan offered in connection with employment, or a government program like Medicare, Medicaid, or the Children's Health Insurance Program (CHIP)

health information management (HIM) professionals that plan information systems, develop health policy, identify current and future information needs, and practice the maintenance and care of health records

Health Information Technology for Economic and Clinical Health (HITECH) Act an act enacted in February 2009 as part of the ARRA that promoted the nationwide implementation of EHR technology

Health Insurance Portability and Accountability Act of 1996 (HIPAA) a comprehensive federal law passed in 1996 to protect all patient-identifiable medical information

health insurance type of insurance that pays for healthcare services that are incurred by the insured person(s)

health insurer–provided PHR a PHR system owned by a health insurance company where the insurer populates information about a subscriber, such as insurance claim information, a list of providers, prescriptions, and benefits coverage

health IT ecosystem a collection of individuals and groups that are interested in health information technology

Health Level Seven International (HL7) the most common communication protocol that focuses on the exchange of clinical and administrative data; also an international group of collaborating healthcare subject-matter experts and information scientists

health maintenance organization (HMO) a type of health insurance plan that usually limits coverage to include care only from doctors who work for or contract with the HMO

health maintenance organization (HMO) Act an act that provided grants to employers who set up HMOs

health record an accumulation of information about a patient's past and present health

Health Resources and Services Administration (HRSA) an agency of the US Department of Health and Human Services; focuses on improving health and health equity through innovative programs and a skilled health workforce and providing access to services to those who are economically or medically vulnerable

health savings account (HSA) a medical savings account available to taxpayers who are enrolled in a high deductible health plan

Healthcare Common Procedure Coding System (HCPCS) a classification system used to code ancillary services and procedures

Healthcare Cost and Utilization Project (HCUP) is a collection of databases that is sponsored by the Agency for Healthcare Research and Quality

healthcare delivery (HCD) system a healthcare facility

healthcare facility an organization, such as a hospital, clinic, dental office, outpatient surgery center, birthing center, or nursing home, that performs healthcare services

healthcare informatics is the study of managing health information

Healthcare Information and Management Systems Society (HIMSS) an organization that focuses on using information technology and management systems to improve the quality and delivery of healthcare

healthcare operations activities including quality assessment and improvement, competency assurance activities, conducting or arranging for medical reviews, audits, or legal services, specified insurance functions, business planning, development, management, and administration and business management and general administrative activities

healthcare treatment when the medical provider who treats the work-related injury or illness is paid directly by the patient's employer's insurer

HealthData.gov provides access to health data with the hope of improving health care quality

HETS (HIPAA Eligibility Transaction System) Medicare eligibility database application

hibernation mode a privacy feature in an EHR system that prevents disclosure of PHI

high deductible health plan a plan that has a higher annual deductible than typical health plans and has a maximum limit on the sum of the annual deductible that an insured must pay for covered expenses

HIPAA X12 837 Health Care Claim generated by the software and then transmitted to appropriate insurance payers

Hippocrates considered one of the most important figures in medical history; he was among the first to describe and document many diseases and medical conditions

History and Physical Examination (H&P) a report that helps identify and treat patient diagnoses; consists of two main elements: a subjective element and an objective element

history the subjective element of an H&P that includes history of present illness, past medical history, allergies, medications currently prescribed to the patient, and family and social histories

hospice care palliative, or short-term, care provided to terminal patients within acute care or home care settings

hospice services care for those who are at the end of life

hospital acquired diagnoses and conditions that developed when the patient was an inpatient in the hospital

hospital chargemaster computer database that compiles all procedures, services, supplies, and drugs that are billed to insurance payers

Hospital Compare part of the CMS's Hospital Quality Initiative; meant to provide data to examine how well a hospital delivers quality care and how health care organizations can improve

hybrid health record a patient record that is stored on paper and electronically

I

implementation the fifth step in the migration plan; this step creates a timeline for the implementation, and is often created to look like a Gantt chart

in-network providers or healthcare facilities that are part of a health plan's group of providers with which it has negotiated a discount

indexes in a database are used to find data without searching every row

individual health insurance plan an insurance plan that an individual purchases for himself or herself and/or his or her family

individually identifiable health information information including demographic data that identifies an individual

informatics is defined as the science of processing data for storage and retrieval

information data collected and analyzed

information governance an effective framework for the access and use of healthcare data including the policies, procedures, and processes for data and information creation, storage, access, use, analysis, archival, and deletion

information processing cycle the sequence of events that includes four components: input, processing, output, and storage

inpatient prospective payment system (IPPS) the first diagnostic-related group (DRG) system that was implemented in 1983 to reimburse acute care hospitals for the treatment of Medicare patients

inpatients patients who occupy a hospital bed for at least one night in the course of treatment, examination, or observation

input device a device used to enter data into an EHR system; includes keyboard, mouse, scanner, microphone, camera, stylus, and touchscreen

input the first component of the information processing cycle; data entered by the user of an EHR system (e.g., the patient's first name, last name, identification number)

insurance audits reviews conducted by insurance companies or auditing companies hired to review coding assignments on behalf of insurance companies

insurance premium the amount that the subscriber pays to the insurance company, usually paid in regular installments, such as monthly, in exchange for insurance coverage

insurance verifier the person who confirms the patient's insurance coverage with the insurance company

integrated care the systematic coordination of health care

integrated health record a health record format that is organized either in chronologic or reverse chronologic order

integrated system the combination of systems an organization already uses and the new EHR system

interface provides communication flow between two or more computer systems

internal data data that is accessed from within the healthcare organization

internal rate of return (IRR) a calculation used to measure the profitability of an investment

International Classification of Diseases (ICD) one of the most widely used classification systems used to code diagnoses and procedures for inpatients and diagnoses for all healthcare providers

interoperability the ability of an EHR system to exchange data with other sources of health information, including pharmacies, laboratories, and other healthcare providers

isolation status the precautions that must be taken by healthcare staff and visitors to avoid the spread of bacterial or viral infections

J

Joint Commission an independent, not-for-profit organization that accredits and certifies a variety of healthcare organizations; formerly known as the Joint Commission on Accreditation of Healthcare Organizations (JCAHO)

K

knowledge-based system that utilizes inference software and databases containing the most current medical, scientific, and research information

L

learning healthcare system (LHS) an approach to improving the quality of health care by using patient clinical data from EHRs to drive medical research, and by using medical research to influence clinical practices

legal data information composed of consents for treatment and authorizations for the release of information

lifetime limit a cap on the total lifetime benefits you may receive from your insurance company

limited data set protected health information from which certain specified direct identifiers of individuals and their relatives, household members, and employers have been removed

local area network (LAN) a group of computers connected through a network confined to a single area or small geographic area such as a building or hospital campus

long-term care facility a facility in which patients typically reside more than 30 days

longitudinal a patient's record that will continue to develop over the course of care

M

manual data collection a process initiated by a staff member upon initial patient contact with a healthcare facility done without the aid of an automatic system

manual method the entry of results that needs to be manually scanned into the EHR for access

master patient index (MPI) a database created by a healthcare organization to assign a unique medical record number to each patient served, thus allowing easy retrieval and maintenance of patient information; also known as a *patient list*

meaningful use the set of standards that governs the use of EHRs and allows eligible providers and hospitals to earn incentive payments by meeting specific criteria

MEDCIN a naming system primarily used in physicians' offices

Medicaid a state-administered health insurance program for low-income families and children, pregnant women, the elderly, people with disabilities, and in some states, other qualified adults

medical coder career that plays a key role in the billing process by coding diagnoses and procedures in preparation for billing claims

medical coding the process of assigning and validating standardized alphanumeric identifiers to the diagnoses and procedures documented in a health record

medical procedure an activity performed on an individual to improve health, treat disease or injury, or identify a diagnosis

Medicare a federal health insurance program for people who are age 65 or older and certain younger people with disabilities

Medicare Part A Hospital Insurance; covers inpatient care in hospitals including critical access hospitals and skilled nursing facilities (not custodial or long-term care)

Medicare Part B Medical Insurance; covers doctors' services and outpatient care

Medicare Part C—Medicare Advantage program that gave more coverage options in the private insurance market and added options such as prescription drug coverage for Medicare subscribers who wished to pay for additional coverage

Medicare Part D a program that helps pay for prescription drugs for Medicare beneficiaries who have a plan that includes Medicare prescription drug coverage

Medicare Prescription Drug Improvement and Modernization Act of 2003 law that added an optional prescription drug benefit to Medicare recipients

Medicare Provider Analysis and Review (MEDPAR) a database that contains inpatient hospital and skilled nursing facility records for all Medicare beneficiaries

Medigap Medicare supplemental insurance

migration plan a plan that provides the framework to identify the basic steps of how the healthcare facility will move from a paper-based record system to an EHR system

mileage reimbursement paid from employers for the mileage cost and for some of the wages they lose while in transit to and from, and during their appointments

Minimum Data Set (MDS) a core set of screening, clinical, and functional status elements required to be completed for all residents of nursing homes certified by Medicare or Medicaid

minimum necessary a concept required by the Privacy Rule that states that covered entities must make reasonable efforts to limit the use, disclosure of, and requests for the minimum amount of protected health information necessary to accomplish the intended purpose

minimum standards a set of requirements for reporting care and treatment

modified wave type of schedule in which patients arrive at planned intervals in the first half hour; then, in the second half hour, the healthcare provider catches up

morbidity consists of illness statistics

mortality consists of death statistics

N

National Committee for Quality Assurance (NCQA) an independent, nonprofit organization that focuses on healthcare quality

National Committee on Vital and Health Statistics (NCVHS) an advisory body to the US Department of Health and Human Services; the NCVHS completed a review of core health data elements and developed a list and definitions of the 42 core elements that can be used in a variety of healthcare settings

National Practitioner Data Bank (NPDB) a database that contains information on medical malpractice payments and actions against healthcare practitioners, providers, and suppliers

Nationwide Health Information Network (NwHIN) a set of standards that enable the secure exchange of health information over the Internet

net present value (NPV) the present value of future cash flows minus the purchase price of goods or services

new patient a patient who has not received any services from a healthcare provider or a provider in the group in the same specialty within the past three years

no interoperability stand-alone systems that do not communicate

no-shows patients who do not show for their scheduled appointments

nomenclature a common system of naming things

noncovered entities entities that do not have to comply with HIPAA Privacy and Security Rules; these include workers' compensation carriers, employers, marketing firms, life insurance companies, pharmaceutical manufacturers, casualty insurance carriers, pharmacy benefit management companies, and crime victim compensation programs

O

objective element the portion of the history and physical report that includes the physical examination

Office for Civil Rights (OCR) the agency responsible for enforcing the HIPAA Privacy and Security Rules

Office of the National Coordinator for Health Information Technology (ONC) the US federal body that recommends policies, procedures, protocols, and standards for interoperability

Omnibus Reconciliation Act of 1980 the act that expanded home health services, also brought Medigap under federal oversight

open hours type of schedule typically used in an urgent care setting in which patients are seen throughout certain time frames or on a first-come, first-served basis

operative report a form of clinical documentation that contains the details of a particular surgery or procedure performed on a patient

opportunity cost the value of a decision

optional data elements the data elements that are optional for the master patient index, and include marital status, telephone number, mother's maiden name, place of birth, advance directive decision-making, organ donor status, emergency contact, allergies, and problem list

out-of-network physicians, hospitals or other healthcare providers who are considered nonparticipants in an insurance plan (usually an HMO or PPO)

out-of-pocket amount expenses for medical care that are not reimbursed by the insurance company; include deductibles, coinsurance, and copayments for covered services plus all costs for services that are not covered

Outcome and Assessment Information Set (OASIS) a group of data elements that represent core items of a comprehensive assessment for an adult home care patient

outpatients patients who do not spend more than 24 hours in a healthcare facility

output device a device that displays the results from EHRs; includes computer monitor, digital device screen, and printer

output the third component of the information processing cycle; data produced that provides meaningful information for the user

P

patient aging report an accounts receivable report that shows how long patients have owed money to the practice

patient day sheet daily reconciliation or balancing sheet used to prevent fraud

patient identification number a unique patient or medical record number

patient ledger a report that reflects the patient's financial status in summary and/or in detail

patient portal a web-based site that gives patients access to their health records

Patient Protection and Affordable Care Act law that expanded health insurance coverage for Americans

payer all insurance payers or patients or specific insurance payer or patient

payer type insurance or patient

payment date from and to

payment day sheet similar to the patient day sheet, except that it only lists the payments made during the 24-hour period

payment the activities of a health plan to obtain premiums, to determine or fulfill responsibilities for coverage and provision of benefits, and to furnish or obtain reimbursement for healthcare delivered to an individual

Permanent Partial Disability Benefits (PPD) paid when medical maximum improvement has been achieved and a worker may be able to work in some capacity, but his or her injury has caused damage for an indefinite period and he or she cannot return to his or her old occupation

Permanent Total Disability Benefits (PTD) paid when the worker's injury permanently prevents him or her from returning to his or her former occupation

personal health record (PHR) an emerging health information technology initiative that gives patients a tool to improve the quality of their healthcare; these records are updated and maintained by the patient

physical examination the objective element of the H&P; this procedure is conducted by the nursing or medical staff and consists of a physical examination of body systems, an assessment of the patient and his or her condition, and a treatment plan

physician query a request, typically from a coder or a case manager, to add documentation to the health record that clarifies a diagnosis or procedure performed

pilot a test run of the EHR system

point of service (POS) plans a hybrid of HMOs and PPOs as the POS plans contain elements from both the HMOs and PPOs

policies principles or guidelines that are agreed upon by the organization

practice management the day-to-day operations of a medical practice

preferred provider organization (PPO) a type of health plan that contracts with medical providers, such as hospitals and doctors, to create a network of participating providers

present on admission (POA) diagnoses and conditions that the patient already had when they were admitted to the healthcare organization

primary sources data and information from the patient's EHR

Problem-Oriented Medical Information System (PROMIS) a software program developed at the University of Vermont under a federal grant in the 1970s

Problem-Oriented Medical Record (POMR) a medical record format that takes a systematic approach to documentation

problem-oriented record (POR) a health record format that focuses on assessment of the clinical documentation by healthcare providers and the creation of a plan that addresses the patient's health concerns

procedures methods used to put policies in action within the health care organization

processing the second component of the information processing cycle; takes data and makes the information usable within the system

production by insurance report reflects the amount of revenue generated by each insurance carrier

production by procedure report reflects the number of procedures performed during a specific time period along with the associated revenue

production by provider report shows how many patients are treated within a specified period of time by each provider in a practice, along with the revenue generated

production reports assists the practice manager with budgeting and revenue management

progress notes the portion of the health record in which healthcare providers of all disciplines document the patient's progress or lack thereof in relation to the established goals of the care plan

protected health information (PHI) all individually identifiable health information held or transmitted by a covered entity or its business associate, in any form or media, whether electronic, paper, or oral

protected health information (PHI) all individually identifiable health information held or transmitted by a covered entity or its business associate, in any form or media, whether electronic, paper, or oral

provider A specific provider or all providers

Q

Quality Improvement Organization (QIO) a group of health experts, providers, and consumers who are dedicated to improving the quality of care for people with Medicare

R

record a collection, usually in writing, of an account or an occurrence

Registered Health Information Administrator (Bachelor's Degree) (RHIA) professional who works as a liaison between healthcare providers, organization staff, payers, and patients; an expert in managing health information and the professionals responsible for managing health information

Registered Health Information Technician (Associate's Degree) (RHIT) professional who performs the technical procedures related to the management of health information, frequently working in positions of medical coding, billing, and data management

registrar the healthcare personnel at the admission or registration desk that is the initial contact for a patient

rehabilitation facility a facility that offers acute care and ambulatory care, typically serving patients recovering from accidents, injuries, or surgeries

reimbursement the act of compensating a person for services rendered

relative value units (RVU) calculated for work RVU, practice expense RVU, and malpractice RVU

remittance advice (RA) report lists the patient's information and amount paid by Medicare or other payer to the physician practice

remote coders coders who work from home

request for proposal (RFP) a document that includes requirements, services, vendor information, and a bid or quote for the EHR system

required standard the portions of the standards with which each covered entity must comply

requirements the first step in the migration plan; this step asks a facility to identify the scope of the project and user needs

resolution agreement a contract signed by the federal government and a covered entity in which the covered entity agrees to perform certain obligations (e.g., staff training regarding privacy and confidentiality, audits of all releases of health information to ensure compliance) and to send reports to the federal government for a certain time period (typically three years)

resource-based relative value scale (RBRVS) used to create the MPFS

resources items necessary to a project, such as equipment and staff

return on investment (ROI) a performance measurement that calculates the benefit or gain of an investment

revenue cycle management all administrative and clinical functions that contribute to the capture, management, and collection of patient service revenue

review of systems (ROS) an examination of each body system that includes physical assessment of general appearance; vital signs; head, ears, eyes, nose, and throat (HEENT); respiratory; cardiovascular; abdominal; gastrointestinal; genitourinary; musculoskeletal; and neurologic

rollout process of introducing an EHR to a facility that occurs in three phases: organizational, training, and operational

S

schedules timeline for a project

secondary data indexes and registries

Security Rule the standards developed to address the security provisions of HIPAA; also known as *Security Standards for the Protection of Electronic Protected Health Information*

Security Standards for the Protection of Electronic Protected Health Information the standards developed to address the security provisions of HIPAA; also known as *Security Rule*

security the standard that prevents data loss and ensures that patient health information is private

self-pay patients patients who do not have any type of insurance coverage and must pay for healthcare services themselves

semantic interoperability level the level that allows the meaning of data to be shared and information interpreted

SNOMED CT a standardized vocabulary of clinical terminology used by healthcare providers for clinical documentation and reporting; considered the most comprehensive healthcare terminology in the world

source-oriented record (SOR) the health record format used most by healthcare facilities; organizes health documents into sections that contain information collected from a specific department or type of service

storage device a place where data for the EHR may be stored, such as on a dedicated server at the healthcare facility or on a server provided by a vendor; if an EHR system is networked, then the storage may exist on the healthcare system's server

storage the fourth component of the information processing cycle; patient information is stored so that it can be retrieved, added to, or modified for later use

strategic plan an organization's process of defining its direction by including goals or objectives and a sequence of steps to achieve each goal and objective

structured data a format in which data is stored in a database rather than in an unstructured or free-form format; examples include date of birth, sex, and race

subjective element the portion of the history and physical report that relies on patient narrative

subscriber the person whose insurance coverage is used for acute or ambulatory care

superbill a document that records the diagnosis and treatment for each patient at each visit; also known as an *encounter form*

syndromic a group of symptoms that, when grouped together, are characteristic of a specific disorder or disease

syntactic interoperability level the level that introduces a common data format for information exchange, but the meaning of the data cannot be interpreted

T

technical interoperability allows systems to exchange bits and bytes of data without any ability to interpret the shared data

template a preformatted file that provides prompts to obtain specific, consistent information

Temporary Partial Disability Benefits (TPD) paid when an employee works in a reduced capacity, but cannot work to the same extent as he or she could before his or her injury or illness

Temporary Total Disability Benefits (TTD) paid when an employee has been injured at work and cannot perform his or her work duties

test the fourth step in the migration plan; this step tests the functionality of the new EHR system

third-party payer an entity other than the patient that is financially responsible for payment of the medical bill

time specified type of schedule used in an acute care setting in which patients are given a specific date and time to arrive at a facility

total cost of ownership a financial estimate that helps determine the direct and indirect costs of the EHR system

TPO acronym for treatment, payment, and healthcare operations

trauma registry includes the collection, storage, and reporting of patient trauma data

treatment plan a plan a healthcare practitioner decides on to treat a patient's diagnoses

treatment the provision, coordination, or management of healthcare and related services for an individual by one or more healthcare providers, including consultation among providers regarding a patient, and referral of a patient by one provider to another

TRICARE a DoD regionally managed healthcare program for active duty and retired members of the uniformed services, their families, and survivors

U

UHDDS core data elements a set of patient-specific data elements outlined by the Uniform Hospital Discharge Data Set (UHDDS) committee

Uniform Ambulatory Care Data Set (UACDS) the data set that ensures that all healthcare settings and providers are gathering identical types of information on each patient

Uniform Hospital Discharge Data Set (UHDDS) a set of items used for reporting inpatient data in acute care hospitals

unstructured data a format in which data is stored in a free-form format rather than in a database; examples include progress notes, test interpretations, and operative reports

upcoding an illegal maneuver that encourages physicians to document simply for the purpose of claiming a higher paying diagnostic-related group (DRG) and, therefore, increased reimbursement

uploading the process of transmitting a file from one computer to another or to a portal

V

Veterans Administration the federal department that provides a government-run military benefit system

W

wave type of schedule in which patients are scheduled to arrive at the beginning of the hour, and the number of appointments is determined by dividing the hour by the length of an average visit or procedure

web-based tethered PHR a PHR system where the health information is attached to a specific organization's health information system

web-based untethered PHR a PHR system that is not attached to a specific organization's health information system

wide area network (WAN) a network that covers a broader area than a LAN, spanning regions, countries, or the world

Work Plan an annual report created by the OIG that establishes areas of healthcare documentation and billing practices to be addressed and audited during the year

work-list reports reports that present the patient accounts for coding in a priority order, beginning with the oldest accounts with the highest balances

Workers' Compensation an insurance plan that employers are required to have to cover employees who get sick or injured on the job

workflow analysis a process that reviews how an organization currently functions and how paper records are used to care for patients

workstation a computer paired with input and output devices

A

abbreviations
    Do Not Use list, 49, 50*f*
    standards for use of, in
      documentation, 49, 50*f*
abuse, unintentional upcoding as, 215
accounting cost, 366
Accreditation Association for Ambulatory
    Health Care (AAAHC), overview of,
    51
accreditation organizations, 51
acronyms, standards for use of, in
    documentation, 49, 50*f*
Activity Feed feature, 83, 83*f*
acute care setting
    characteristics of, 45
    health record content for, 45–46
    patient care in, 107–108
    patient registration/admission,
      114–115
Add Chart Note, 95, 95*f*
addressable standards, 171, 171*f*
Add Superbill dialog box, 89
administrative data, 34–35, 35*f*
administrative features of EHR navigator,
    81–94
    Billing feature, 89–91, 89*f*–91*f*
    Charts feature, 92, 92*f*–93*f*
    Documents feature, 93–94, 93*f*–94*f*
    Home menu, 81, 81*f*
    Messages function, 84, 85*f*
    Patient Tracker, 82, 82*f*
    Reports feature, 82–84, 83*f*, 84*f*
    Schedule feature, 86–88, 86*f*–88*f*
administrative management
    acute care setting and, 107–108,
      108*t*
    adding documents to patient record,
      121–125
    admission and registration, 110,
      111*f*
    advance directive, 105, 107, 124,
      124*f*
    ambulatory care setting and, 108,
      108*t*
    check-in process, 110
    consent forms, 123
    core and optional data elements,
      113
    enterprise master patient index
      (EMPI), 114
    established patient admission, 117
    financial agreements, 122
    healthcare settings and, 107–109
    initial patient contact, 109–110,
      109*f*
    insurance information, 118–120
    master patient index (MPI),
      110–114

new patient admission, 116
Notice of Privacy Practices for
    Protected Health Information
    form, 107
overview of, 106–107
patient identifiers, 112
patient registration/admission,
    114–115
privacy notices, 107, 121–122
Administrative Safeguards of Security
    Rule, 169
Administrative Simplification Provisions,
    155, 155*f*
admission, patient
    acute care registration, 114
    ambulatory care setting, 115
    entry into healthcare system, 110
admission assessment, 186, 187*t*
admission date, 107–108
Admission Face Sheet, 35*f*
admission/registration clerks, 227
advance directive, 105
    adding to EHR, 124
    registration and, 107
    sample of, 124*f*
adverse drug interactions, CDSS to
    prevent, 298
Affordable Care Act (ACA), insurance
    reforms from, 230
Agency for Healthcare Research and
    Quality (AHRQ), 52, 277–278
alert fatigue, 298
alerts, in clinical decision support system
    (CDSS), 297–298, 297*t*
Allergies feature, in patient portal, 335,
    335*f*
Allowed amount, 231
ambulatory care setting
    characteristics of, 46
    health record content for, 46–47
    patient care in, 108
    patient registration/admission, 115
American College of Surgeons (ACS), 31
American Dental Association (ADA),
    209
American Health Information
    Management Association (AHIMA)
    core data elements, 113
    core data set, 39
    credentialing programs of, 21
    Information Governance Principles
      for Healthcare (IGPHC),
      281–282
    MyPHR website, 318, 318*f*
    optional data elements, 113
    overview of, 51–52
    PHR definition, 315*t*
American Medical Association (AMA),
    208

American Recovery and Reinvestment
    Act of 2009 (ARRA), 4
    incentives for EHR adoption, 33
amyotrophic lateral sclerosis (ALS), 230
annual limit, 231
Anthem, 173
appointment scheduling. *See* scheduling
Appointments feature, in patient portal,
    338–339
    Cancel My Appointments feature,
      339, 339*f*
    Request My Appointment feature,
      339, 339*f*
    View My Appointment feature,
      338, 338*f*
Archived Messages, 84, 85*f*
Assignment of Benefits form, 122, 122*f*
Association for Healthcare
    Documentation Integrity (AHDI),
    51–52
auditing
    by insurance companies, 216
    internal and external coding audits,
      216–217
    Recovery Audit Contractor (RAC)
      program, 216–217
automated data collection, 183, 272
automatic method of clinical results
    reporting, 193

B

backup system, requirements for, 98
behavioral health setting, 109
Benefit year, 231
Bertillon, Jacques, 202, 206
Bertillon Classification of Causes of Death,
    202, 206
best-of-breed EHR system, 362, 368
big data, 282
billing. *See also* reimbursement
    charge entry, 239
    claim scrubbing, 246–247
    cloned progress notes and issues of
      reimbursement, 189
    CMS-1450/UB-04 form, 241, 242*f*
    CMS-1500 form, 239, 241*f*
    co-payment, 231
    deductible, 232
    837 Claim file, 240
    electronic billing, 239
    electronic superbill, 239
    encounter form, 239, 240*f*, 244
    Explanation of Benefits (EOB), 232
    HIPAA X12 837 Health Care
      Claim, 240
    improved accuracy and efficiency
      with EHR system, 243–244
    insurance terminology, 230–232

Photo Credits

2 ©iStockphoto/sqback, ©iStockphoto/UygarGeographic; 3 ©Shutterstock/ilterriorm, ©Shutterstock/Rene Jansa; 4 ©iStockphoto/dra_schwartz; 6 ©Shutterstock/Monkey Business Images; 10 Courtesy of Steve Hart, Senior IT Consultant, HL7 2.X Certified, http://www.hartsteve.com; 16 ©Cartoonstock/Bacall, Aaron; 18 ©iStockphoto/Pamela Moore; 28 ©Shutterstock/sheff, ©Shutterstock/PENGYOU91, ©Shutterstock/SPb photo maker; 29 ©Shutterstock/Marc Dietrich, ©Shutterstock/Feng Yu, ©Shutterstock/yanugkelid; 30 ©iStockphoto/spxChrome; 31 ©iStock/imagestock, ©Shutterstock/Smart7; 33 ©National Academies Press; 36 ©Shutterstock/alexskopje; 45 ©iStockphoto/babyblueut; 46 ©iStockphoto/BanksPhotos; 48 ©iStockphoto/Snowleopard1; 50 Courtesy of the Joint Commission; 55 ©iStockphoto/joeynick, Wikipedia/Intelati; 56 ©iStock/macrovector; 57 ©iStockphoto/alexsl; 58 ©iStock/macrovector; 66 ©Shutterstock/alexmillos, ©Shutterstock/Andrey_Popov; 67 ©Shutterstock/megainarmy; 70 ©Shutterstock/planet5D LLC; 71 ©Shutterstock/Ohmega1982; 98 Courtesy of Practice Fusion; 104 ©shutterstock/ideyweb, ©iStockphoto/Franck-Boston; 105 ©shutterstock/Christine Langer-Pueschel, ©shutterstock/Anan Kaewkhammul; 106 ©iStockphoto/JerryPDX; 107 ©Shutterstock/Monkey Business Images; 109 ©iStockphoto/101dalmatians, ©iStockphoto/SolStock; 115 ©iStockphotos/Mypurgatoryyears; 130 ©Shutterstock/wavebreakmedia, ©iStockphoto/exdez, ©iStockphoto/Spiderstock; 132 ©iStockphoto/DenGuy; 136 ©iStockphoto/Mark Bowden; 137 ©Shutterstock/Monkey Business Images; 140 ©iStockphoto/annedde; 144 ©iStockphoto/vm; 152 ©Shutterstock/Africa Studio, ©Shutterstock/PhotoMediaGroup; 153 ©iStock/dra_schwartz, ©iStockphoto/DNY59; 157 ©Shutterstock/zimmytws; 158 ©iStockphoto/leezsnow; 164 ©cartoonstock/mban1505; 165 ©Shutterstock/nyasha; 169 ©Shutterstock/Robert A. Levy Photography, LLC; 170 ©Shutterstock/eyjafjallajokull; 171 Public Domain; 180 ©Shutterstock/Radu Razvan; 181 ©shutterstock/Daboost, ©Shutterstock/Brian A Jackson; 183 ©iStockphoto/Sportstock; 184 ©iStockphoto/LajosRepasi; 190 ©George Brainerd; 193 ©iStockphoto/GlobalStock; 194 ©2012 R.J. Romero, ©iStockphoto/PhotoEuphoria; 202 ©2012 R.J. Romero, ©Shutterstock/PRILL; 203 ©Shutterstock/KITSANANAN; 204 ©iStockphoto/pkline; 209 ©iStockphoto/bjones27; 211 ©Shutterstock/Keith Bell; 217 ©Shutterstock/elwynn; 224 ©Shutterstock/Cartoon Resource, ©iStock/PeopleImages; 225 ©iStock/JohnnyLye; 228 ©iStock/Weekend Images Inc.; 229 ©iStock/uschools; 234 ©iStock/fstop12; 235 ©iStock/ginosphotos; 240 Public domain; 241 Public domain; 243 Public domain; 244 ©iStockphoto/row lbodvar; 266 ©Mike Konopacki and the California Nurses Association, ©iStock/Hilch; 269 ©Shutterstock/Andrey_Popov; 270 ©iStock/mirceax, ©iStock/kali9; 271 Public domain; 279 ©iStock/KatarzynaBialasiewicz; 280 ©iStock/simonkr; 292 Courtesy of Darline Foltz; 293 ©Shutterstock/Bombaert Patrick, ©Shutterstock Pete Saloutos, ©Shutterstock/Feng Yu; 294 ©Shutterstock/iofoto, ©iStockphoto/svetikd; 298 ©iStockphoto/stevecoleimages; 299 ©iStockphoto/Sproetniek; 301 ©Shutterstock/StockLite; 312 ©iStockphoto/exdez, ©iStockphoto/dra_schwartz; 313 ©iStock/hudiemm; 319 ©iStockphoto/andhedesigns; 320 ©iStockphoto/Christopher Futcher; 321 MyHealtheVet Website; 350 ©Shutterstock/My Life Graphic; 351 ©iStockphoto/XonkArts, National Learning Soncortium; 355 ©iStockphoto/Steve Debenport; 357 ©Shutterstock/Monkey Business Images; 359 ©Shutterstock/zimmytws; 361 ©2012 R.J. Romero; 362 ©Shutterstock/dotshock; 366 ©Shutterstock/Denise Lett